1999
YEAR BOOK OF
SPORTS MEDICINE®

Statement of Purpose

The YEAR BOOK Service

The YEAR BOOK series was devised in 1901 by practicing health professionals who observed that the literature of medicine and related disciplines had become so voluminous that no one individual could read and place in perspective every potential advance in a major specialty. In the final decade of the 20th century, this recognition is more acutely true than it was in 1901.

More than merely a series of books, YEAR BOOK volumes are the tangible results of a unique service designed to accomplish the following:

- to *survey* a wide range of journals of proven value
- to *select* from those journals papers representing significant advances and statements of important clinical principles
- to provide *abstracts* of those articles that are readable, convenient summaries of their key points
- to provide *commentary* about those articles to place them in perspective

These publications grow out of a unique process that calls on the talents of outstanding authorities in clinical and fundamental disciplines, trained literature specialists, and professional writers, all supported by the resources of Mosby, the world's preeminent publisher for the health professions.

The Literature Base

Mosby and its editors survey approximately 500 journals published worldwide, covering the full range of the health professions. On an annual basis, the publisher examines usage patterns and polls its expert authorities to add new journals to the literature base and to delete journals that are no longer useful as potential YEAR BOOK sources.

The Literature Survey

The publisher's team of literature specialists, all of whom are trained and experienced health professionals, examines every original, peer-reviewed article in each journal issue. More than 250,000 articles per year are scanned systematically, including titles, text, illustrations, tables, and references. Each scan is compared, article by article, with the search strategies that the publisher has developed in consultation with the 270 outside experts who form the pool of YEAR BOOK editors. A given article may be reviewed by any number of editors, from one to a dozen or more, regardless of the discipline for which the paper was originally published. In turn, each editor who receives the article reviews it to determine whether or not the article should be included in the YEAR BOOK. This decision is based on the article's inherent quality, its probable usefulness to readers of that YEAR BOOK, and the editor's goal to represent a balanced picture of a given field in each volume of the YEAR BOOK. In addition, the editor indicates when to include figures and tables from the article to help the YEAR BOOK reader better understand the information.

Of the quarter million articles scanned each year, only 5% are selected for detailed analysis within the YEAR BOOK series, thereby assuring readers of the high value of every selection.

The Abstract

The publisher's abstracting staff is headed by a seasoned medical professional and includes individuals with training in the life sciences, medicine, and other areas, plus extensive experience in writing for the health professions and related industries. Each selected article is assigned to a specific writer on this abstracting staff. The abstracter, guided in many cases by notations supplied by the expert editor, writes a structured, condensed summary designed so that the reader can rapidly acquire the essential information contained in the article.

The Commentary

The YEAR BOOK editorial boards, sometimes assisted by guest commentators, write comments that place each article in perspective for the reader. This provides the reader with the equivalent of a personal consultation with a leading international authority—an opportunity to better understand the value of the article and to benefit from the authority's thought processes in assessing the article.

Additional Editorial Features

The editorial boards of each YEAR BOOK organize the abstracts and comments to provide a logical and satisfying sequence of information. To enhance the organization, editors also provide introductions to sections or individual chapters, comments linking a number of abstracts, citations to additional literature, and other features.

The published YEAR BOOK contains enhanced bibliographic citations for each selected article, including extended listings of multiple authors and identification of author affiliations. Each YEAR BOOK contains a Table of Contents specific to that year's volume. From year to year, the Table of Contents for a given YEAR BOOK will vary depending on developments within the field.

Every YEAR BOOK contains a list of the journals from which papers have been selected. This list represents a subset of the approximately 500 journals surveyed by the publisher and occasionally reflects a particularly pertinent article from a journal that is not surveyed on a routine basis.

Finally, each volume contains a comprehensive subject index and an index to authors of each selected paper.

The 1999 Year Book Series

Year Book of Allergy, Asthma, and Clinical Immunology: Drs. Rosenwasser, Boguniewicz, Borish, Routes, Spahn, and Weber

Year Book of Anesthesiology and Pain Management®: Drs. Tinker, Abram, Chestnut, Roizen, Rothenberg, and Wood

Year Book of Cardiology®: Drs. Schlant, Collins, Gersh, Graham, Kaplan, and Waldo

Year Book of Chiropractic®: Dr. Lawrence

Year Book of Critical Care Medicine®: Drs. Parrillo, Balk, Calvin, Franklin, and Shapiro

Year Book of Dentistry®: Drs. Meskin, Berry, Jeffcoat, Leinfelder, Roser, Summitt, and Zakariasen

Year Book of Dermatology and Dermatologic Surgery™: Drs. Thiers and Lang

Year Book of Diagnostic Radiology®: Drs. Osborn, Birdwell, Dalinka, Groskin, Maynard, Pentecost, Ros, Smirniotopoulos, and Young

Year Book of Emergency Medicine®: Drs. Wagner, Dronen, Davidson, King, Niemann, and Hamilton

Year Book of Endocrinology®: Drs. Bagdade, Braverman, Fitzpatrick, Horton, Kannan, Landsberg, Molitch, Morley, Odell, Poehlman, and Rogol

Year Book of Family Practice®: Drs. Berg, Bowman, Davidson, Dexter, and Scherger

Year Book of Gastroenterology: Drs. Aliperti and Fleshman

Year Book of Hand Surgery®: Drs. Amadio and Hentz

Year Book of Medicine®: Drs. Klahr, Frishman, Malawista, Mandell, Jett, Young, Barkin, and Bagdade

Year Book of Neonatal and Perinatal Medicine®: Drs. Fanaroff, Maisels, and Stevenson

Year Book of Nephrology, Hypertension, and Mineral Metabolism: Drs. Schwab, Bennett, Emmett, Hostetter, and Moe

Year Book of Neurology and Neurosurgery®: Drs. Bradley and Gibbs

Year Book of Nuclear Medicine®: Drs. Gottschalk, Blaufox, Coleman, Strauss, and Zubal

Year Book of Obstetrics, Gynecology, and Women's Health®: Drs. Mishell, Herbst, and Kirschbaum

Year Book of Oncology®: Drs. Ozols, Eisenberg, Glatstein, Loehrer, and Urba

Year Book of Ophthalmology®: Drs. Wilson, Augsburger, Cohen, Eagle, Grossman, Laibson, Maguire, Nelson, Penne, Rapuano, Sergott, Spaeth, Tipperman, Ms. Gosfield, and Ms. Salmon

Year Book of Orthopedics®: Drs. Morrey, Beauchamp, Currier, Tolo, Trigg, and Swiontkowski

Year Book of Otolaryngology–Head and Neck Surgery®: Drs. Paparella, Holt, and Otto

Year Book of Pathology and Laboratory Medicine®: Drs. Raab, Cohen, Dabbs, Olson, and Stanley

Year Book of Pediatrics®: Dr. Stockman

Year Book of Plastic, Reconstructive, and Aesthetic Surgery®: Drs. Miller, Bartlett, Garner, McKinney, Ruberg, Salisbury, and Smith

Year Book of Psychiatry and Applied Mental Health®: Drs. Talbott, Ballenger, Frances, Lydiard, Meltzer, Jensen, and Tasman

Year Book of Pulmonary Disease®: Drs. Jett, Castro, Maurer, Peters, Phillips, and Ryu

Year Book of Rheumatology, Arthritis, and Musculoskeletal Disease™: Drs. Panush, Hadler, Hellmann, LeRoy, Pisetsky, and Simon

Year Book of Sports Medicine®: Drs. Shephard, Drinkwater, Eichner, Torg, Alexander, and Mr. George

Year Book of Surgery®: Drs. Copeland, Bland, Deitch, Eberlein, Howard, Luce, Seeger, Souba, and Sugarbaker

Year Book of Urology®: Drs. Andriole and Coplen

Year Book of Vascular Surgery®: Dr. Porter

Table of Contents

Journals Represented

Mosby and its editors survey approximately 500 journals for its abstract and commentary publications. From these journals, the editors select the articles to be abstracted. Journals represented in this YEAR BOOK are listed below.

Acta Orthopaedica Scandinavica
Acta Radiologica
Age and Ageing
American Family Physician
American Journal of Cardiology
American Journal of Clinical Nutrition
American Journal of Emergency Medicine
American Journal of Epidemiology
American Journal of Gastroenterology
American Journal of Obstetrics and Gynecology
American Journal of Orthopedics
American Journal of Physical Medicine & Rehabilitation
American Journal of Physiology
American Journal of Preventive Medicine
American Journal of Public Health
American Journal of Sports Medicine
Annals of Emergency Medicine
Annals of Internal Medicine
Archives of Physical Medicine and Rehabilitation
Arthroscopy
British Journal of Sports Medicine
British Medical Journal
Clinical Biomechanics
Clinical Orthopaedics and Related Research
European Heart Journal
European Respiratory Journal
Foot & Ankle International
Heart
Injury
International Journal of Obesity
International Journal of Sports Medicine
Journal of Applied Physiology: Respiratory, Environmental and Exercise
    Physiology
Journal of Athletic Training
Journal of Biomechanics
Journal of Bone and Joint Surgery (American Volume)
Journal of Bone and Mineral Research
Journal of Computer Assisted Tomography
Journal of Gerontology
Journal of Neurology, Neurosurgery and Psychiatry
Journal of Orthopaedic Research
Journal of Orthopaedic and Sports Physical Therapy
Journal of Pediatric Orthopaedics
Journal of Rheumatology
Journal of Sports Medicine and Physical Fitness
Journal of Sports Sciences

Journal of the American Academy of Orthopaedic Surgeons
Journal of the American College of Cardiology
Journal of the American Medical Association
Journal of the National Cancer Institute
Journal of the Neurological Sciences
Lancet
Medical Journal of Australia
Medicine and Science in Sports and Exercise
Neurology
Neurosurgical Focus
New England Journal of Medicine
New Zealand Medical Journal
Orthopedics
Pediatrics
Physical Therapy
Physician and Sportsmedicine
Public Health Reports
Spine
Sports Medicine
Stroke
Thorax

STANDARD ABBREVIATIONS

The following terms are abbreviated in this edition: acquired immunodeficiency syndrome (AIDS), cardiopulmonary resuscitation (CPR), central nervous system (CNS), cerebrospinal fluid (CSF), computed tomography (CT), deoxyribonucleic acid (DNA), electrocardiography (ECG), health maintenance organization (HMO), human immunodeficiency virus (HIV), intensive care unit (ICU), intramuscular (IM), intravenous (IV), magnetic resonance (MR) imaging (MRI), and ribonucleic acid (RNA).

NOTE

The YEAR BOOK OF SPORTS MEDICINE is a literature survey service providing abstracts of articles published in the professional literature. Every effort is made to assure the accuracy of the information presented in these pages. Neither the editors nor the publisher of the YEAR BOOK OF SPORTS MEDICINE can be responsible for errors in the original materials. The editors' comments are their own opinions. Mention of specific products within this publication does not constitute endorsement.

To facilitate the use of the YEAR BOOK OF SPORTS MEDICINE as a reference tool, all illustrations and tables included in this publication are now identified as they appear in the original article. This change is meant to help the reader recognize that any illustration or table appearing in the YEAR BOOK OF SPORTS MEDICINE may be only one of many in the original article. For this reason, figure and table numbers will often appear to be out of sequence within the YEAR BOOK OF SPORTS MEDICINE.

Publisher's Preface

Mosby, Inc. would like to extend our sincere thanks to Dr. Randy Eichner and Dr. Barbara Drinkwater. Drs. Eichner and Drinkwater will step down from the editorial board effective with the 2000 edition of the YEAR BOOK OF SPORTS MEDICINE. They have been devoted editors of the YEAR BOOK for 11 and 6 years, respectively, and will be missed.

Introduction

As the millennium approaches, the pace of research in sports medicine continues unabated, and it is a wonderful asset to have such a talented pool of associates to select the key pieces of new information in sports medicine for presentation as succinct structured abstracts, complete with their editorial insights. I would also like to pay a warm tribute to Jaime Pendill and her team for the prompt and efficient manner in which they have handled the complex mechanics of preparing this volume.

What are the current trends in sports medicine? A welcome development in many of the surgical reports presented in this volume is a focus on long-term outcomes. This year, the spotlight on injuries in individual sports focuses in particular on snowboarding, with other articles discussing the risks associated with rock-climbing, wrestling, tennis, golf, rowing, in-line skating and snowmobiling. One article compares injury patterns of elite hockey players between on-ice and in-line skating. Winter conditions are shown not to eliminate the danger of injury from lightning. Hyperbaric oxygen is suggested in the treatment of muscle stretch injuries. Arthroscopic repair of rotator cuff injuries and the possible complications of this procedure continue to attract attention. Ninety cases of throwing fracture of the humeral shaft are analyzed. Methods for the early detection of osteochondritis dissecans in the capitellum of young baseball players are discussed. The use of cadaver models examine gleno-humeral motion after simulated capsulolabral injury, is discussed. Cadavers also proved helpful in a study determining optimal techniques for the emergency removal of football equipment following spinal injury. Several articles highlight the risk of spinal injuries during rugby football. The application of fast-spin echo imaging in examining the articular cartilages of the knee is studied. One survey explores the extent of the problem of septic arthritis of the knee following anterior cruciate ligament reconstruction. Interest in the ability to regenerate knee cartilages from mesenchymal progenitor cells continues. The trend to lesser use of formal hospital facilities is instanced by a home-based program for rehabilitation following anterior cruciate ligament reconstruction.

Active living is shown to be as effective as a formal exercise program in enhancing fitness over a six-month period. As assessed by doubly-labeled water, physcial activity is indicated better by measurements of maximal oxygen intake and fat-free mass than by questionnaire data. Regular physical activity does not do much to enhance various measures of reaction speed, but there is a substantial decrease in age-specific mortality associated with an enhancement of fitness. Active individuals are also at a lower risk of injury, and have a much lower prevalence of functional limitations over an 8-year follow up; over a 12-year follow-up, those who are active show a lesser mortality and fewer demands for medical and personal care. Anthropological arguments support the current emphasis on moderate physical activity as the optimal prescription for overall health, with active living as effective as structured activities. Several reports show the primary care practitioners are effective in promoting increased physical activity, although the cost of their motivational efforts is by no means negligible. A large epidemiological study provides new data on the aerobic power of elderly subjects up to 85 years of age. Hospital admission is shown to be a frequent precipitating cause of inability to walk independently in older individuals. Even healthy young adults divert 14% to 16% of their cardiac output to the chest muscles during maximal effort. The physiological basis of dyspnea appears to differ in patients as hypercarbia begins to develop. New approaches to the treatment of exercise-induced bronchospasm include the blockage of the enzymes forming leukotrienes and an assault on the corresponding receptors; exercise-induced bronchospasm is also associated with an increase in the excretion of prostaglandin metabolites. Adverse effects of ozone on pulmonary function can be countered by giving antioxidant vitamins. A high proportion of older endurance athletes, such as orienteers, develop isolated paroxysms of atrial fibrillation; nevertheless, the mortality of endurance competitors is only a fifth of that for the general population, and it seems sufficient to control the disordered cardiac rhythm by antiarrythmic drugs, rather than prohibiting involvement in endurance competition. Adoption of a healthy lifestyle reduces the prospect of future cardiac events for as long as five years, with associated improvements in coronary vascular dimensions. Technicians who are well-trained can monitor exercise stress tests as effectively as a cardiologist. Regardless of age, women are three times less likely than men to undergo an exercise stress test. The diagnostic value of a stress test is increased if it is combined with psychological stress; incorporation of right ventricular leads increases sensitivity but not specificity. Differentiation of myocardial infarction from muscle microtraumata is helped by the combined determinations of creatine kinase MB isoenzymes and leukocyte differential counts. A careful meta-analysis confirms that an exercise program can do much to enhance functional capacity in patients with peripheral vascular disease. The effects of exercise training on the severity and duration of upper respiratory illnesses are explored, and a number of articles provide new insights into exercise-associated changes in immune function.

A large volume of research on fluid replacement continues. Men appear to use more carbohydrate than women during endurance exercise. Ski jumpers are identified as a further class of athletes who engage in major weight-reduction programs. Glycopenia can develop with rapid weight loss in wrestling, impairing cognitive function, and glucose supplements also enhance the technical skills of tennis players. However, carbohydrate supplements are shown to be ineffective in preventing the drop in plasma amino acid concentrations that some have associated with immunosuppression. The hypoglycemia associated with a precompetition meal can be avoided if carbohydrate is taken as sweetened oat flour with a moderate glycemic index and a high fiber content. Absorption of fluid from the first 0.5 meters of duodenum and jejunum does not differ between pure water and glucose/salt mixtures. Training shifts metabolism from carbohydrate to fat, and in the first few days a part of this benefit may be caused by plasma volume expansion. A recent review article confirms the temporary suppression of appetite associated with a brisk bout of exercise, a fact that can be exploited in a fat loss program. Sustained weight loss is most commonly achieved on a self-help basis, rather than through organized programs. A Step 2 diet is shown to be ineffective in correcting lipid profile unless accompanied by exercise. A method for measuring individual heat stress from a combination of rectal temperature and heart rate is described; a new portable electrical conductivity meter also allows assessments of chronic dehydration in the field. Dehydration reduces muscle endurance by as much as 15%. Creatine supplements speed the resynthesis of phosphocreatine and extend the time to fatigue in older adults.

Collateral blood flow in ischemic limbs can be enhanced by both exercise and the administration of basic fibroblast growth factor, with synergism between the two stimuli. Angioplasty is shown to enhance exercise tolerance less in patients who continue to smoke. The level of physical activity found in the average active woman does not appear sufficient to offer significant protection against breast cancer. A brief stress test to 85% of heart rate maximum is enough to cause temporary impairment of cognition in patients with chronic fatigue syndrome. When mice are run for the equivalent of a marathon, the replication of viruses in alveolar macrophages is substantially increased, with parallel changes in interferon production.

Among female athletes, the issue of energy balance continues to be a concern, and new evidence presented here illustrates both the adverse impact of inadequate nutrition on bone mineral density, and the protective effect of high intensity resistance exercise. Gender differences in the biomechanics of walking are highlighted, and it is demonstrated that anterior cruciate ligament reconstruction has a long-term impact on the biomechanics of walking. Several longitudinal studies report age-related changes in muscle strength and flexibility. The impact of aging on muscle fiber characteristics is contrasted between the masseter muscle and the biceps brachii, and age-related changes in the ability to side-step are documented.

This introduction provides just a tantalizing preview of the many exciting articles summarized in the current edition of the YEAR BOOK OF SPORTS MEDICINE. I trust that you will enjoy reading about these new developments as much as I have.

Roy J. Shephard, M.D., Ph.D., D.P.E.

Prescribing Exercise for Female Patients

ROY J. SHEPHARD, M.D., PH.D., D.P.E.
Faculty of Physical Education & Health, University of Toronto, Toronto Rehabilitation Centre, Toronto, Ontario, and Health Sciences Program, Brock University, St. Catharines, Ontario.

This article reviews gender differences influencing the prescription of exercise for middle-aged and older female patients, looking at what epidemiologists have sometimes classified as "secondary" and "tertiary" preventive programs (ie, programs that are begun before and after an overt clinical event such as the onset of anginal pain).[1] Information on the biological characteristics of female athletes is growing rapidly, but there is still a dearth of information on how the average woman responds to exercise, physical conditioning, and cardiac rehabilitation programs.[2] Nevertheless, women make up some 15% of those who attend cardiac rehabilitation programs.[3] The annual economic burden due to heart disease in US women has been estimated at $20 billion[4]; moreover, the prevalence of ischemic heart disease is currently declining much less rapidly in women than in men, and by the age of 70 years as many as 20% of women are affected by coronary vascular disease.[5]

Exercise prescriptions based on the responses of male patients may be inappropriate for women, decreasing motivation and even presenting physical danger, since there are important gender-related differences in the physiologic and psychological reactions to both acute exercise and training. Clinical manifestations of ischemic heart disease develop in women at a much older age than they do in men. The typical female cardiac patient is thus initially seen with symptoms of angina pectoris, rather than with myocardial infarction, and the careful clinician will be aware of many gender-specific features of diagnosis and treatment.

Responses to Exercise

Current data indicate that there are substantial gender differences in exercise responses between male and female patients, but it is less clear whether these differences have a biological, constitutional basis, or whether they are caused by sociocultural factors that discourage the involvement of women in many forms of vigorous physical activity.

Physical Work Capacity

Physical work capacity overlaps widely between men and women. In consequence, although the average woman scores poorly relative to her male counterpart on many of our current tests, a well-trained female can outperform many men of similar age, particularly in terms of aerobic power, balance, and flexibility.

Gender-related differences in physical work capacity can be detected among quite young children, but these differences first become large enough to assume practical significance at the age of puberty. Relative to men of similar age, young women are 4% to 8% shorter, with a 20% to

30% lower body mass, a 30% greater body fat content, a 30% to 40% lower lean tissue mass, and a 10% lower hemoglobin concentration.[6,7] Women also have a smaller heart volume, even after adjusting for differences in body size,[8] and perhaps because of the smaller cardiac mass, the peak systolic and diastolic pressures are lower in women than in men.[9]

The difference in stature is indisputably biological. The leverage of the arm and leg muscles is reduced by the shorter limb length; this makes rapid, repetitive movements more difficult, but facilitates fine, highly coordinated motor tasks. The woman's lower hemoglobin level also has a strong biological component, reflecting low levels of circulating androgens and menstrual blood loss. Gender differences in body fat content, muscle development, and bone strength are again partly determined by biological factors, but here the magnitude of the observed differences also reflects gender stereotypes that have held girls to less active roles throughout their developmental years.[10,11] The progressive diminution of gender-related differences in physical work capacity in recent years is most easily explained by the progressive elimination of barriers to female participation in vigorous physical activity.

Because women have a lower hemoglobin level, they can carry less oxygen per liter of cardiac output than men and their maximal oxygen transport is correspondingly handicapped. Body fat content further reduces, relative to men, their oxygen transport per unit of body mass. Weak skeletal muscles limit tolerance of heavy work, and attempts to match the muscle force developed by a male peer cause a larger and more rapid rise of systemic blood pressure, a higher heart rate, a heavier afterloading of the left ventricle, and a greater increase of cardiac work rate. Because afterloading tends to be greater, the increase of ejection fraction during progressive, maximal exercise is smaller in women than in men.[8,12-15]

Exercise Electrocardiogram

More women than men report exercise-induced chest pain and show "ischemic" electrocardiograms (ECGs),[16-18] but it remains controversial whether there is a higher incidence of false-positive reports, or whether the clinical diagnosis of ischemic heart disease is more easily overlooked in women.

A quarter of women aged 20 to 39, half of those 40 to 59, and two thirds of those over the age of 60 have ECGs that (by male criteria) would be diagnosed as myocardial ischemia.[12] However, specificity of an "ischemic" ECG relative to such diagnostic "gold standards" as angiography is poor in women (59% to 66%[17,19]); only 4.6% of women with ischemic ECGs progress to overt cardiac disease in 5 years, compared with 18% of men.[20] In women, the further investigation of apparent ischemia with thallium scintigraphy may also be difficult, since the scintigraphic signals are attenuated by the overlying breast fat.[18,21] However, exercise echocardiography is reported as having a greater sensitivity and specificity for the diagnosis of coronary artery disease than the exercise ECG record.[22]

The majority of women with "positive" ECGs show no angiographic evidence of coronary vascular narrowing, although a poor exercise ejection fraction may suggest a relative myocardial ischemia,[16] perhaps due to small vessel disease, which is not readily detected by means of angiography. A second factor is the low prevalence of coronary disease in women. As Bayes theorem makes clear, this inevitably compromises the ability of the exercise ECG (or, indeed, any other diagnostic test) to detect clinically significant coronary vascular disease. A further issue is the cross-sectional thickness of the ventricular wall, which is substantially less in a woman than in a man. A greater tension per unit cross-section of ventricular wall is thus developed during vigorous exercise, and the intramural tension may rise to a sufficient level to occlude the penetrating coronary vessels. Tension within the ventricular wall is proportional to the average ventricular diameter. Thus, a woman's situation is exacerbated by a lesser catecholamine-mediated increase of ventricular contractility than would occur in a male patient[23]; exercise induces a greater increase of ventricular dimensions, and in consequence the wall tension is higher than in a man.[13] Other possible disadvantages in the female patient include evaluation by exercise test protocols that are designed for men, a heavy afterloading of the left ventricle because limb blood flow is impeded by skeletal muscle weakness, and a depressant effect of estrogens on myocardial contractility.[23]

Environmental Factors

Women react less favorably than men when exercising in either cold or hot and dry environments, because women have a larger body surface area-to-mass ratio and thus a greater heat exchange with the environment.[24] In a very cold environment there are additional handicaps; women's peak rate of heat production is lower,[25] and they are less able to generate heat by non-shivering thermogenesis.[26]

Despite a thicker layer of subcutaneous fat, women lose heat faster than men do in a cold environment. Under hot and dry conditions, they gain heat more rapidly than do men.[27] They may also sweat less readily than men,[28] although when making experimental comparisons of heat tolerance, it is often difficult to decide whether female and male subjects have been appropriately matched for initial training status, another variable that influences tolerance of stressful environments.

Biomechanical Factors

There are gender-related differences in motor coordination and the oxygen cost of many everyday tasks, but these seem related mainly to differences in body size, center of gravity, joint flexibility, angles of limb carriage, and the individual's experience in the performance of specific activities.

The tables of oxygen costs used in prescribing exercise have generally been developed with male subjects in mind, and they do not necessarily apply to women, even if standardized per unit of body mass (for example, by expression as MET units). In contrast, exercise prescriptions based on a heart rate range or a rating of perceived exertion generally impose a similar relative stress on women and men.

Metabolic Factors

Depot fat seems to be mobilized less readily in women than in men. This may reflect a woman's need to conserve energy for the demands of pregnancy and lactation.[29-32] On the other hand, women have a much higher HDL cholesterol level than do men.[33]

The bones are both lighter and less densely calcified in women, and one might anticipate an increased risk of fractures during the performance of various sports. However, in practice this danger is offset by patterns of play that are based on skill rather than physical aggression and a lighter body mass than in the average man.

Response to Training

Effects of Training

A woman's responses to equivalent amounts of aerobic training are similar to those anticipated in men, but in general women prefer walking, swimming, and aerobic dance rather than the vigorous competitive physical activities favored by many men.[34] Training induces a 5 to 10 mm Hg decrease in resting blood pressures in both normotensive and hypertensive subjects,[35,36] and insulin responsiveness is also increased after a period of conditioning.[37,38]

As in men, training decreases the exercise blood pressure and heart rate, reducing the cardiac work rate and thus the oxygen demand of the myocardium at any given power output. Further, a lengthening of the diastolic phase of the cardiac cycle improves myocardial perfusion, particularly in the sub-endocardial zone, where most of the flow occurs during diastole. However, there have been suggestions that women show less improvement of left ventricular filling dynamics than do their male counterparts.[39]

It is unclear whether the intrinsic magnitude of the aerobic training response is equivalent for women and for men, because of difficulties in matching initial fitness levels. Female cadets at West Point Military Academy showed larger gains of maximal oxygen intake than did their male counterparts, but the authors of this study attributed the difference to a poorer initial physical condition of the female recruits.[40]

Women who engage in resistance exercise do not develop the massive muscle hypertrophy that is seen in men,[41,42] probably because circulating androgen concentrations are low in women. Nevertheless, weight-lifting programs can induce increases of strength which have considerable practical value to older female patients, primarily through such mechanisms as improved neuromuscular coordination.

Training also reduces body fat content less readily in women than in men, probably because the secretion of prolactin conserves the depot fat of a female against the metabolic needs of pregnancy and lactation. However, body fat content can decrease in response to adequate and sustained programs of exercise,[43,44] with resultant improvements in blood lipids (particularly increases in HDL2-cholesterol and A-2 apoprotein).[44-48] Women who have a distorted body image may couple a high level of habitual physical activity with an inadequate food intake, leading to manifestations of anorexia nervosa.

Motives for Exercising

Perceived motives for exercise reveal some important gender differences, and these differences are important to program design and exercise prescription.

Men indicate four main reasons for program enrollment: a desire to improve fitness or health, the availability of the exercise facility, a desire to "assist science" (in experimental studies), and recreational or hedonistic.[49] Women indicate at least six motivating factors: to improve health or fitness, the availability of programs and facilities adapted to their needs, to enhance well-being, to assist science, recreational/hedonistic, and a desire to socialize or make friends.[49,50]

Women value detailed exercise programming. In contrast, men are attracted by the convenience and quality of the facility and by respect for the operating personnel.[51] Women wish to lose weight[34] and improve health, but men place more value on the relief of tension and "feeling better."[52] Women often enter an exercise program with a lesser sense of self-efficacy than their male peers,[53] and are more concerned about pain and fatigue arising from the exercises.[54] Perhaps because women tend to emphasize the social aspects of an exercise program at the expense of strenuous physical effort, involvement has only a limited impact on other forms of health behavior. Over the first year of one worksite fitness program, men showed a 2.4-year decrease in their biological age (as assessed from their risk-taking behavior). In contrast, women showed only a 0.1-year reduction in biological age.[55]

In healthy individuals, program compliance was similar in men and women,[56] but in post-coronary patients there was a 19% dropout rate among the women, compared with 8% in men.[57] One might anticipate that gender differences in compliance would reflect largely the physiologic and psychological problems that women encounter if they enter exercise programs that have been tailored to the desires and abilities of men.[4] However, characteristics of the female drop-out do not seem strongly related to program content; they include high anger scores on the Profile of Mood States and a poor flexibility on the sit and reach test.[56]

Health Benefits of Regular Exercise

The health benefits of regular exercise have been examined less frequently in women than in men.[58,59] One meta-analysis of the response to cardiac rehabilitation programs found data for female subjects in only 4 of 43 studies.[60] Questionnaire reports suggest that there is little association between physical activity and protection against cardiac disease in women,[61,62] but this may be because activity patterns have been ascertained by means of questionnaires that were designed for men; such instruments may fail to elicit forms of physical activity that are more common in women (for example, care for dependents). Different (and sometimes simpler) questionnaires[63-65] and fitness scores[66] show that women can decrease their risks of cardiac disease by adopting a physically active lifestyle.

Responses After Myocardial Infarction

Acute Exercise

Because a woman's heart is small, a given-size of infarct destroys a larger fraction of ventricular muscle than in a man. A given decrease in aerobic power also has greater functional significance, since the average woman has a smaller functional reserve prior to development of a myocardial infarction.

Loss of lean tissue during hospitalization exacerbates problems associated with the weak musculature of a female patient. If a woman returns to heavy physical activity too rapidly post-infarction, the rise of blood pressure during exercise bouts is likely to provoke acute ischemia and related disturbances of myocardial function.[67,68] Only a half of women who report typical angina, and less than a fifth of those with atypical chest pain, show significant coronary obstruction at routine angiography.[4] However, such observations are usually made with the patient at rest after a period of abstinence from cigarettes. A higher proportion of abnormalities would be anticipated if observations could be made during normal daily life.

In those who develop chest pain, exercise causes a decrease of ejection fraction three times more often in women than in men.[68] This suggests that the acute effect of exercise in the female patient is a compromise of myocardial oxygen supply or contractile function through such factors as vascular spasm, microvascular narrowing, weak skeletal muscles, a large increase of heart rate and blood pressure, and a high cardiac work rate. However, the exercise-induced change in ejection fraction has less diagnostic significance in women than in men,[69,70] perhaps because women have a hyperdynamic pattern of left ventricular function.[71]

Immediate Risks of Exercise

The first symptoms of coronary heart disease appear 10 years later in women than in men. Even at this stage, a woman is much less likely to be referred for angiography and coronary vascular surgery[72-74] and is at greater risk of death in hospital immediately following an acute incident.

Diagnosed coronary heart disease does not peak in women until around 75 years of age. The initial presentation is commonly angina pectoris, rather than infarction, and the full picture of myocardial infarction does not develop until 20 years later than in a man.[4] Thus, many female patients have become frail and dependent, with a very low level of habitual physical activity even before the diagnosed ischemic episode; indeed, the infarct may be an incidental finding during a routine ECG or even at postmortem examination.

Attempts to implement exercise rehabilitation programs for the female patient are hampered by chest pain, frailty, and other concomitants of advanced aging. Concomitant morbidity, including rheumatoid or osteoarthritis, poor pulmonary function, a deterioration of vision, neurologic problems, nutritional deficiencies, and a distorted perception of exertion—all tend to curtail physical activity sessions before an adequate training response has been achieved.[75]

A high proportion of elderly women report an exercise-induced pain that has many of the characteristics of angina pectoris. Some also show congestive failure, secondary to previous undiagnosed myocardial infarction.[76] In the first few weeks after myocardial infarction, death is twice as common in women as in men, and 39% of women (as compared with 31% of men) are likely to die over the first year of rehabilitation.[77] However, because women usually pursue exercise less aggressively than do men, the proportion of exercise-induced deaths is smaller in women than in men.[78]

Exercise After Angioplasty

Gains from postsurgical rehabilitation seem similar in both sexes,[79] possibly because initial gender-related impairments of left ventricular function are corrected during hospital treatment.

Responses to Training After a Cardiac Incident

Investigators have had difficulty in demonstrating the beneficial impact of exercise upon mortality and morbidity, even in large samples of male post-coronary patients. It is thus not surprising that we lack definitive randomized controlled studies based on the much smaller and older pool of female patients. Kavanagh[3] claimed that the effectiveness of cardiac rehabilitation was unaffected by gender, but many authors now suggest that women have a less favourable immediate response than men after myocardial infarction.

Morbidity and Mortality

Many studies have found equal or better short-term[80-82] and long-term[83-89] prognoses in women than in men after myocardial infarction. But in support of an authoritative review,[90] several recent reports have demonstrated that women have a higher age-adjusted in-hospital myocardial infarction mortality rate than do men (17% vs 12%[91]), with more post-infarct complications, comorbid events that limit exercise participation,[92,93] and a higher mortality rate over the next 1 to 4 years.[94-99]

An older age and a greater prevalence of hypertension[94] both contribute to a poor prognosis in female patients. However, much of the argument regarding a better or poorer prognosis in women probably turns around difficulties in diagnosis, and the extent of allowances that are made for risk factors such as diabetes mellitus.[100-103] Other subtle biological and cultural factors contribute to a poorer outcome in women. Sometimes, myocardial health has already been compromised by previous, undetected infarctions.[76] A given lesion also has greater functional impact in a woman, because the heart is smaller than in a man.

Program Participation

It can be difficult to implement an effective program of exercise-based rehabilitation if a woman is frail and elderly before infarction. A high proportion of women experience anginal pain, and this makes vigorous exercise an uncomfortable experience.

Whereas most men are willing to take 3 to 4 weeks of graded rest after myocardial infarction, women have been socialized to feel guilty if they are not attending to household chores.[104] They do not regard such activities as demanding exercise, and thus return to quite heavy housework, including lifting and reaching above their heads, as soon as they leave the hospital. In consequence, they become physically fatigued, and this discourages subsequent participation in a structured exercise program.

Cardiac rehabilitation programs often require thrice weekly attendance at a distant exercise facility. Female patients may lack personal transportation to reach the facility, and domestic duties often preclude their attendance at the typical 6 to 7 PM post-coronary exercise class. Assuming that practical obstacles to participation can be overcome, program compliance is still strongly influenced by the individual's mood state; women with myocardial infarction more frequently suffer from depression, anxiety, and feelings of guilt than do their male peers.[105-107] They are thus less likely to be recruited to an exercise program, and show a poorer compliance than men.[95,104] Personnel operating cardiac rehabilitation programs for female patients must therefore devote more time to recruiting and motivating class members.[108]

Program Response

One report claimed that over a typical rehabilitation program, women showed a similar increase in functional capacity to men, despite poorer program compliance.[109] Presumably, a poor initial fitness level gives greater scope to enhance physical work capacity in the female patient.

The value of estrogen replacement therapy as an adjunct to rehabilitation is discussed below. Smoking cessation programs, treatment of hyperlipidemia, and the control of hypertension probably contribute to the success of exercise-centered rehabilitation programs much as they do in men.

Return to Work

Women typically have a longer period of poor health than do men after myocardial infarction, and fewer women than men ultimately return to paid work.[105,110]

An early return to work is often associated with denial of disease and type A behavior,[111,112] which are less common characteristics in female than in male patients. Depression is also more prevalent in women than in men. The low initial work capacity of a woman is also more easily pushed below the minimum job requirement by a combination of illness and hospitalization.[113]

Women in traditional marriages may have fewer incentives to return to paid work. Outside employment may provide no more than discretionary income, and paid work must be combined with responsibilities as a home-maker.[105] In contrast, single women have a strong interest in returning to work because their financial resources are limited.[105]

Hormonal Factors

Gender-related differences in the hormonal milieu and mineral reserves may make a woman's heart less vulnerable to cardiovascular disease than that of a man.[115] Certainly, the risk of infarction rises steeply as the protective action of estrogens is lost following the menopause.[116-118] Angina pectoris often antedates infarction in women, suggesting that female patients either escape or retard the fatal consequences of atheroma for many more years than their male counterparts.[114] However, this is difficult to evaluate, given reports of a gender-related differential in access to medical services.[72-74] Other factors—both constitutional and cultural—may also keep middle-aged women from making sudden competitive physical efforts and engaging in the aggressive, hostile behavior that convert "silent" atheroma to an overt heart attack.

Use of estrogen contraceptives increases the risk of a cardiovascular incident prior to the menopause. However, after menopause or oophorectomy, therapeutic estrogen reduces the risk of cardiovascular death.[119-121] One potential mechanism for the protective action of estrogen is through an increase in HDL-cholesterol levels, although changes in lipid profile do not seem sufficient to account for all of the protection that postmenopausal women gain from hormone replacement therapy.

Risk Factors in Women

Estrogens

In young women, myocardial infarction is strongly related to the administration of estrogens, whether as contraceptive agents (relative risk about 15) or in other types of treatment (relative risk about 9). However, the increase of cardiovascular risk disappears rapidly once estrogen treatment has stopped.[121] Protection may be derived from the administration of estrogens after the menopause.

Cigarette Smoking

Cigarette smoking carries a risk ratio of 5 in female patients,[122-125] and the risk of a recurrent infarction remains elevated if the patient continues to smoke.[126-130] The risk from the premenopausal administration of estrogens is also exacerbated by smoking.

As in men, smoking causes tachycardia (with a resultant increase in cardiac work rate), coronary vascular spasm, poor left ventricular function, and a reduced efficacy of anti-anginal drugs.[131-134] These responses exacerbate myocardial ischemia, and favor a recurrence of clinical disease of the myocardium.

Cardiovascular Abnormalities

Ventricular premature beats are not an independent risk factor in women,[135] but hypertension is a significant cardiac risk factor.[124] Women commonly have a better left ventricular ejection fraction than men when they are discharged from hospital,[104] but perhaps because of the prevalence of hypertension, they seem more vulnerable to the development of congestive heart failure.[107]

A substantial proportion of women who complain of chest pain remain free of clinically diagnosed myocardial infarction for many years, and angina seems a less significant risk factor for women than for men.[76,136] However, it is difficult to dissociate this gender difference from (1) differential patterns of diagnosis and treatment and (2) a greater prevalence of pain without angiographic evidence of coronary artery narrowing in female patients.[4,137]

Metabolic Factors

An adverse lipid profile remains a cardiac risk factor for women, as in men,[138-139] despite gender differences in average normal values. Triglycerides are also an independent cardiac risk factor in women.[62,140] Obesity does not appear to be a direct risk factor in women,[124] but it limits functional capacity in patients with weakened hearts, and it predisposes to maturity-onset diabetes mellitus. Women with diabetes mellitus have about twice the risk of dying of a heart attack as do men, and the risk of death from a cerebrovascular accident is also greater than in men.[126,141,142] A combination of diabetes mellitus and hypertension increases the risk of sudden death,[144] perhaps because the cardiac work rate is greater under such conditions.

Gender Differences in Treatment

Men are more likely than women to die outside of a hospital.[144] Because of their younger age at the time of the clinical incident, men are more likely to have a heart attack develop when working or playing in circumstances where prompt access to emergency treatment is lacking. More women than men are referred for coronary artery bypass surgery,[145,146] although they seem less likely to have undergone prior noninvasive testing or angiography than male patients.[72,73,147-150] Women also take longer to reach a hospital after myocardial infarction; they are less likely to be admitted[151] and are less likely to be referred to cardiac rehabilitation programs or tertiary care hospitals.[152] There are also gender-related differences in symptom-denial, self-medication, willingness to call a physician, and the service rendered, all of which should be considered when planning preventive programs.

Risk Factors After Myocardial Infarction and Coronary Vascular Surgery

The progression of atherosclerosis is, in general, similar in women and in men.[153] However, there is little information on the nature of cardiac risk factors in women after they have sustained a cardiac incident. Despite the need for such research,[154] there are major practical problems in recruiting adequate subject numbers to conduct appropriate investigations. One study found that after myocardial infarction, the only predictors of increased risk were continued cigarette smoking and diabetes mellitus.[126] In female patients, exercise-induced chest pain or ST segmental depression is not associated with an adverse prognosis if arteriography shows a near normal coronary vascular supply.[12,155] However, the adverse impact of persistent congestive failure is about twice as great in women as in men.[107]

Benefit from β-blocking agents seems smaller in women than in men.[156,157] Low-dose aspirin[158,159] and streptokinase[159,160] are also useful adjuvants to an exercise rehabilitation program.

The perioperative mortality rate of angioplasty is higher in women than in men, possibly because women's coronary vessels are smaller,[107] although other factors also contribute to a poor early prognosis in women. The operation less frequently relieves chest pain, complicating exercise rehabilitation programs.[4,161] Women also have a greater short-term risk of bradycardia, hypotension, and coronary dissection than men, and account should be taken of such potential complications when planning exercise programs. In a long-term perspective, the risk of restenosis is lower in women than in men.[162]

Implications for Management of the Female Patient

The primary objectives after either myocardial infarction or coronary vascular surgery include the relief of symptoms, a reduction of morbidity and early mortality, and an optimization of the quality of life for the patient's remaining years. Encouragement of exercise compliance is important to both function and survival.

Prescribed exercise must recognize gender differences in acute and chronic responses to physical activity. Programs for women should be arranged in a format and at a time that encourages attendance and active participation (based on female aptitudes and motives for exercising). Women in general have a greater desire for the "safety" of monitoring, peer support, social interactions, and emotional support.[163] Feelings of depression, anxiety, guilt, and a poor quality of life are more common in female than in male patients,[107,164] in part because women have a higher incidence of associated diseases and a greater chance of widowhood.[165] Thus, women have a greater need for associated psychotherapy sessions. Participants must learn the normalcy of a depressed mood-state following myocardial infarction, and spouses should be educated regarding physical and emotional problems of the recovery process. If vigorous physical activity is limited by anginal pain, appropriate medication should be provided, and an interval training regimen should be substituted for continuous aerobic exercise. Because the incidence of coronary vascular spasm is high, nitrites and calcium-channel blocking drugs may be particularly effective in helping women to begin exercising. Both beta-blockers[166] and ACE inhibitors[167] can be useful adjuncts to rehabilitation. However, nonspecific beta-blocking drugs should be given with care, since the vulnerability to cold-induced vasospasm is greater in women than in men.

Correction of obesity will increase relative aerobic power and relative strength, thus increasing the patient's functional capacity and quality of life.[162] As with male patients, low-fat diets and pharmacologic treatment can make useful contributions to the slowing of atherosclerosis.[168-170] There is a particular need to strengthen skeletal muscles in older women, given their low initial strength. Finally, it may be important to teach women techniques to reduce the energy costs of household work, thus extending the range of activities that they can undertake in the face of limited cardiovascular function.[108]

Continuing risk factors (smoking, use of oral contraceptives, diabetes, and hypertension) should be corrected where possible. Regular monitoring and counseling are important to success. One study found adequate treatment of hypertension in only 27% of women after myocardial infarction,[171] with a higher mortality in untreated individuals. Others have noted the improved prognosis with smoking cessation,[127-130] but also the unfortunate tendency to recidivism among smokers after recovery from myocardial infarction.[3,172]

Estrogen replacement therapy may help postmenopausal patients, perhaps by boosting levels of HDL-cholesterol.[120,121,173] If given alone to premenopausal women, there is an offsetting increase in the risk of uterine and breast cancers,[174] and it remains unclear how far coronary protection is attenuated if estrogen is administered in combination with progesterone. Exercise may encourage smoking withdrawal, although the socially focused activities popular with many women have less impact than a demanding aerobic-type endurance training program. The intake of saturated fats should be reduced, although women respond less favorably than men to a change in diet, particularly if they have the apoE 3/2 phenotype. The HDL-cholesterol level falls, and the LDL/HDL ratio rises to male levels.[175]

Conclusions

The interaction between cardiac risk factors and gender-related differences in responses to exercise and training must be considered carefully when designing cardiac rehabilitation programs for women. Nevertheless, programs offer substantial therapeutic benefit if women are given strong encouragement to participate in a program that is designed specifically to meet their needs.

Dr. Shephard's studies are supported, in part, by research grants from the Toronto Rehabilitation Centre and Canadian Tire Acceptance Limited.

References

1. Mausner JS, Bahn AK: *Epidemiology: An Introductory Text.* Philadelphia, WB Saunders, 1974.

2. Thomas RJ, Houston-Miller N, Lamendola C, et al: National survey on gender differences in cardiac rehabilitation programs. *J Cardiopulm Rehabil* 16:401-412, 1996.
3. Kavanagh T: *The Healthy Heart Programme.* Toronto, Van Nostrand, 1985.
4. Packard B: Clinical aspects of coronary heart disease in women, in Wenger NK and Hellerstein HK (eds): *Rehabilitation of the Coronary Patient,* ed 3. New York, Churchill Livingstone, 1992, pp 217-230.
5. Newnham H: Women's hearts are hard to break. *Lancet* 346:13-16, 1997.
6. Klafs CE, Lyon MJ: *The female athlete: A coach's guide to conditioning and training.* St. Louis, Mosby, 1978.
7. Wells CL: *Women, sport and performance.* Champaign, IL, Human Kinetics Publishers, 1985.
8. Hanley PC, Zinsmeister AR, Clements IP, et al: Gender-related differences in cardiac response to supine exercise assessed by radionuclide angiography. *J Am Coll Cardiol* 13:624-629, 1989.
9. Daida H, Allison TG, Squires RW, et al: Peak exercise blood pressure stratified by age and gender in apparently healthy subjects. *Mayo Clin Proc* 71:445-452, 1996.
10. Hall MA: Sport and physical activity in the lives of Canadian women, in: Gruneau RG and Albinson JG (eds): *Canadian Sport: Sociological Perspectives.* London, Addison-Wesley, 1976, pp 170-199.
11. Loy JW, McPherson BD, Kenyon G: *Sport and Social Systems.* London, Addison-Wesley, 1978.
12. Houghton JL, Price C, Chatterjee B, et al: Short term prognosis in females with no or insignificant coronary disease and a diagnostic exercise test. *J Cardiopulm Rehabil* 10:58-64, 1990.
13. Franquiz, JM, Alvarez A, Fernandez R, et al: Effect of gender on the left ventricular response to supine exercise in healthy subjects. *J Cardiopulm Rehabil* 12:183-187, 1992.
14. Higginbotham MB, Morris KG, Coleman E, et al: Sex-related differences in normal cardiac responses to upright exercise. *Circulation* 70:357-366, 1984.
15. Merz CNB, Moriel M, Rozanski A, et al: Gender-related differences in exercise ventricular function among healthy subjects and patients. *Am Heart J* 131:704-709, 1996.
16. Cumming GR, Dufresne C, Samm J: Exercise e.c.g. changes in normal women. *Can Med Assoc J* 109:108-111, 1973.
17. Sidney KH, Shephard RJ: Training and ecg abnormalities in the elderly. *Br Heart J* 39:1114-1120, 1977.
18. Chaitman BR, Bourassa MG, Lam J: Non-invasive diagnosis of coronary heart disease in women, in Eaker ED, Packard B, Wenger NK, et al (eds): *Coronary Heart Disease in Women.* New York, Haymarket Doyma, 1987, p 222.
19. Sullivan AK, Holdright DR, Wright CA, et al: Chest pain in women: Clinical, investigative, and prognostic features. *Br Med J* 308:883-886, 1994.
20. Manca C, Dei Cas L, Albertini D, et al: Different prognostic value of exercise electrocardiogram in men and women. *Cardiology* 63:312-319, 1978.
21. Jones RH, McEwan P, Newman GE, et al: Accuracy of diagnosis of coronary artery disease by radionuclide measurement of left ventricular function during rest and exercise. *Circulation* 64:586-601, 1981.
22. Williams MJ, Marwick TH, O'Gorman D, et al: Comparison of exercise echocardiography with an exercise score to diagnose coronary artery disease in women. *Am J Cardiol* 74:435-438, 1994.
23. Glazer MD, Hurst JW: Coronary atherosclerotic heart disease: Some important differences in men and women. *Am J Noninvasive Cardiol* 1:61-67, 1987.
24. Kollias J, Bartlett L, Bergsteinova V, et al: Metabolic and thermal responses of women during cooling in water. *J Appl Physiol* 36:577-580, 1974.
25. Graham TE: Alcohol ingestion and sex differences on the thermal responses to mild exercise in a cold environment. *Hum Biol* 55:463-476, 1983.
26. Shephard RJ: Metabolic adaptations to exercise in the cold: An update. *Sports Med* 1993; In press.

27. Drinkwater B: Women and exercise: Physiological aspects. *Ex Sport Sci Rev* 12:21-51, 1984.
28. Frye AJ, Kamon E: Responses to dry heat of men and women with similar aerobic capacities. *J Appl Physiol* 50:65-70, 1981.
29. Murray SJ, Shephard RJ, Greaves S, et al: Effects of cold stress and exercise on fat loss in females. *Eur J Appl Physiol* 55:610-618, 1986.
30. Brownell KD, Bachorik PS, Ayerle RS: Changes in plasma lipid and lipoprotein levels in men and women after a program of moderate exercise. *Circulation* 65:477-484, 1982.
31. Goldberg L, Elliot DL: The effect of exercise on lipid metabolism in men and women. *Sports Med* 4:307-321, 1987.
32. Després JP, Bouchard C, Savard R, et al: Effects of exercise training and detraining on fat cell lipolysis in men and women. *Eur J Appl Physiol* 53:25-30, 1984.
33. Rifkind BM, Tamir I, Heiss G, et al: Distribution of high density and other lipoproteins in selected LRC prevalence study populations: A brief survey. *Lipids* 14:105-112, 1979.
34. Williford HN, Scharff-Olson M, Blessing DL: Exercise prescription for women. Special considerations. *Sports Med* 15:299-311, 1993.
35. Tipton CM: Exercise, training and hypertension: An update. *Exerc Sport Sci Rev* 19:447-506, 1991.
36. Gibbons LW, Blair SN, Cooper KH, et al: Association between coronary heart disease risk factors and physical fitness in healthy adult women. *Circulation* 67:977-983, 1983.
37. King DS, Galsky GP, Staten MA, et al: Insulin action and secretion in endurance-trained and untrained humans. *J Appl Physiol* 63:2247-2252, 1987.
38. Holloszy JO, Schultz J, Kusni J, et al: Effects of exercise on glucose tolerance and insulin resistance: Brief review and some preliminary results. *Acta Med Scand Suppl* 711:55-65, 1986.
39. Spina RJ, Miller TR, Bogenhagen WH, et al: Gender-related differences in left ventricular filling dynamics in older subjects after endurance exercise training. *J Gerontol* 51A:B232-B237, 1996.
40. Daniels WL, Kowal DM, Vogel JA, et al: Physiological effects of a military training program on male and female cadets. *Aviat Space Environ Med* 50:562-566, 1979.
41. Brown CH, Wilmore JH: The effects of maximal resistance training on the strength and body composition of women athletes. *Med Sci Sports Exerc* 6:174-177, 1974.
42. Oyster N: Effects of heavy-resistance weight training program on college women athletes. *J Sports Med Phys Fitness* 19:79-83, 1979.
43. Lewis S, Haskell WL, Wood PD, et al: Effects of physical activity on weight reduction in obese middle-aged women. *Am J Clin Nutr* 29:151-156, 1976.
44. Owens JF, Mathews KA, Wing RR, et al: Can physical activity mitigate the effects of aging in middle-aged women? *Circulation* 85:1265-1270, 1992.
45. Durstine JL, Pate RR, Sparling PB, et al: Lipid, lipoprotein, and iron status of elite women distance runners. *Int J Sports Med* 8:119S-123S, 1987.
46. Rotkis T, Boyden TW, Parmenter RW, et al: High density lipoprotein cholesterol and body composition of female runners. *Metabolism* 30:994-995, 1981.
47. Hardman AE, Hudson A, Jones PR, et al: Brisk walking and plasma high density lipoprotein cholesterol concentration in previously sedentary women. *BMJ* 299:1204-1205, 1989.
48. Haskell WL: Exercise-induced changes in plasma lipids and lipoproteins. *Prev Med* 13:23-36, 1984.
49. Sidney KH, Shephard RJ: Attitudes toward health and physical activity in the elderly. Effects of a physical training programme. *Med Sci Sports Exerc* 8:246-252, 1977.
50. Sidney KH, Niinimaa V, Shephard RJ: Attitudes towards exercise and sports: Sex and age differences, and changes with endurance training. *J Sports Sci* 1:195-210, 1983.
51. Morgan PP, Shephard RJ, Finucane R, et al: Health beliefs and exercise habits in an employee fitness programme. *Can J Appl Sport Sci* 9:87-93, 1984.

52. Godin G, Shephard RJ: Psychosocial predictors of exercise intentions among spouses. *Can J Appl Sport Sci* 10:36-43, 1985.
53. Godin G, Shephard RJ: Gender differences in perceived physical self-efficacy among older individuals. *Percept Motor Skills* 60:599-602, 1985.
54. Moore SM, Kramer FM: Women's and men's preferences for cardiac rehabilitation program features. *J Cardiopulm Rehabil* 16:163-168, 1996.
55. Shephard RJ, Corey P, Cox MH: Health Hazard Appraisal: The influence of an employee fitness program. *Can J Publ Health* 73:183-187, 1982.
56. Ward A, Morgan WP: Adherence patterns of healthy men and women enrolled in an adult exercise program. *J Cardiac Rehabil* 4:143-152, 1984.
57. Oldridge NB, LaSalle D, Jones NL: Exercise rehabilitation of female patients with coronary artery disease. *Am Heart J* 100:755-757, 1980.
58. Healy B: The Yentl syndrome. *N Engl J Med* 325:274-276, 1991.
59. Gurwitz JH, Col NF, Vaorn J: The exclusion of the elderly and women from clinical trials in myocardial infarction. *JAMA* 268:1417-1422, 1992.
60. Powell KE, Thompson PD, Caspersen CJ, et al: Physical activity and the incidence of coronary heart disease. *Ann Rev Publ Health* 8:253-287, 1987.
61. Kannel WB, Sorlie P: Some health benefits of physical activity: The Framingham study. *Arch Int Med* 139:857-861, 1979.
62. Lapidus L, Bengtsson C: Socioeconomic factors and physical activity in relation to cardiovascular disease and death: A 12-year follow-up in a study of women in Gothenburg, Sweden. *Br Heart J* 55:295-301, 1986.
63. Magnus K, Matroos A, Strackee J: Walking, cycling or gardening with or without seasonal interruption, in relation to acute coronary events. *Am J Epidemiol* 110:724-733, 1979.
64. Scragg R, Stewart A, Jackson R, et al: Alcohol and exercise in myocardial infarction and sudden coronary death in men and women. *Am J Epidemiol* 126:77-85, 1987.
65. O'Connor GT, Buring JE, Goldhaber SZ, et al: Physical exercise and non-fatal myocardial infarction. *Am J Epidemiol* 126:741A-742A, 1987.
66. Blair SN, Kohl HW, Paffenbarger RS, et al: Physical fitness and all-cause mortality: A prospective study of healthy men and women. *JAMA* 262:2395-2401, 1989.
67. Berger HJ, Sands MJ, Davies RJ: Exercise left ventricular performance in patients with chest pain, ischemic appearing exercise electrocardiograms and angiographically normal coronary arteries. *Ann Intern Med* 94:186-191, 1981.
68. Gibbons RJ, Lee KL, Cobb F, et al: Ejection fraction response to exercise in patients with chest pain and normal coronary arteriograms. *Circulation* 64:952-957, 1981.
69. Jones RH, McEwan P, Newman GE, et al: Accuracy of diagnosis of coronary artery disease by radionuclide measurement of left ventricular function during rest and exercise. *Circulation* 64:586-601, 1981.
70. Moriel M, Rozanski A, Klein J, et al: The limited efficacy of exercise radionuclide ventriculography in assessing prognosis of women with coronary artery disease. *Am J Cardiol* 76:1030-1035, 1995.
71. Buonanno C, Rossi AL, Dander B, et al: Left ventricular function in men and women. *Eur Heart J* 3:525-528, 1982.
72. Ayanian JZ, Epstein AM: Differences in the use of procedures between women and men hospitalized for coronary heart disease. *N Engl J Med* 325:221-225, 1991.
73. Steingart RM, Packer M, Hamm P, et al: Sex differences in the management of coronary artery disease. *N Engl J Med* 325:226-230, 1991.
74. Petticrew M, McKee M, Jones J: Coronary artery surgery: are women discriminated against? *BMJ* 306:1164-1166, 1993.
75. Shephard RJ. Habitual physical activity levels and the perception of exertion in the elderly. *J Cardiopulm Rehabil* 9:17-23, 1989.
76. Lerner DJ, Kannel WB: Patterns of coronary heart disease morbidity and mortality in the sexes: A 26-year follow-up of the Framingham population. *Am Heart J* 111:383-390, 1986.
77. Kannel WB, Abbott RD: Incidence and prognosis of myocardial infarction in women, in Eaker ED, Packard B, Wenger NK, et al (eds): *Coronary Heart Disease in Women.* New York, Haymarket Doyma, 1987, p 208.

78. Romo M: Factors relating to sudden death in acute ischaemic heart disease. A community study in Helsinki. *Acta Med Scand* 547S:1-92, 1972.

79. Hanson P, Stevens R, Berkoff H, et al: Exercise capacity and cardiovascular responses to serial exercise testing in men and women after coronary bypass graft surgery. *J Cardiopulm Rehabil* 5:389-397, 1985.

80. Helmers C: Short and long-term prognostic indices in acute myocardial infarction. *Acta Med Scand* 555:1S-86S, 1974.

81. Norris RM, Caughey DE, Deeming LW, et al: Coronary prognostic index for predicting survival after recovery from acute myocardial infarction. *Lancet* 2:485-488, 1970.

82. Elveback LR, Connolly DC: Coronary heart disease in residents of Rochester, Minnesota: V. Prognosis of patients with coronary heart disease based on initial manifestations. *Mayo Clin Proc* 60:305-311, 1985.

83. Martin CA, Thompson PL, Armstrong BK, et al: Long-term prognosis after recovery from myocardial infarction: A nine year follow-up of the Perth Coronary Register. *Circulation* 68:961-969, 1983.

84. Ditttrich H, Gilpin E, Nicod P, et al: Acute myocardial infarction in women: Influence of gender on mortality and prognostic variables. *Am J Cardiol* 62:1-7, 1988.

85. Johansson S, Bergstrand R, Ulvenstam G, et al: Sex differences in preinfarction characteristics and long-term survival among patients with myocardial infarction. *Am J Epidemiol* 119:610-623, 1984.

86. Merrilees MA, Scott PJ, Norris RM: Prognosis after myocardial infarction: Results of 15-year follow-up. *BMJ* 288:356-359, 1984.

87. Saito M, Fukami KI, Hiramori K, et al: Long term prognosis of patients with acute myocardial infarction: Is mortality and morbidity as low as the incidence of ischemic heart disease in Japan? *Am Heart J* 113:891-897, 1987.

88. Wong ND, Cupples LA, Ostfeld AM, et al: Risk factors for long-term coronary prognosis after initial myocardial infarction: The Framingham Study. *Am J Epidemiol* 130:469-480, 1989.

89. Galatius-Jensen S, Launbjerg J, Mortensen LS, et al: Sex-related differences in short and long-term prognosis after acute myocardial infarction: 10 year follow-up of 3,073 patients in database of first Danish verapamil infarction trial. *BMJ* 313:137-140, 1996.

90. Wenger NK: Coronary disease in women. *Ann Rev Med* 36:285-294, 1985.

91. Walling A, Tremblay GJL, Jobin J, et al: Evaluating the rehabilitation potential of a large population of post-myocardial infarction patients: Adverse prognosis for women. *J Cardiopulm Rehabil* 8:99-106, 1988.

92. Wenger NK, Speroff L, Packard B: Cardiovascular health and disease in women. *N Engl J Med* 329:247-256, 1993.

93. Wilkinson P, Laji K, Ranjadayalan K, et al: Acute myocardial infarction in women: Survival analysis in first six months. *BMJ* 309:566-590, 1994.

94. Puletti M, Sunseri L, Curione M, et al: Acute myocardial infarction: Sex-related differences in prognosis. *Am Heart J* 108:63-66, 1984.

95. Tofler GH, Stone PH, Muller JE, et al: Effects of gender and race in prognosis after myocardial infarction: Adverse prognosis for women, particularly black women. *J Am Coll Cardiol* 9:473-482, 1987.

96. Greenland P, Reicher-Reiss H, Goldbourt U, et al: In-hospital and 1-year mortality in 1,524 women after myocardial infarction. Comparison with 4,315 men. *Circulation* 83:484-491, 1991.

97. Madsen JK, Thomsen BL, Sorensen JN, et al: Risk factors and prognosis after discharge for patients admitted because of suspected acute myocardial infarction with and without a confirmed diagnosis. *Am J Cardiol* 59:1064-1070, 1987.

98. Thygesen K, Dalsgaard P, Nielsen BL: Prognosis after first myocardial infarction. *Acta Med Scand* 195:253-259, 1974.

99. Juergens JL, Edwards JE, Achor RWP, et al: Prognosis of patients surviving first clinically diagnosed myocardial infarction. *Arch Int Med* 105:444-450, 1960.

100. Savage MP, Kroleski AS, Kenien GG, et al: Acute myocardial infarction in diabetes mellitus and significance of congestive heart failure as a prognostic factor. *Am J Cardiol* 62:665-669, 1988.
101. Smith JW, Marcus FI, Serokman K, et al: Prognosis of patients with diabetes mellitus after acute myocardial infarction. *Am J Cardiol* 54:718-721, 1984.
102. Jaffe AS, Spadaro JJ, Schectman K, et al: Increased congestive heart failure after myocardial infarction of modest extent in patients with diabetes mellitus. *Am Heart J* 108:31-37, 1984.
103. Tansey MJB, Opie LH, Kennelly BM: High mortality rates in obese women diabetics with acute myocardial infarction. *BMJ* (I):1624-1626, 1977.
104. Boogaard MAK, Briody ME: Comparison of the rehabilitation of men and women post-myocardial infarction. *J Cardiopulm Rehabil* 5:379-388, 1985.
105. Chiricos TN, Nickel JL: Work disability from coronary heart disease in women. *Women Health* 9:55-74, 1984.
106. Wenger NK: Coronary disease in women. *Ann Rev Med* 36:285-294, 1985.
107. Fisher LD, Kennedy JW, Davis KB, et al: Association of sex, physical size and operative mortality after coronary by-pass in the Coronary Artery Surgery Study (CASS). *J Thorac Cardiovasc Surg* 84:334-341, 1982.
108. Wenger NK: Elderly coronary patients, in Wenger NK and Hellerstein HK (eds): *Rehabilitation of the Coronary Patient*. New York, Churchill-Livingstone, 1992, p 415.
109. O'Callaghan WG, Teo KK, O'Riordan J, et al: Comparative response of male and female patients with coronary artery disease to exercise rehabilitation. *Eur Heart J* 8:649-651, 1984.
110. Maeland JG, Havik OE: Return to work after myocardial infarction: The influence of background factors, work characteristics and illness severity. *Scand J Soc Med* 14:183-195, 1986.
111. Burgess AW, Lerner DJ, D'Agostino RB, et al: A randomized control trial of cardiac rehabilitation. *Soc Sci Med* 24:359-370, 1987.
112. Degré-Coustry C, Grevisse M: Psychologic problems in rehabilitation after myocardial infarction. Non-institutional approach. *Adv Cardiol* 29:126-131, 1982.
113. Smith GR, O'Rourke DF: Return to work after a first myocardial infarction. A test of multiple hypotheses. *JAMA* 1673-1677, 1988.
114. Kannel WB, Brand FN: Cardiovascular risk factors in the elderly, in Andres R, Bierman EL, Hazzard WR (eds): *Principles of Geriatric Medicine*. New York, McGraw Hill, 1985, pp 104-119.
115. Anderson TW: The vulnerable myocardium. *Lancet* 2:1084-1085, 1973.
116. Szadjerman M, Oliver MP: Spontaneous premature menopause, ischemic heart disease and serum lipids. *Lancet* 1:962-965, 1963.
117. Rosenberg L, Hennekens CH, Rosner B, et al: Early menopause and the risk of myocardial infarction. *Am J Obstetr Gyn* 139:47-51, 1981.
118. Gordon T, Kannel WB, Hjortland MC, et al: Menopause and coronary heart disease. *Ann Intern Med* 89:157-161, 1978.
119. Bush TL, Barrett-Connor E, Cowan LD, et al: Cardiovascular mortality and non-contraceptive use of estrogen in women: Results from the Lipid Research Clinics Program Follow-up Study. *Circulation* 75:1102-1109, 1987.
120. Sullivan JM, Vander-Zwaag R, Hughes JP, et al: Estrogen replacement therapy and coronary artery disease. Effect on survival in postmenopausal women. *Arch Intern Med* 150:2557-2562, 1990.
121. Royal College of General Practitioners: *Oral Contraceptives and Health*. London, Pitman, 1974.
122. Mann JI, Vessey MP, Thorogood M, et al: Myocardial infarction in young women with special reference to oral contraceptive practice. *BMJ* 2:241-245, 1975.
123. Jick H, Dinan B, Herman R, Rothman KJ: Myocardial infarction and other vascular diseases in young women. Role of estrogens and other factors. *JAMA* 240:2548-2552, 1978.
124. Rosenberg L, Miller DR, Kaufman DW, et al: Myocardial infarction in women under 50 years of age. *JAMA* 250:2801-2806, 1983.

125. Freedman DS, Gruchow HW, Walker JA, et al: Cigarette smoking and non-fatal myocardial infarction in women: Is the relation independent of coronary artery disease? *Br Heart J* 62:273-280, 1989.

126. Khaw K-T, Barrett-Connor E: Prognostic factors for mortality in a population-based study of men and women with a history of heart disease. *J Cardiopulm Rehabil* 6:474-480, 1986.

127. Johansson S, Bergstrand R, Pennert K, et al: Cessation of smoking after myocardial infarction in women: Effects on mortality and reinfarctions. *Am J Epidemiol* 121:823-831, 1985.

128. Perkins J, Dick TB: Smoking and myocardial infarction: Secondary prevention. *Postgrad Med J* 61:295-300, 1985.

129. Salonen JT: Stopping smoking and long-term mortality after acute myocardial infarction. *Br Heart J* 43:463-469, 1980.

130. Mulcahy R: Influence of cigarette smoking on morbidity and mortality after myocardial infarction. *Br Heart J* 49:410-415, 1983.

131. Rode A, Ross R, Shephard RJ: Smoking withdrawal program. *AMA Arch Env Health* 24:27-36, 1972.

132. Winniford MD, Jansen DE, Reynolds GA, et al: Cigarette smoking-induced coronary vasoconstriction in atherosclerotic heart disease and prevention by calcium antagonists and nitroglycerin. *Am J Cardiol* 59:203-207, 1987.

133. Deanfield JE, Shea MJ, Wilson RA, et al: Direct effects of smoking on the heart: Silent ischemic disturbances of coronary flow. *Am J Cardiol* 57:1005-1009, 1986.

134. Mauoad J, Fernandez F, Hebert JL, et al: Cigarette smoking during coronary angiography: Diffuse or focal narrowing (spasm) of the coronary arteries in 13 patients with angina at rest and normal coronary angiograms. *Cathet Cardiovasc Diagn* 12:366-375, 1986.

135. Moss AJ, and Multicenter Postinfarction Research Group: Gender differences in the mortality risk associated with ventricular arrhythmias after myocardial infarction, in Eaker ED, Packard B, Wenger NK (eds): *Coronary Heart Disease in Women*. New York, Haymarket Doyma, 1987, p 204.

136. Elveback LR, Connolly DC: Coronary heart disease in residents of Rochester, Minnesota. V. Prognosis of patients with coronary heart disease based on initial manifestation. *Mayo Clin Proc* 60:305-311, 1985.

137. Harris T, Cook EF, Kannel WB, et al: Proportional hazards analysis of risk factors for coronary heart disease in individuals aged 65 or older. The Framingham Heart Study. *J Am Geriatr Soc* 36:1023-1028, 1988.

138. Kannel WB, Feinleib M: Natural history of angina pectoris in the Framingham study. Prognosis and survival. *Am J Cardiol* 29:154-163, 1972.

139. Harris F, Cook EF, Kannel WB, et al: Proportional hazards analysis of risk factors for coronary heart disease in individuals aged 65 or older. The Framingham Heart Study. *J Am Geriatr Soc* 36:1023-1028, 1988.

140. Johansson S, Bondjers G, Fager G, et al: Serum lipids and apolipoprotein levels in women with acute myocardial infarction. *Arteriosclerosis* 8:742-749, 1988.

141. Westlund K: *Mortality of Diabetics*. Oslo, Universitetsforlaget, 1969.

142. Tansey MJB, Opie LH, Kennelly BM: High mortality in obese women diabetics with acute myocardial infarction. *BMJ* 1:1624-1629, 1977.

143. Kannel WB, Sorlie P, Castelli WP, et al: Blood pressure and survival after myocardial infarction: The Framingham study. *Am J Cardiol* 45:326-330, 1980.

144. Gillum RF: Sudden coronary death in the United States: 1980-1985. *Circulation* 79:756-765, 1989.

145. Fisher LD, Kennedy JW, Davis KB, et al: Association of sex, physical size, and operative mortality after coronary artery bypass in the Coronary Artery Surgery Study (CASS). *J Thor Cardiovasc Surg* 84:334-341, 1982.

146. Findlay IN, Cunningham D, Dargie HJ: The rights of woman. *Br Heart J* 71:401-403, 1994.

147. Jaglal SB, Slaughter PM, Baigrie RS, et al: Good judgment or sex bias in the referral of patients for the diagnosis of coronary artery disease? An exploratory study. *Can Med Assoc J* 152:873-880, 1995.

148. Pfeffer MA, Braunwald E, Moye LA, et al: Effect of captopril on mortality and morbidity in patients with left ventricular dysfunction after myocardial infarction: Results of the survival and ventricular enlargement trial. *N Eng J Med* 327:669-677, 1992.

149. Lauer MS, Pashkow FJ, Snader CE, et al: Gender and referral for coronary angiography after treadmill thallium testing. *Am J Cardiol* 78:278-283, 1996.

150. Tobin JN, Wassertheil-Smoller S, Wexler JP, et al: Sex bias in considering coronary bypass surgery. *Ann Intern Med* 107:19-25, 1987.

151. Clarke KW, Gray D, Keating NA, et al: Do women with myocardial infarction receive the same treatment as men? *BMJ* 309:563-566, 1994.

152. Blackburn GG, Sprecher DL, Apperson-Hansen C: Gender bias restricts cardiac rehabilitation entry for women. *Circulation* 94:I-582A, 1996.

153. Campeau L, Enjalbert M, Lesperance J, et al: The relation of risk factors to the development of atherosclerosis in saphenous vein by-pass grafts and the progression of disease in the native circulation: A study 10 years after aorto-coronary bypass surgery. *N Engl J Med* 311:1329-1332, 1984.

154. Khaw KT: Where are the women in studies of coronary heart disease? *BMJ* 306:1145-1146, 1993.

155. Kemp HC, Kronmal RA, Vliestra RE, et al: Seven year survival of patients with normal or near normal coronary arteriograms. *J Am Coll Cardiol* 7:479-483, 1986.

156. Shekelle RB, Gale M, Norusis M: Type A score (Jenkins Activity Survey) and risk of recurrent coronary heart disease in the aspirin myocardial Infarction Study. *Am J Cardiol* 56:221-225, 1985.

157. Pedersen TR: Six-year follow-up of the Norwegian Multicenter Study on Timolol after acute myocardial infarction. *N Engl J Med* 313:1055-1058, 1985.

158. Beta-blocker Heart Attack Trial Research Group: A randomized trial of propranolol in patients with acute myocardial infarction. I. Mortality results. *JAMA* 247:1707-1717, 1982.

159. ISIS-2 (Second International Study of Infarct Survival) Collaborative Group: Randomized trial of intravenous streptokinase, oral aspirin, both or neither among 17,187 cases of suspected acute myocardial infarction: ISIS-2. *Lancet* ii:349-353, 1988.

160. Italian Group for the Study of Streptokinase in Myocardial Infarction (GISSI): Effectiveness of intravenous thrombolytic treatment in acute myocardial infarction. *Lancet* i:397-401, 1986.

161. Stanton BA, Zyzanski SJ, Jenkins CD, et al: Recovery after major heart surgery: Medical, psychological, and work outcomes, in Becker R (ed): *Psychopathological and Neurological Dysfunctions Following Open-Heart Surgery*. Heidelberg, Springer Verlag, 1982, p 217.

162. Cowley MJ, Mullin SM, Kelsey SF, et al: Sex differences in early and long-term results of coronary angioplasty in the NHLBI PTCA Registry. *Circulation* 71:90-97, 1985.

163. Moore SM: Women's views of cardiac rehabilitation programs. *J Cardiopulm Rehabil* 16:123-129, 1996.

164. Deshotels A, Planchock N, Dech Z, et al: Gender differences of quality of life in cardiac rehabilitation patients. *J Cardiopulm Rehabil* 15:143-148, 1995.

165. Loose MS, Fernhall B: Differences in quality of life among male and female cardiac rehabilitation participants. *J Cardiopulm Rehabil* 15:225-231, 1995.

166. Yusuf S, Peto R, Lewis J, et al: Beta blockade during and after myocardial infarction: An overview of the randomized trials. *Progr Cardiovasc Dis* 27:335-371, 1985.

167. CONSENSUS Trial Study Group: Effects of enalapril on mortality in severe congestive heart failure: Results of the Cooperative North Scandinavian Enalapril Survival Study (CONSENSUS). *N Engl J Med* 316:1429-1435, 1987.

168. Blankenhorn DH, Alaupovic P, Wickham E, et al: Prediction of angiographic change in native human coronary arteries and aortocoronary bypass grafts. Lipid and nonlipid factors. *Circulation* 81:470-476, 1990.

169. Ornish D, Brown SE, Scherwitz LW, et al: Can lifestyle change reverse coronary heart disease? The Lifestyle Heart Trial. *Lancet* 336:129-133, 1990.

170. Blankenhorn DH, Nessim SA, Johnson RL, et al: Beneficial effects of combined colestipol-niacin therapy on coronary atherosclerosis and coronary venous bypass grafts. *JAMA* 257:3233-3240, 1987.

171. Connolly DC, Elveback LR, Oxman HA: Coronary heart disease in residents of Rochester, Minnesota, 1950-1975. III. Effect of hypertension and its treatment on survival of patients with coronary artery disease. *Mayo Clin Proc* 58:249-254, 1983.

172. Young DT, Kottke TE, McCall MM, et al: A prospective controlled study of in-hospital myocardial infarction rehabilitation. *J Cardiac Rehabil* 2:32-36, 1982.

173. Stampfer MJ, Coldlitz GA, Willett WC, et al: Postmenopausal estrogen therapy and cardiovascular disease: Ten year follow up from nurses' health study. *N Engl J Med* 325:756-762, 1991.

174. American Medical Association Council on Scientific Affairs (Kaplan NM, Chair): Estrogen replacement in the menopause. *JAMA* 249:359-367, 1983.

175. Cobb MM, Teitlebaum H, Risch N et al: Influence of dietary fat, Apolipoprotein E, phenotype and sex on plasma lipoprotein levels. *Circulation* 86:849-857, 1992.

1 Sport-specific Injuries, Prevention, Treatment, Head, Neck and Spine

Prevention of Sports Injuries
Hergenroeder AC (Baylor College of Medicine, Houston)
Pediatrics 101:1057-1063, 1998   1–1

Objective.—Annually, 3 million children and adolescents in the United States are injured playing sports. Management of these musculoskeletal injuries should be integrated into the training of pediatricians. A review of the epidemiology of sports injuries in children, injury prevention, rehabilitation, and the psychosocial aspects of sports participation are presented for pediatricians.

Role of the Pediatrician.—A 1994 survey of pediatric chief residents found that only 26% of programs had a sports medicine elective and only 55% offered clinical experience in managing musculoskeletal injuries.

Epidemiology of Sports Injuries.—Approximately 25% to 30% of sports injuries occur in organized sports and 40% occur during unorganized sports. Football and wrestling have the highest injury rates. Boys and girls have similar injury rates although knee injuries are more common in girls. There are few fatalities.

Injury Prevention by Removing Environmental Risks.—Safety regulations, safer equipment, and removal of dangerous equipment can reduce injury rates.

Potential Mechanisms for Reducing Injuries.—Preseason medical evaluations, medical coverage at sports events, proper coaching, adequate hydration, proper officiating, and proper equipment and field/surface playing conditions can reduce injuries.

Injury Prevention in the Individual Patient.—Proper rehabilitation of injuries, warm-up and cool-down periods, enforced wearing of protective equipment, and appropriate support of weak or unstable joints will help prevent injuries.

Rehabilitation of Musculoskeletal Injuries.—Limiting additional injury and controlling pain and swelling; improving strength, flexibility, and range of motion; increasing strength, flexibility, endurance, and proprioception to near-normal levels; and returning to sports in a stepwise manner can prevent reinjury.

Playing With Pain.—Athletes should not exercise or participate in sports if it is painful.

Conclusion.—Pediatricians must receive appropriate training to manage sports-related injuries in children and to prevent further injuries. Medical coverage should be provided at sports events; athletes and coaches should be educated about injury prevention and rehabilitation; and equipment and surfaces should be designed to prevent injuries.

▶ This article encourages pediatricians to become involved in sports medicine and describes methods to accomplish this. The author outlines mechanisms for injury prevention, treatment, and rehabilitation of young patients, and discusses the psychological impact sports may have on children and adolescents.

F.J. George ATC, PT

Retrospective Report on the Effectiveness of a Polyurethane Football Helmet Cover on the Repeated Occurrence of Cerebral Concussions
Torg JS, Harris SM, Rogers K, et al (Hahnemann Univ, Philadelphia)
Am J Orthop 28:128-132, 1999   1–2

Background.—Many football players use a polyurethane helmet cover to prevent the recurrence of cerebral concussion. However, whether these devices are effective is not known. Users of the helmet covers were surveyed, and the results of published and unpublished studies were reviewed to determine the effectiveness of polyurethane helmet covers in preventing cerebral concussion recurrence.

Methods.—Surveys were sent to 245 purchasers of the polyurethane helmet cover; 155 responded, a 63.3% rate. Of that total, 126 said they had worn the device in the past season. Most of them (119, or 94.4%) were using it because they had previously had at least 1 concussion; two thirds of the 119 respondents were high school football players. The survey asked for detailed information on the user's concussions during the 4 years before and during the helmet's use. Respondents were grouped according to the number of concussions they had experienced before using the helmet cover, either 1 (n = 41), 2 (n = 41), 3 (n = 19), or 4 or more (n = 18). Then the concussion recurrence rate was calculated based on the number of respondents in each group who experienced a concussion while using the helmet cover.

Findings.—In the groups with 1, 2, 3, or at least 4 concussions before use of the helmet cover, reconcussion occurred in 1, 2, 3, and 5 respondents, respectively. This gave concussion recurrence rates of 2.4%, 7.3%, 15.8%, and 33.3%, respectively. Thus, the more concussions an athlete had experienced before using the helmet cover, the more concussions he experienced while using the helmet cover. These findings were also present in the literature.

Conclusions.—The natural history of reconcussion might just be that repeated concussion leaves the athlete more prone to subsequent concussions. Thus, the use of a polyurethane helmet cover may not protect against reconcussion; certainly, its effectiveness is not proven. The authors neither recommend nor disapprove of the helmet cover but do recommend that it not be routinely used prophylactically but be reserved for use by athletes with previous concussions.

▶ This article has been included for informational purposes only. To be emphasized, the helmet cover should not be routinely used prophylactically. Fine et al have reported to the American Orthopedic Society for Sports Medicine the apparent beneficial results of the device found in a prospective randomized study among high school football players. The question that this study raises is whether the device does have a protective effect or whether the recurrence of concussion represented the "natural history."

J.S. Torg, M.D.

Use of Simple Measures of Physical Activity to Predict Stress Fractures in Young Men Undergoing a Rigorous Physical Training Program
Shaffer RA, Brodine SK, Almeida SA, et al (Naval Health Research Ctr, San Diego, Calif)
Am J Epidemiol 149:236-242, 1999   1–3

Background.—Lower extremity stress fractures are among the more severe injuries associated with excessive training. A screening tool for identifying persons at increased risk for such injury would be useful in determining appropriate exercise levels.

Methods and Findings.—A screening tool was developed using data on 1,286 military recruits. The screening tool was then tested and refined among another 1,078 recruits. The modified algorithm consisted of 5 physical activity questions and a 1.5 mile run time. There was a strong association between measures of physical activity and aerobic fitness and the occurrence of stress fracture. Twenty-two percent of recruits at high risk for stress fractures sustained more than 3 times as many such fractures as those at low risk.

Conclusion.—Poor physical fitness and low levels of physical activity before entry into the military increase the risk of stress fractures during rigorous physical training of recruits. Such physical activity and fitness measures can be quantified into a simple screening algorithm.

▶ The conclusion that physical fitness screening combined with an appropriate "preconditioning" program can prevent stress fractures is not supported by the data.

J.S. Torg, M.D.

Effectiveness of Active Physical Training as Treatment for Long-standing Adductor-related Groin Pain in Athletes: Randomised Trial
Hölmich P, Uhrskou P, Ulnits L, et al (Amarger Univ, Copenhagen; Herlev Univ, Denmark; Glostrup Univ, Denmark; et al)
Lancet 353:439-443, 1999   1–4

Background.—Groin pain is a common problem for athletes in many sports. Although many disorders can cause groin pain, 1 of the most frequent causes is injury to the adductor muscle. Previous research has shown that exercises designed to strengthen a muscle might protect it from injury. A physiotherapy program that included active training for the adductor muscle was evaluated to determine whether it would reduce pain in athletes with long-standing adductor-related groin pain.

Methods.—The subjects were 68 male athletes who had experienced sports-related groin pain for 2 median of 40 weeks. None of them had inguinal or femoral hernia; prostatitis; urinary tract disease; vertebral pain; fracture of the pelvis or lower extremities; nerve entrapment of the ilioinguinal, genitofemoral, or lateral femoral cutaneous nerves; hip-joint disease; or bursitis of the hip or groin. All the subjects experienced at least 2 of the following symptoms suggestive of adductor involvement: a characteristic symptom history (eg, groin pain with coughing or sneezing), pain upon palpation of the symphysis joint, increased scintigraphic activity in the pubic bone, and osteitis pubis around the symphysis joint. Subjects were randomly assigned to an active training (AT) program (n = 34) or a physiotherapy (PT) program that did not involve active training (n = 34). The AT program was targeted at improving strength and coordination of the muscles that act on the pelvis (especially the adductor). Both programs were followed for 8 to 12 weeks, and subjects were evaluated 4 months after the end of treatment to determine groin symptoms and their current athletic involvement.

Findings.—Four months after the end of treatment, significantly more subjects in the AT group had excellent outcomes (23 vs 4 subjects) and were able to return to athletic participation without groin pain. Multiple regression analysis indicated that subjects were much more likely to have unilateral rather than bilateral groin pain (odds ratio 6.6 vs bilateral pain). After adjustment for unilateral groin pain in the model, subjects in the AT group were markedly less likely to experience pain (odds ratio 12.7 vs PT group). Subjects in the AT group also rated their improvement significantly better than did subjects in the PT group.

Conclusions.—An active training program to strengthen and improve coordination of the pelvic muscles (especially the adductor muscle) was effective in treating long-standing adductor-related groin pain. Whether such an active training program could prevent adductor-related groin pain is worth investigation.

▶ Groin pain from a variety of causes can be a major and disabling problem. Characteristically, it involves participants in ice hockey and soccer. Although this article does not identify specific pathologic involvement, the inclusion criteria included at least 2 of the following: characteristic history, pain on palpation of the symphysis, increased radioactive activity in the pubic area, and radiologic signs of osteitis pubis. In addition to the uncertainty as to what exactly this program is treating, it remains unclear why an active program with specific exercises improving strength and coordination of muscles acting on the pelvis was significantly better than a conventional physical therapy program.

J.S. Torg, M.D.

Hyperbaric Oxygen in the Treatment of Acute Muscle Stretch Injuries: Results in an Animal Model
Best TM, Loitz-Ramage B, Corr DT, et al (Univ of Wisconsin, Madison)
Am J Sports Med 26:367-372, 1998   1–5

Objective.—Hyperbaric oxygen (HBO) therapy has been used as a treatment for various types of injuries, including burns, crush injuries, osteomyelitis, and compartment syndromes. Initial studies suggest that it may be of benefit for patients with muscle-tendon and ligament injuries; however, there are no definitive data to confirm these benefits. The effects of HBO therapy were studied in a rabbit model of acute muscle stretch injury.

Methods.—A standardized partial stretch injury of the tibialis anterior muscle-tendon unit was created in 18 rabbits. The opposite limb was left uninjured as a control. Starting 24 hours after injury, 1 group of animals received HBO therapy, consisting of exposure to oxygen levels greater than 95% at a pressure of 2.5 atm, 60 min/day for 5 days. The other group received no treatment. Tissue healing and functional and morphological indicators of recovery were assessed after 7 days.

Results.—The functional deficit after 7 days was significantly reduced in HBO-treated animals. The percentage of ankle isometric torque on the injured side, compared with the uninjured side, was 15% in the HBO group versus 48% in the uninjured group. Surgical wound healing was also quicker in the HBO group. On histologic analysis, the HBO-treated specimens had reduced cellularity and fiber damage (Fig 2).

Conclusion.—This animal model suggests that HBO therapy may help to hasten recovery after muscle stretch injury. Both functional and morphological recovery appear to be significantly improved after 1 week of treatment. Further laboratory and clinical studies are needed to define treatment strategies and assess the mechanism of HBO's effect.

▶ The mechanism by which hyperbaric oxygen affects soft-tissue trauma has not been defined. However, some studies suggest that hyperbaric oxygen treatment decreases the inflammatory response, limits edema, and improves microvasculature to involved tissue. It does appear, though, that

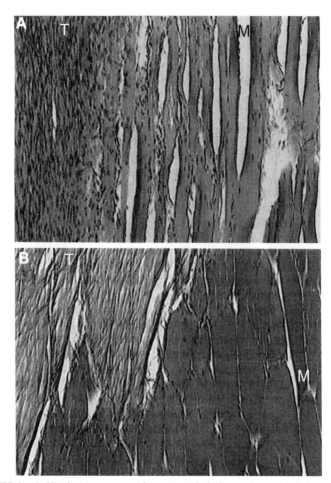

FIGURE 2.—**A,** Histologic appearance of an untreated tibialis anterior muscle 7 days after stretch injury showing persistent muscle fiber rupture and retraction from the tendon. Note the persistent hypercellularity in both the tendon and the muscle. **B,** Histologic appearance of an HBO-treated tibialis anterior muscle 7 days after stretch injury showing less fiber disruption and more complete healing. Note the relative lack of cellularity. Abbreviations: *T,* tendon; *M,* intact muscle fibers; (hematoxylin-eosin stain; original magnification, ×100). (Courtesy of Best TM, Loitz-Ramage B, Corr DT, et al: Hyperbaric oxygen in the treatment of acute muscle stretch injuries: Results in an animal model. *Am J Sports Med* 26:367-372, 1998.)

interest in hyperbaric oxygen for the treatment of athletic injuries has followed a popularity course similar to that of di-methyl sulfoxide—specifically, initial popularity engendered by fringe practitioners with interest dissipating shortly thereafter.

J.S. Torg, M.D.

The Effect of Anabolic Steroids and Corticosteroids on Healing of Muscle Contusion Injury
Beiner JM, Jokl P, Cholewicki J, et al (Yale Univ, New Haven, Conn)
Am J Sports Med 27:2-9, 1999   1–6

Background.—Contusions and strains make up about 90% of all sports-related injuries. Because of its effect on nitrogen and protein balance and the stimulation of cell synthesis, an anabolic steroid may be useful in the treatment of contusion injuries. The effects of nandrolone, an anabolic steroid, and methylprednisolone acetate, a corticosteroid, on muscle healing were studied in a rat model.

Methods.—Rat muscle was injured using a drop-mass technique. Active contractile tension was measured in each muscle, and histologic analysis was performed to determine healing.

Findings.—On day 2, rats given the corticosteroid had significant improvement in twitch and tetanic strength compared with control rats. By day 7, this effect was reversed, the corticosteroid muscles being significantly weaker than the control muscles. There was still no significant effect in the anabolic steroid group. On day 14, total degeneration was observed in the corticosteroid muscles, with disorganized muscle fiber architecture. The anabolic steroid muscles were significantly stronger in twitch. A similar trend was evident in tetanus compared with control muscles.

Conclusion.—This rat model suggests that corticosteroids may be beneficial in the short term but result in irreversible damage to muscle healing in the long term. Anabolic steroids may facilitate the healing of muscle contusion injury by speeding the recovery of force-generating capacity. Further research is warranted.

▶ Certainly the pharmacology of corticosteroids has been clearly delineated to have a catabolic effect on tissue healing. Corticosteroids, because of their anti-inflammatory effect, do, however, have a limited place in management of soft-tissue injuries. The fact that anabolic steroids facilitate healing of muscle tissue should come as no surprise. What this article does provide is enlightened thinking with regard to the potential use of these pharmaceutical agents in the management of soft-tissue injuries in humans.

                                                                        J.S. Torg, M.D.

Pharmacologic Considerations in the Treatment of Injured Athletes With Nonsteroidal Anti-inflammatory Drugs
Houglum JE (South Dakota State Univ, Brookings)
J Athletic Train 33:259-263, 1998   1–7

Background.—A thorough understanding of the general pharmacologic principles of nonsteroidal anti-inflammatory drugs (NSAIDs) may help clinicians optimize the use of these drugs in the treatment of athletic injuries. These principles include the onset and duration of drug action, potency, half-life, steady state, and the effect of exercise and disease on absorption, metabolism, and excretion of NSAIDs.

Review.—The primary mechanism of NSAID action is through inhibition of arachidonic acid metabolism. This has implications for potential adverse effects and drug interactions, particularly those associated with increased blood clotting time, reduced kidney function, and the occurrence of gastrointestinal discomfort. Extent of injury, drug dosing, duration of therapy, and the specific agent used can affect the efficacy of NSAIDs in increasing the rate of healing and in relieving pain and inflammation. Only 1 NSAID at a time should be used by a patient. In addition, NSAIDs should be taken with food. Clinicians should delineate outcomes and consider each patient's physical condition and medical history before prescribing NSAIDs.

▶ The general theme of this article is that there should be a clear understanding of basic pharmacologic principles to obtain optimal therapeutic outcome while minimizing undesirable side effects. Specifically, when the therapeutic result is achieved, the drug should be discontinued. Although this is an obvious concept to the physician, it is not necessarily so to the patient. Also, the use of 2 or more drugs in combination provides no increased therapeutic benefit and may increase toxic effects. Also, potential side effects should always be a consideration when prescribing these agents.

J.S. Torg, M.D.

The Effects of Platelet-derived Growth Factor-BB on Healing of the Rabbit Medial Collateral Ligament: An In Vivo Study
Hildebrand KA, Woo SL-Y, Smith DW, et al (Univ of Pittsburgh, Pa)
Am J Sports Med 26:549-554, 1998   1–8

Background.—A biologic technique was used to improve healing in the medial collateral ligament using growth factors found in healing tissue. In a previous in vitro study, the authors showed that platelet-derived growth factor-BB promoted fibroblast proliferation and that transforming growth factor-β_1 promoted matrix synthesis. These growth factors were used in vivo to determine whether they could improve healing in the medial collateral ligament, whether the effect would be dose-dependent, and whether combinations of growth factors would be more effective than individual growth factors.

Methods.—Various doses of growth factors were administered with a fibrin sealant delivery vehicle to 37 rabbits in ruptured right medial collateral ligaments. Rabbits were divided into 5 groups. Two groups were given a high or low dose of platelet-derived growth factor-BB, 2 groups were given a high or low dose of platelet-derived growth factor-BB plus a high or low dose of transforming growth factor-β_1, and 1 group was given fibrin sealant only. Rabbits were sacrificed at 6 weeks, and biomechanical and histologic analysis of the healing ligament was performed.

Results.—In femur-medial collateral ligament-tibia complexes of knees given the higher dose of platelet-derived growth factor-BB, values for ultimate load, energy absorbed to failure, and ultimate elongation were 1.6, 2.4, and 1.6 times greater than in the same complexes in the control group. The addition of transforming growth factor-β_1 did not increase the structural properties of the complex any further.

Discussion.—The use of platelet-derived growth factor-BB may improve healing in the medial collateral ligament. The use of this growth factor may also improve healing in other ligaments, tendons, and biologic ligament grafts.

▶ This excellent study was the recipient of the 1997 O'Donoghue Sports Injury Research Award presented by the American Orthopedic Society for Sports Medicine. Although the study is believed to have demonstrated the ability of platelet-derived growth factor-BB to improve the biomechanical properties of the healing medial collateral ligament in the early phases of ligament repair in rabbits, there does not appear to be an immediate clinical application of the method.

J.S. Torg, M.D.

Pathomechanics of Closed Rupture of the Flexor Tendon Pulleys in Rock Climbers
Marco RAW, Sharkey NA, Smith TS, et al (Univ of California, Davis)
J Bone Joint Surg [Am] 80-A:1012-1019, 1998   1–9

Objective.—More than one fourth of advanced rock climbers have damage to the flexor tendon pulley system of the hand. These injuries occur as the climbers attempt to support their entire weight with one or two fingers, using a crimp grip, in which the proximal interphalangeal joints are flexed 90 degrees or more and the distal interphalangeal joints are slightly hyperextended. The pulleys can be injured whenever the flexed finger is subjected to a large, rapidly applied external force that loads it into sudden extension. A cadaver study was performed to examine the mechanism of closed rupture of the flexor tendon pulleys in rock climbers.

Methods.—The study used 21 fingers of 7 nonpaired cadaver forearms; the subjects' mean age at death was 74 years. The fingers were tested under simulated in vivo loading conditions, with the flexor digitorum superficialis and profundus tendons attached to force transducer–equipped computer-controlled linear stepper motors. The force necessary to achieve tendon avulsion or osseous failure was recorded, along with tendon excursion and force at the fingertip (Fig 3). A fiberoptic camera was used to examine pulley damage and tendon bowstringing.

Results.—Two of 21 fingers fractured before pulley rupture occurred. In 89% of the remaining cases, isolated rupture of the A2 or A4 pulley was

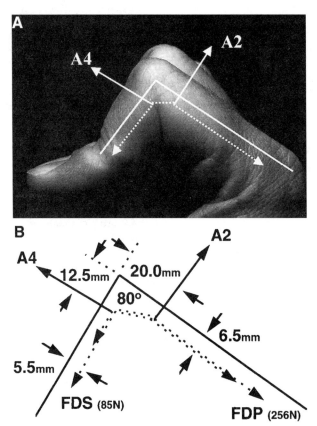

FIGURE 3.—Photograph (A) and corresponding schematic diagram (B) illustrating the two-dimensional static analysis that was used to estimate perpendicular forces in the A2 and A4 pulleys at the instant of the initial rupture of a pulley. The distances from the centers of rotation to the centers of the pulleys and from the centers of the phalanges to the centers of the tendons were measured in a representative test (index) finger and were used as inputs in the analysis, as were the mean forces in the tendons that were recorded during bench-top testing. With use of this analysis, the perpendicular forces in the A2 and A4 pulleys at the time of the initial rupture were estimated to be 241 and 250 newtons, respectively. *Abbreviations: FDS*, flexor digitorum superficialis; *FDP*, flexor digitorum profundus. (Courtesy of Marco RAW, Sharkey NA, Smith TS, et al: Pathomechanics of closed rupture of the flexor tendon pulleys in rock climbers. *J Bone Joint Surg [Am]* 80A:1012-1019, 1998.)

the initial failure event; the A4 pulley usually ruptured first. Only after rupture of 2 consecutive pulleys—either the A2 and A3 or the A3 and A4—did subtle bowstringing of the flexor digitorum profundus occur. Bowstringing did not occur if just 1 pulley ruptured, and it did not become obvious until all 3 pulleys had ruptured. The A1 pulley never ruptured.

Conclusions.—The mechanism of a common rock-climbing injury, closed flexor tendon pulley rupture, is reported. Whereas tendon bowstringing across the proximal interphalangeal joint has been considered diagnostic for isolated rupture of the A2 pulley, the new results suggest that isolated A2 rupture is rare. Instead, the presence of bowstringing likely signals extensive damage to the flexor tendon pulley system. Isolated damage to the A4 pulley can occur.

▶ An excellent study; however, not without several problems. The average age of the cadaveric specimens was 74 years, certainly not to be considered in the rock-climbing activist group. Also, the mean compressive force produced at the fingertips in the experimental design was only one third that required to suspend the average-sized individual. Also, the authors point out that "the connective tissue in our specimens was assumed to be much weaker than that in healthy young adults." However, the observations of this study were similar to the operative findings of Bowers et al.[1] who reported that injuries for flexion tendon pulleys associated with the bowstringing had damaged the A2, A3, and A4 pulleys.

J.S. Torg, M.D.

Reference

1. Bowers WM, Kuzma GR, Bynum DK, et al: Closed traumatic rupture of finger flexor pulleys. *J Hand Surg [Am]* 19A:782-787, 1994.

Injuries in Collegiate Wrestling
Jarrett GJ, Orwin JF, Dick RW (Univ of Wisconsin, Madison; Natl Collegiate Athletic Assoc Injury Surveillance System, Overland Park, Kan)
Am J Sports Med 26:674-680, 1998   1–10

Objective.—Data on musculoskeletal injury rates in collegiate wrestling compiled from 1985 through 1996 by the National Collegiate Athletic Association Injury Surveillance System were reviewed.
Methods.—Data are collected through a random annual sample of 15% to 20% of schools sponsoring a particular sport; participation is voluntary.

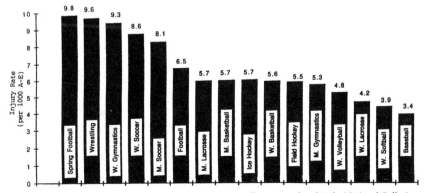

FIGURE 1.—Total (practice and game) injury rate across all sports analyzed in the National Collegiate Athletic Association Injury Surveillance System through the 1995 to 1996 season. *Abbreviation: A-E,* athlete-exposures. (From Jarrett GJ, Orwin JF, Dick RW: Injuries in collegiate wrestling. *Am J Sports Med* 26:674-680, 1998. Courtesy of the National Collegiate Athletic Association Injury Surveillance System.)

Injury was defined as an occurrence during participation in a sports activity or competition that required medical attention and resulted in 1 or more days of restriction from participation. The average number of wrestling teams studied was 45.

Results.—The combined practice and competition injury rate over the study period was 9.6/1,000 athlete-exposures, with wrestling resulting in the second highest injury rate (Fig 1). The knee (21%), shoulder (14%), and ankle (9%) were the most common body parts injured in both practice and competition and during preseason and regular season, with lower rates during postseason. The most common types of injuries during practice and competition, respectively, were sprains (26.1% and 33.4%), infection (17.4% and 0%), and strains (16.2% and 17.8%). The most common mechanisms of injury in practice and competition, respectively, were body contact (53.6% and 64.4%), contact with mat (22.3% and 22.4%), and no contact (16.3% and 7.8%). Injury rates for different weight classes were similar.

Conclusion.—Knee, shoulder, and ankle injuries were the most common and the most serious and should be addressed. The injury rate during competition was significantly higher than during practice; it was higher during preseason and regular season than during postseason. Injury rates for different weight classes were similar.

▶ I take exception to the conclusion that in collegiate wrestling "most injuries were not serious, and catastrophic injuries were exceedingly rare." Sixteen percent of institutions sponsoring intercollegiate wrestling were included in the study. It is inferred that 38% of the injuries resulted in 1 or more weeks of athletes being disabled by their activity and that these were not serious, with only 6% resulting in surgery. In that injury severity is not presented on the basis of pathoanatomical criteria, we really do not know whether any or all of these injuries were serious or not serious. To be mentioned is the fact that there has recently been a rash of dehydration deaths in National Collegiate Athletic Association wrestling, each of which was, of course, certainly catastrophic.

J.S. Torg, M.D.

Golf Injuries: An Overview
Thériault G, Lachance P (Laval Univ, Ste-Foy, Québec)
Sports Med 26:43-57, 1998   1–11

Objective.—Golf is a popular sport in many countries. Most golfers who practice the sport as a recreational activity are motivated by the health and leisure aspect or by contact with the natural environment. Most golfers who are injured are hurt during the swing.

Biomechanics of the Golf Swing.—The golf swing is divided into 6 phases: ball address, backswing, forward swing and acceleration, ball impact, early follow-through, and late follow-through.

TABLE 3.—Main Causes of Golf Injuries

Overuse
Technical errors during the swing
Physical fitness deficiencies
  aerobic
  muscular strength
  flexibility
No pre-game warm-up
Carelessness towards other players or lack of etiquette
Natural environmental conditions (uneven course surface, wet
grass, thunderstorm, etc.)

(Courtesy of Thériault G, Lachance P: Golf injuries: An overview. *Sports Med* 26:43-57, 1998).

Epidemiology of Golf Injuries.—Injuries in amateur golfers result in inability to play golf an average of 5.2 weeks a year. Injury rates for men and women are similar. Golfers with a lower handicap and who are older than 50 have a higher injury prevalence, whereas those who have golfed 3 years or more have a lower injury prevalence. The average injury rate per amateur golfer is 1.28–1.31; per professional golfer it is approximately 2. The leading causes of golf injuries are overuse and poor technique (Table 3).

Golf Injury Profiles and Characteristics.—Injuries are fairly evenly distributed across all body segments, although professional golfers tend to have more wrist/hand, lumbar spine, and shoulder injuries, whereas amateur golfers tend to have more dorsolumbar and elbow injuries. Men tend to have more spinal injuries whereas women tend to have more upper limb injuries. Amateur golfers have more overuse injuries, particularly of the upper limbs, and sustain more than 50% of their injuries at midseason. Injuries to all anatomic segments show a 70% to 75% recuperation rate within 6 months.

Specific Golf Injuries and Their Treatment.—Early immobilization of the hand and wrist for 1–2 weeks is necessary to treat golfer's elbow or wrist injuries. Application of ice, anti-inflammatory medication, and physical therapy are important, and gradual rehabilitation for a minimum of 2–4 weeks is crucial. Most dorsolumbar injuries can be treated with rest, anti-inflammatory medication, physical therapy, traction or manipulation, and rehabilitation. Shoulder injuries are treated with rest, anti-inflammatory medication, and physical therapy, followed by correction of faulty technique. Surgical subacromial decompression may be necessary.

Prevention.—Better technical skills, good physical conditioning, and proper equipment can prevent injuries.

Conclusion.—Golf carries a moderate risk of injury resulting mainly from poor technique, poor conditioning, or overuse. Improving skills, conditioning, and equipment can prevent injuries. Early proper treatment and good rehabilitation can prevent reinjury.

▶ The authors state that many golf injuries can be prevented through proper conditioning, warm-up, and correct biomechanical swing. There are a number of athletic trainers and physical therapists now working in conjunction with professional golf instructors to analyze a person's golf swing. They evaluate any physical limitations which may prevent a correct biomechanical swing. A rehabilitation program is designed to correct these physical limitations and to prevent injury and improve one's score.

F.J. George A.T.C., P.T.

Rib Stress Fractures in Elite Rowers: A Case Series and Proposed Mechanism

Karlson KA (Univ of Michigan, Ann Arbor)
Am J Sports Med 26:516-519, 1998   1–12

Objective.—The causes of stress fractures in elite rowers were reviewed retrospectively.

Methods.—Ten elite rowers (3 men) with 14 stress fractures were interviewed. Sex, date of injury, side rowed, weight class, fracture location, training phase, and method of diagnosis were evaluated.

Results.—There were 3 lightweight men, 2 lightweight women, and 5 heavyweight women. Fractures occurred on the antero- to posterolateral aspects of ribs 5–9. Fractures were diagnosed by bone scan (n = 11), plain radiographs (n = 2), and clinical observation (n = 1). Nine fractures occurred in the winter during high-volume rowing with a high load per stroke. Five fractures occurred during a race. Onset was slow, with several days to weeks of discomfort followed by sharp pain that worsened at the end of the arm pull-through phase. There were 3 scullers, 3 sweep rowers, and 4 rowers who were both. Seven of 9 stress fractures in sweep rowers occurred on the side closer to the oar. The incidence of stress fracture may be reduced by decreasing the force of pull on the rib by the serratus anterior muscle, the external oblique muscle, or both (Fig 2).

Conclusion.—Rib stress fractures appear to be the result of the pull of the serratus anterior and external oblique muscles on the rib, which causes repetitive bending of the rib. A modified rowing technique can decrease the risk of stress fracture.

▶ Stress injuries in the rib area are becoming more prevalent in rowers. The author demonstrates a modified finish position to decrease the forces on the serratus anterior and external oblique muscles. This finish is recommended for long-distance or endurance rowing and is not necessary for sprinting or racing. Coaches must stress good rowing form to prevent injuries and lighten the load on the oar during training.

F.J. George, A.T.C., P.T.

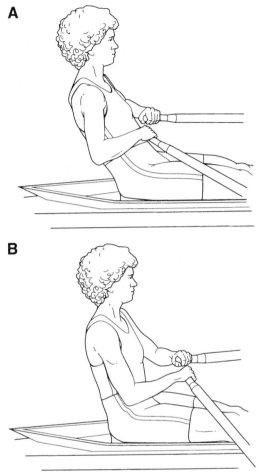

FIGURE 2.—**A,** Standard layback and arm position at the finish of the rowing stroke. **B,** Modified finish position to decrease forces exerted on the rib by the serratus anterior and external oblique muscles. (Courtesy of Karlson KA: Rib stress fractures in elite powers: A case series and proposed mechanism. *Am J Sports Med* 26:516-519, 1998).

Common Sports Injuries in Young Tennis Players

Bylak J, Hutchinson MR (Univ of Illinois at Chicago)
Sports Med 26:119-132, 1998   1–13

Objective.—The physical characteristics of young tennis players result in different patterns of injury than in adults. Prevention of overuse injuries should be the prime focus for younger tennis players. A review of common injuries in young players and their evaluation, treatment, and rehabilitation were presented, and preventive physical conditioning was discussed.

Demands and Musculoskeletal Adaptations.—Physical demands vary with skill level and duration of playing time. The ability to withstand forces on joints, high strength, and flexibility are required to prevent muscle weakness and imbalance as well as sprain and strain injuries.

Epidemiology of Injuries.—Leg injuries are twice as common as upper extremity injuries. Overuse injuries result in tendinitis, chronic muscle strain, and stress fractures. Females are at higher risk of injury than males and have a higher percentage of leg and knee injuries.

Overuse Injuries.—Evaluation of overuse injuries should include evaluation and treatment of all adjacent areas. The most common upper extremity injuries involve the shoulder, elbow, and wrist and are treated conservatively with rest, cryotherapy, anti-inflammatory drugs, steroid injections for persistent elbow pain, and rehabilitation. Chronic or acute lower extremity injuries are treated with ice, support, massage, anti-inflammatory drugs, and exercises that increase flexibility in the case of strains; and rest, anti-inflammatory drugs, and cryotherapy for tendinitis. Foot stress fractures are treated conservatively; plantar fasciitis, blisters, and tennis toe are treated with proper footwear, stretching, and possibly a short course of anti-inflammatory drugs. Knee injuries, which are common, are treated with cryotherapy, anti-inflammatory drugs, rest, and rehabilitation.

Acute Injuries.—Acute injuries are less common in young athletes and generally include ankle and knee sprains; these are treated conservatively but carefully to avoid high re-injury rates. Contusions, abrasions, and fractures are managed according to the diagnosis.

Rehabilitation.—A complete program should include an acute phase, a recovery phase, and a maintenance phase.

Preventive Conditioning.—Motor balance, flexibility, and strength training geared to the demands of the sport are necessary.

Conclusion.—The physical demands of tennis are now well understood, evaluation and treatment have become more complete, and rehabilitation is comprehensive and well-structured. Proper conditioning can prevent most injuries, and proper treatment can improve deficits before injuries become chronic.

▶ This is basically a review article describing a litany of injuries common to young athletes in general. Interestingly, the somewhat rare subungual hematoma has been renamed "tennis toe." However, it is pointed out that some injuries with eponyms such as tennis elbow, tennis leg, and tennis shoulder are less commonly seen in the younger player.

J.S. Torg, M.D.

Injury Risk in First-Time Snowboarders Versus First-Time Skiers

O'Neill DF, McGlone MR (Plymouth Sports & Orthopaedic Clinic, NH)
Am J Sports Med 27:94-97, 1999   1–14

Background.—As the popularity of snowboarding increases, so do the injury rates. The risk of injury among first-time snowboarders was compared with that among first-time skiers.

Methods.—Injury patterns in more than 22,000 first-time snowboarders and skiers between 1994 and 1996 were studied. All had enrolled in Learn to Snowboard and Learn to Ski programs at 2 major northeastern ski resorts.

Findings.—Four percent of first-time snowboarders and 4% of first-time skiers sustained an injury. Snowboarders had a greater percentage of upper extremity injuries, and skiers had a greater percentage of lower extremity injuries. The incidence of emergent injuries necessitating immediate care—such as fracture, concussion, dislocation, and lost teeth—was significantly greater in snowboarders than in skiers.

Conclusion.—Snowboarding is associated with a significantly higher rate of emergent injuries than skiing. The use of helmets and wrist guards should decrease this rate. First-time snowboarders and skiers are at a much greater risk for injury than participants at higher skill levels.

▶ It is well documented that snowboard injuries among both the experienced and the inexperienced, for the most part, involve the upper extremity. An important statistic derived from this study was a concussion rate of 15% of the total snowboarding injuries studied. Clearly, the use of a helmet while persuing this activity is, so to speak, a no-brainer.

J.S. Torg, M.D.

Shoulder Injuries From Alpine Skiing and Snowboarding: Aetiology, Treatment and Prevention

Kocher MS, Dupré MM, Feagin JA Jr (Harvard Med School, Boston; Jackson Hole Ski Resort, Jackson, Wyo; Duke Univ, Durham, NC)
Sports Med 25:201-211, 1998   1–15

Objective.—The number of skiing and snowboarding injuries has been decreasing, but the percentage of shoulder injuries has been proportionately increasing. Shoulder injury patterns were reviewed, diagnosis and treatment were discussed, and prevention methods were suggested.

Shoulder Injury Patterns.—Alpine skiing shoulder injuries account for 4% to 11% of skiing injuries and 22% to 41% of upper extremity injuries. The injury rate is 0.2 to 0.5 per 1,000 skier-days. The most common injuries are rotator cuff strains, anterior glenohumeral dislocations or subluxations, acromioclavicular separations, and clavicle fractures. With snowboarding, 8% to 16% of all injuries and 20% to 34% of upper extremity injuries involve the shoulder. The injury rate is 4 to 16 injuries/ 1,000 skier-days.

Diagnosis and Treatment.—Diagnoses are based primarily on mechanism, direction, extent, and history of injury and on radiographic evidence. Injuries occur most frequently during falls. Neurovascular examination should be performed in the case of glenohumeral instability.

Prevention.—Education, experience, and proper conditioning can lower the risk of injury. Good quality, safe equipment including protective equipment are important preventive measures. Good ski conditions and better-designed lifts can lower injury rates.

▶ This is a comprehensive review of the subject matter. The original article is recommended for the interested reader.

J.S. Torg, M.D.

The Snowboarder's Foot and Ankle

Kirkpatrick DP, Hunter RE, Janes PC, et al (North County Orthopaedic Surgery and Sports Medicine, Queensburg, NY; Orthopaedic Associates of Aspen and Gleenwood, Colo; Summit-Vail Orthopaedics and Sports Medicine, Frisco; et al)
Am J Sports Med 26:271-277, 1998   1–16

Background.—The popularity of snowboarding is increasing. Definite patterns of injury have been reported in ankle trauma sustained during snowboarding. Fractures of the lateral process of the talus, a fracture pattern previously believed to be rare, have been noted. The type and distribution of foot and ankle snowboarding injuries were determined in a prospective study.

Methods and Findings.—Data on 3,213 snowboarding injuries occurring between 1988 and 1995 were analyzed. Four hundred ninety-one (15.3%) were ankle injuries, and 58 (1.8%), foot injuries. Forty-four percent of the ankle injuries were fractures, and 52% were sprains. Fifty-seven percent of the foot injuries were fractures, and 28% were sprains. The remainder were soft tissue injuries, contusions, or abrasions. Boot type was uncorrelated with overall foot or ankle injury rate. Significantly fewer ankle sprains occurred in patients wearing hybrid boots, and fewer fractures of the talar lateral process occurred in patients wearing soft boots. The number of fractures of the talar lateral process was surprisingly high, consisting of 2.3% of all snowboarding injuries, 15% of all ankle injuries, and 34% of all ankle fractures. Many of these fractures were not apparent on plain radiographs. CT was needed to diagnose these fractures (Fig 3C).

Conclusions.—Clinicians must maintain a high index of suspicion of anterolateral ankle pain in snowboarders. Subtle fractures that may need surgical treatment should not be mistaken for anterior talofibular ligament sprains.

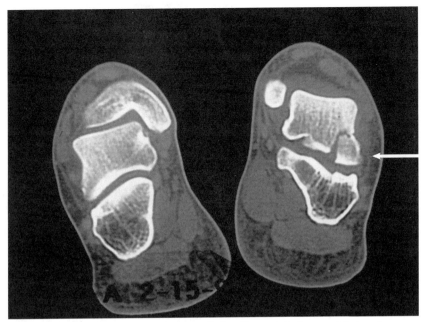

FIGURE 3C.—A CT scan of the ankle shows a displaced interarticular fracture of the lateral processes (*arrow*); the opposite foot shows normal anatomy. (Courtesy of Kirkpatrick DP, Hunter RE, Janes PC, et al: The snowboarder's foot and ankle. *Am J Sports Med* 26:271-277, 1998.)

▶ This is a timely article with an important message. Specifically, physicians must suspect this fracture in a snowboarder with lateral ankle pain. Late diagnosis or misdiagnosis of fractures of the lateral process is associated with significant morbidity.

J.S. Torg, M.D.

Injuries Associated With Snowmobiles, Alaska, 1993-1994

Landen MG, Middaugh J, Dannenberg AL (Ctrs for Disease Control and Prevention, Atlanta, Ga; Alaska Division of Public Health, Anchorage)
Public Health Rep 114:48-52, 1999   1–17

Background.—Snowmobile use is increasingly popular in the United States. Injuries associated with snowmobile use in Alaska in 1993 and 1994 were investigated.

Methods and Findings.—Injury deaths and hospitalizations associated with snowmobiles were compared with those associated with on-road motor vehicles. Data were obtained from the Department of Public Safety, the Department of Transportation, and medical examiner records for the years 1993 and 1994. In those years, rates of injury death and hospitalization associated with snowmobiles were greater than with on-road motor vehicles. A total of 26 deaths resulted from snowmobile injuries. Seven persons drowned after breaking through ice, and 8 were ejected from snowmobiles. Fifty-eight percent of the injury deaths involved a natural entity, such as a boulder, ravine, or river. Blood alcohol concentrations were available for 17 decedents, 65% of whom had alcohol levels of 100 mg/dL or greater.

Conclusion.—Natural obstacles and alcohol intoxication appear to contribute to the high risk of injury death from snowmobile use. Possible injury control strategies would include trail development and improvement.

▶ The fact that in northern Alaska snowmobile injuries outnumber on-road motor vehicle injuries is further accentuated by the fact that the "snowmobile season" is 6 months, as opposed to 12 months for on-road vehicles, and miles driven are considerably less. Active preventive measures suggested include snowmobiler education, helmet use, mandatory snowmobile registration, and driver licensure. All appear to be in order.

J.S. Torg, M.D.

The Effectiveness of Ski Bindings and Their Professional Adjustment for Preventing Alpine Skiing Injuries

Finch CF, Kelsall HL (Deakin Univ, Burwood, Victoria, Australia; Dept of Human Services, Melbourne, Victoria, Australia)
Sports Med 25:407-416, 1998   1–18

Objective.—Studies examining the effectiveness of ski bindings and their adjustment for prevention of injuries were reviewed.

Methods.—Fifteen studies were identified through Medline and SPORT Discus CD-ROM searches. The strength of scientific evidence, rated from the strongest to the weakest, included controlled evaluations (n = 1), epidemiologic evidence (n = 5), laboratory-based or equipment testing (n = 13), and anecdotal or informed/expert opinion (n = 15).

Results.—Standard release settings that have been established depend on the relationship between the binding-release force and the tibial plateau width and ISO standards determined by the weight method. Maladjustment influences binding-release performance. Sports and equipment rental shops are responsible for making correct adjustments for each individual. Multidirectional release sensitivities are needed in bindings. Biomechanical studies have led to the development of 2 prototype binding systems in which heel release is activated by the anterior-posterior bending moment at the sole in one and by a twisting motion that is modulated according to the level of 1 of the vastii muscles of the quadriceps group. Failure of 1 or both bindings to release was associated with increased risk of injury (odds ratio, 3.3 and 2.3, respectively). A prospective cohort study found that 95% of all bindings tested had at least 1 fault and an average of 3.4 faults per binding unit. Skiers with more information were more likely than skiers with no information to appreciate the need for professional binding adjustment. Many binding-release systems for children were poorly adjusted and of poor quality.

Recommendations.—Multidirectional-release bindings must be developed. Ski binding designs must be continually evaluated. Case-control studies should be conducted on different methods of binding adjustments. Binding adjustments in adults and children should be reevaluated regularly. The standards for children's bindings and boots need to be reviewed and upgraded. Stores and rental agents should use mechanical testing devices. International standards for binding adjustments need to be applied. The role of education in, and the best method for, encouraging professional binding adjustments should be studied.

▶ The value of this article is its conclusion that "currently used bindings are insufficient for the multi-directional release required to reduce the risk of injury to the lower extremity, especially the knee." Thus, despite advances in binding technology, rupture of the anterior cruciate ligament remains a bane of the skier and a boon to the orthopedic surgeon.

J.S. Torg, M.D.

Comparison of Injury Patterns in Elite Hockey Players Using Ice Versus In-line Skates
Hutchinson MR, Milhouse C, Gapski M (Univ of Illinois, Chicago)
Med Sci Sports Exerc 30:1371-1373, 1998   1–19

Background.—Many articles have been published on the injuries and risks associated with in-line skating. However, no one has compared injury patterns in hockey players performing on in-line skates versus ice skates. An injury surveillance study was reported.

Methods and Findings.—Two hockey teams performing on in-line skates and 1 team performing on ice skates were studied. A total of 215 games and 1,122 athletic exposures were evaluated. One hundred forty-two injuries necessitating physician attention occurred. Forty-six of these injuries caused loss of playing time. The total injury rates were similar between in-line and ice skaters, at 139 and 119 per 1,000 athletic exposures, respectively. However, injuries tended to be more severe in the ice hockey players. The mean lost playing time was 8.3 games among players performing on ice skates and 6.5 games among those on in-line skates. Ice skates were associated with an increase in the number of lacerations; in-line skates were associated with an increased number of injuries from checking and a reduced number of injuries from skate equipment. Ice skaters had a greater risk of head and neck injuries than the in-line skaters.

Conclusions.—Injury patterns, compared by anatomic location, mechanism of injury, and type of injury, were similar between these in-line and ice hockey players. Ice hockey was associated with more severe injuries than hockey played on in-line skates.

▶ The fact that ice hockey was associated with more severe injuries is explained on the basis of several differences between the 2 sports: Ice hockey players achieve greater speeds with increased kinetic energy; the beaded puck used in roller hockey is slower; the rules are more strictly enforced; and, of course, blades are absent. This is an interesting study, but I am not sure I see the clinical relevance.

J.S. Torg, M.D.

The New Zealand Rugby Injury and Performance Project: V. Epidemiology of a Season of Rugby Injury
Bird YN, Waller AE, Marshall SW, et al (Univ of Otago, Dunedin, New Zealand; Univ of North Carolina, Chapel Hill)
Br J Sports Med 32:319-325, 1998   1–20

Background.—In rugby union, a full-body contact game, many injuries result from extrinsic forces. The incidence, nature, and circumstances of injuries in a cohort of rugby union players during 1 season were described.

Methods and Findings.—Three hundred fifty-six male and female rugby players were studied prospectively during the 1993 competitive club season. Data were obtained on 4,403 player-games and 8,653 player-practices. Six hundred seventy-one injuries occurred, 569 related to rugby. The injury rate ratio for games versus practices was 8.3. Injury rates were 10.9 per 100 player-games among men and 6.1 among women. Injury rates also varied depending on position, with male locks and female inside backs having the greatest rates (13.0 and 12.3 injuries per 100 player-games, respectively) in their sexes. The body region most commonly injured in both games and practices was the leg. Sprains and strains were the most common injury type. In games, the phase of play in which most injuries occurred was the tackle, followed by rucks and mauls. Thirteen percent of injuries sustained during games were the result of foul play.

Conclusions.—Rugby injury is common, varying according to grade and sex. Identifying the causes of injuries occurring in the tackle and the causes of leg injuries is an important consideration for the prevention of rugby injury, as is the issue of foul play.

▶ A 72% injury rate for a competitive season is certainly impressive. As the authors point out, many of the findings are consistent with those of previous studies. The article also offers little new information with regard to injury prevention. Most of the players who sustained a concussion were not wearing protective equipment, either in the form of a helmet or a mouth guard. It is then noted that "it has not been determined if the use of headgear in rugby protects against concussion." It would appear that the rugby enthusiasts have much to do with regard to injury prophylaxis.

J.S. Torg, M.D.

Predictors of Injury Among Adult Recreational In-Line Skaters: A Multicity Study

Seldes RM, Grisso JA, Pavell JR, et al (Univ of Pennsylvania, Philadelphia; New York Univ; Baylor Univ, Houston)
Am J Public Health 89:238-241, 1999   1–21

Background.—In-line skating is one of the fastest growing recreational sports in the United States. The prevalence of injury, risk factors for injury, safety gear use, and the skating habits of adult recreational in-line skaters were investigated.

Methods and Findings.—A total of 1,014 skaters from 6 major United States cities were selected randomly for inclusion in the study. Nine hundred sixty-four skaters were interviewed. Only 6% of the skaters consistently wore all 4 types of recommended safety gear. The more experienced skaters were more likely to perform tricks, wear less safety gear, and sustain injuries.

Conclusion.—The use of safety gear by adult recreational in-line skaters is alarmingly low. Educational programs on safe skating should target this at-risk population, especially the more experienced in-line skaters, who are less likely to wear safety gear, more likely to perform tricks, and are at increased risk for injury.

▶ It was interesting that the skating locations most associated with prevalence of injury were areas of railings, ramps, and ledges, as opposed to streets. Also, attempting to perform stunts and tricks was a predictor of injury, regardless of skill level or experience.

J.S. Torg, M.D.

Injury and Training Characteristics of Male Elite, Development Squad, and Club Triathletes

Vleck VE, Garbutt G (Staffordshire Univ, Stroke-on-Trent, England)
Int J Sports Med 19:38-42, 1998   1–22

Background.—Overuse injuries are more common in triathletes than traumatic injuries. The intrinsic and extrinsic factors associated with overuse injury are examined in 3 groups of triathletes of different abilities.

Methods.—The subjects were male triathletes training at triathalon distances (swimming 1.5 km, cycling 40 km, running 10 km). Twelve British National Elite Squad, 17 National Development Squad, and 87 club triathletes completed questionnaires about their training distance, duration, and number of sessions during a race training week without taper. They also answered detailed questions about injuries over the previous 5 years, which activities they were performing when they occurred, anatomical site of the injuries, and number of training days lost. A severity index was calculated for each site of injury by multiplying the prevalence of that injury in each of the 3 groups by the average time lost from training because of injury at that site for all groups. The subjects also provided information about intrinsic (eg, health status, symptoms of overtraining, psychological state) and extrinsic (eg, years of competitive experience, level of competition) risk factors for injury.

Findings.—The training mileage, number of training sessions, and duration of sessions differed among the 3 groups of triathletes. However, the prevalence of overuse injury did not differ significantly among the elite, development, and club groups (75%, 75%, and 56.3%, respectively). These 3 groups experienced 2.9, 2.2, and 1.9 sites of injury, respectively, with the most common sites being the knee (14.2% to 21.9%), lower back (15.8% to 17.9%), and Achilles tendon (10.3% to 17.9%). Injuries at these sites were also the most severe. In all 3 groups, significantly more overuse injuries occurred during running than cycling: elite group, 62.1% versus 34.5%; development group, 64.3% vs 25.0%; club group, 58.7% vs 15.9%. The number of overuse injuries that occurred during running correlated significantly with the total triathlon training distance, the cycling distance, the cycling pace, the swimming distance, the total number of triathlon workouts, and the total number of running sessions within a race training week. The number of overuse injuries that occurred during cycling correlated significantly with the time spent running and the time spent cycling within a race training week. However, none of the intrinsic or extrinsic risk factors examined correlated significantly with the prevalence of overuse injury.

Conclusions.—Overuse injuries of the knee, lower back, and ankle/foot are common in triathletes. Most of these occur while running, although the nature of the training program means that the influence of other disciplines cannot be discounted. No relationship was found between the number of overuse injuries and the subject's psychological state, general health, or symptoms of overtraining.

▶ Although it appears obvious that the number of overuse injuries sustained should correlate with the time spent running and cycling, this article does raise other questions: What are the links among injury, speed, recovery session duration, and mileage? Another question concerns the apparent lack of links among psychological state, overtraining symptoms, and injury prevalence.

J.S. Torg, M.D.

A Comparative Mechanical Analysis of the Pointe Shoe Toe Box: An In Vitro Study

Cunningham BW, DiStefano AF, Kirjanov NA, et al (Union Mem Hosp, Baltimore, Md; St Joseph Hosp, Towson, Md; Ballet Theatre of Annapolis, Md)
Am J Sports Med 26:555-561, 1998   1–23

Background.—In ballet, dancing en pointe requires the ballerina to stand on her toes, which are protected only by a cardboard shell in the toe box of the pointe shoe. This cardboard shell is saturated with glue, and during breaking-in of the shoe, the toe box softens and conforms to the foot, but the glue bonds are destroyed in the process. For this reason, pointe shoes last for only a short time and are no longer used when the toe box becomes too soft to adequately support the foot. Most of the research about the pointe shoe has focused on determining toe pressures generated while dancing en pointe and on the prevention of dance injuries. There is no information on the comparative mechanical properties of different pointe shoes.

Methods.—The comparative static stiffness, static strength, and fatigue properties (number of cycles to failure) of 5 brands of pointe shoes were determined (Fig 1). The toe box dimensions and inner volume of the shoes were calculated to determine whether shoe dimension and mechanical properties were correlated. Local dancers were surveyed to determine the shoe characteristics that dancers prefer.

Results.—Under axial loading conditions, the Leo's shoe had the greatest level of stiffness and the Freed shoe had the least strength. Under vertical loading conditions (Fig 3), the Leo's shoe and Freed shoe had the greatest level of stiffness and the Gaynor Minden shoe and Freed shoe had the greatest strength. The greatest differences among the 5 brands of shoes

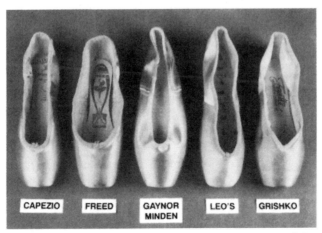

FIGURE 1.—Five different brands of pointe shoes were evaluated: Capezio, Freed, Gaynor Minden, Leo's, and Grishko. All shoes were unused before mechanical testing and were not retested. (Courtesy of Cunningham BW, DiStefano AF, Kirjanov NA, et al: A comparative mechanical analysis of the pointe shoe toe box. *Am J Sports Med* 26:555-561, 1998.)

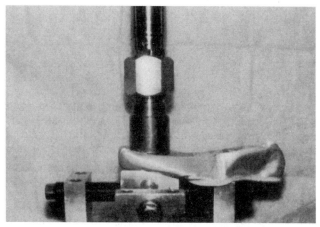

FIGURE 3.—A view of the pointe shoe oriented for vertical compressive loading. The applied load was delivered to the distal plantar surface of the toe box. (Courtesy of Cunningham BW, DiStefano AF, Kirjanov NA, et al: A comparative mechanical analysis of the pointe shoe toe box. *Am J Sports Med* 26:555-561, 1998.)

were seen with fatigue testing. The Gaynor Minden had the highest fatigue life. There appeared to be no relationship between shoe dimension and mechanical properties. The top 5 shoe characteristics preferred by the dancers were fit, comfort, box/platform shape, vamp shape, and durability. The dancers also indicated that the best shoe is one that feels right and allows artistic maneuvers, not necessarily the strongest shoe.

Discussion.—These results provide dancers with an understanding of the comparative mechanical properties of pointe shoes. Stiffness, strength, and fatigue life vary according to shoe type. These results indicate that there should be an optimal load-sharing environment among the pointe shoe, foot, and ankle, regardless of the shoe used.

▶ It is interesting to note that the most durable and mechanically sound shoe is not always the preferred shoe of the dancer. The static testing demonstrated large variations when comparing the vertical and axial results. As the authors point out, the shoes were significantly stiffer and stronger under axial loading than under vertical loading conditions, highlighting the importance of foot and ankle support when the dancer is en pointe versus standing in demi-pointe.

J.S. Torg, M.D.

Rider Injury Rates and Emergency Medical Services at Equestrian Events

Paix BR (Royal Adelaide Hosp, Australia)
Br J Sports Med 33:46-48, 1999   1–24

Background.—Injury and death rates among horse riders are high. Injuries among cross country event riders, a subgroup of riders at high risk, were reported.

Methods and Findings.—Data on injuries occurring during 35 equestrian events in South Australia between 1990 and 1998 were collected. Of 4,220 competitors in the events, 37 sustained injuries, for an overall incidence of 0.88% per competitor per event. Twelve of 26 riders taken to the hospital were subsequently admitted. Nineteen of the 37 injured riders sustained head and neck injuries. Other common injuries were lower-limb fractures, occurring in 3 riders; rib fractures in 3; and soft-tissue injuries of the thoracolumbar spine in 5. One injury was fatal, and 1 was life threatening; both occurred when the horse cartwheeled over a jump and fell on the rider. All 37 injured riders sustained their injuries during the cross country phase of the event, usually as a result of falling from the horse or falling with the horse. Usually the injuries occurred during jumps over an obstacle.

Conclusions.—Injury rates are especially high among event riders. One rider in this series died from injuries. Injury rates were greatest among riders competing at the highest levels. Skilled emergency medical services are needed at equestrian events.

▶ As the author states, the literature is clear that horse riding is a dangerous pastime. In addition to facial abrasions and upper-extremity fractures, reported are (1) a ruptured aorta, liver, and diaphragm; (2) numerous closed head injuries without loss of consciousness and; (3) life-threatening medical emergencies including chest pain, bee-sting allergy, and severe asthma. The conclusion that "there is a need for skilled emergency medical services at equestrian events" is well taken.

J.S. Torg, M.D.

Snowboarding Injuries

Young CC, Niedfeldt MW (Med College of Wisconsin, Milwaukee)
Am Fam Physician 59:131-136, 1999   1–25

Background.—Snowboarding has become a popular winter sport. Injuries associated with this sport were discussed.

Snowboarding Injuries.—Previous research indicates that nearly one fourth of snowboarding injuries occur during a person's first experience. Nearly one half occur during the first season of snowboarding. Falling is the leading cause of snowboarding injuries, followed by jumping. The latter may be associated with head, facial, spinal, and abdominal injuries.

Collisions cause 5% to 10% of injuries. Severe injuries necessitating tertiary trauma canter care occur rarely. Severe injury is most commonly caused by colliding with a tree. Fifty-four percent of severe injuries involve the head, 32% involve the abdomen, 32% involve bones, and 16% involve the thorax. Falls occurring when the snowboarder is waiting in line for a ski lift are likely to result in knee injury, because of the torque force on the locked leg. In general, the average distribution of snowboarding injuries are in the wrist (23%), ankle (16.7%), knee (16.3%), head (9.2%), shoulder (8.3%), trunk (7.8%), elbow (4.4%) and other (6.5%). Compared with alpine skiers, snowboarders are more likely to have upper-extremity injuries but less likely to have knee injuries. Snowboarder's ankle, a lateral talus fracture, must be considered in snowboarders with severe ankle "sprains" unresponsive to treatment.

▶ Clearly, snowboarding is becoming an immensely popular activity. Apparently, 54% of severe injuries involve the head. This suggests that helmets, if nothing more, should certainly be worn. However, whatever protective value helmets may offer remains to be seen.

J.S. Torg, M.D.

Disruption of the Finger Flexor Pulley System in Elite Rock Climbers
Gabl M, Rangger C, Lutz M, et al (Univ Hosp of Traumatology, Innsbruck, Austria; Univ Hosp of Radiology, Innsbruck, Austria)
Am J Sports Med 26:651-655, 1998   1–26

Background.—The popularity of rock climbing is increasing. Unfortunately, training and climbing expose the musculoskeletal system to increased risk for injury. Isolated injuries of the finger pulley system have recently been described in climbers. The diagnosis and treatment of disruptions of the finger pulley system were reported.

Methods.—Thirteen elite rock climbers were treated for isolated disruptions of the pulleys of the long fingers. Diagnosis and treatment were based on the clinical finding and MRI verification of bowstringing. Eight patients with bowstringing indicating incomplete disruption of the major pulley A2 were treated nonsurgically (group A), and 5 with bowstringing indicating complete disruption of the pulley A2 underwent reconstruction after conservative treatment failed (group B). Mean follow-up was 31 months.

Findings.—Loss of extension in the proximal interphalangeal joint was 5.6 degrees in group A and 4 degrees in group B. Finger section circumference was increased 4.2 and 4.8 mm, respectively. Grip strength declined 20 N and 12 N, respectively. Four group A patients and 1 group B patient had bowstringing at clinical assessment. Follow-up MRI showed no changes in bowstringing in group A patients but a decrease in all group B patients. Both groups had good subjective outcomes (Fig 1).

Conclusions.—Bowstringing of the flexor tendons of rock climbers should suggest disruption of the finger pulley system. This diagnosis can be

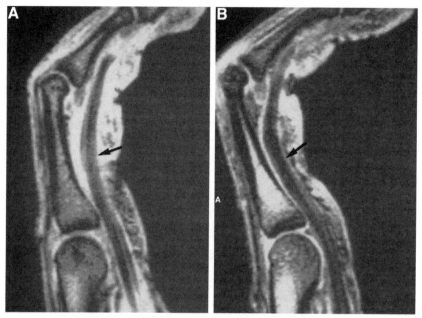

FIGURE 1.—**A,** Sagittal MRI of the right ring finger demonstrates bowstringing of the flexor tendons (*arrow*), indicating complete disruption of the pulley A2. **B,** MRI of an intact pulley system in an uninjured finger. (Courtesy of Gabl M, Rangger C, Lutz M, et al: Disruption of the finger flexor pulley system in elite rock climbers. *Am J Sports Med* 26:651-655, 1998.)

verified by MRI. Surgical repair or reconstruction should be considered when the amount of bowstringing on sagittal MRI extends proximal to the base of the proximal phalanx of the involved finger.

▶ Disruption of the finger flexor pulley systems has been previously reported by several authors. This report of Gabl et al is interesting because they have established criteria on the basis of sagittal MR. Specifically, "bowstringing extending to less than the base of the proximal phalanx of the involved finger as seen on sagittal MRI indicates incomplete disruption of the pulley A2, and bowstringing extending proximal to the base of the proximal phalanx of the involved finger indicates complete disruption of pulley A2." It is recommended that the former be treated nonoperatively, the latter surgically. In this group of patients, a free tendon graft was used to surgically reconstruct the pulleys, resulting in good function of the flexor tendon and reduced bowstringing in 4 of 5 patients.

J.S. Torg, M.D.

Lightning Injuries During Snowy Conditions

Cherington M, Breed DW, Yarnell PR, et al (St Anthony Hosp, Denver; Natl Ctr for Atmospheric Research, Boulder, Colo)
Br J Sports Med 32:333-335, 1998   1–27

Objective.—Few skiers or snowmobilers are struck by lightning. The case of a ski patrol member on a snowmobile struck by lightning was reported, and the conditions necessary for lightning during snow conditions were described.

> *Case Report.*—Man, 38, on a ski rescue mission above the timberline in graupel or snow pellet conditions with lightning, was struck by lightning at 4:30 PM on June 8, 1997, at a temperature of 3.3°C while transporting a skier with a broken neck on a fiberglass toboggan he was towing. The man regained consciousness after a moment and noticed numbness in his left arm and leg; he had difficulty swallowing and speaking for a few minutes. He called for help, which arrived in 15 minutes. The man had garbled speech and was photosensitive. He was wearing a helmet. His neurologic examination results were normal except for swollen eyelids without ecchymosis, chemotic conjunctivae in both eyes, and a stromal swelling reaction in the inferior half of each eye. The diagnosis was electrical burns of both corneas and anterior segments, and the patient was treated with 1% eye drops and topical steroid drops. His photophobia and pain resolved. By 3 months, his corneas were clear. Anterior and posterior cortical cataracts developed in both eyes. His vision was corrected to 20/20.

Discussion.—The patient described here and another skier, who died after being struck by lightning, were struck during spring but in winter-like conditions. The helmet and wet ski suit worn by the ski patroller may have protected him against worse injuries. Tympanic membrane rupture and ophthalmic sequelae are common after lightning strikes. Cataracts are common complications that may develop after months or years. Positively charged ice crystals colliding with negatively charged graupel may have precipitated the lightning strike. The different sized particles falling at different speeds resulted in an accumulated charge in a cloud. Strong updrafts allow supercooled droplets to exist and collect and become unstable when temperatures are warm. Positive lightning flashes are more damaging because they are larger and longer lasting.

Conclusion.—Convective clouds and graupel or snow pellet conditions increase the risk of lightning strikes to skiers and snowmobilers in the spring months.

▶ Lightning injuries during snowy conditions are, to say the least, exceedingly rare. However, the authors' point that outdoor activists should be aware of at least 2 suspicious clues: the appearance of convective clouds and the presence of graupel or snow pellets during precipitation is well taken. It should be pointed out that convective clouds are also known as cumulus clouds and are characterized by enhanced vertical growth and cauliflower-like puffs. Also, apparently these clouds have a higher percentage of positive lightning flashes as opposed to the more common negative lightning flashes in summer. As the authors point out, positive flashes have larger and longer currents and are more damaging.

J.S. Torg, M.D.

Concussion Incidence in Elite College Soccer Players
Boden BP, Kirkendall DT, Garrett WE Jr (Duke Univ, Durham, NC)
Am J Sports Med 26:238-241, 1998   1–28

Background.—The potential for head injuries among soccer players has been widely debated. Previous studies have attributed neuropsychological deficits in soccer players to the cumulative effects of heading, but have not evaluated concussion rates. The incidence of concussion in elite college soccer players was assessed.

Methods.—Seven men's and 8 women's varsity soccer teams in the Atlantic Coast Conference were studied. The incidence of concussion during 2 seasons was documented.

Findings.—Twenty-nine concussions were diagnosed in 26 athletes (17 men and 12 women). The concussions resulted from contact with an opponent's head in 28% of the cases, elbow in 14%, knee in 3%, and foot in 3%; with the ball in 24%; with the ground in 10%; with concrete sidelines in 3%; with the goalpost in 3%; and with a combination of objects in 10%. Sixty-nine percent of the concussions occurred during games. None of the concussions was sustained during intentional heading of the ball. The basic incidence was 0.96 per team per season, with an overall incidence of 0.6 and 0.4 per 1,000 athlete-exposures for men and women, respectively. Seventy-two percent of the concussions were grade 1 and 28% were grade 2.

Conclusions.—Concussion apparently occurs more commonly in soccer than has been believed. Such acute head injuries may result in long-term neuropsychologic changes.

▶ By some accounts, an elite male soccer player has a 50% probability of suffering a concussion if he plays for 10 years. Also, several studies suggest—and other studies refute—that cumulative head injury leads to neuropsychological impairment. No study is definitive, but concern exists about the results of concussions in soccer. This article suggests that concussions are indeed common in soccer, apparently not from routine heading of the ball, but from colliding with another player's head or being hit in the head by a ball kicked hard from close range. Concussions also occur when players fall and hit their heads on the ground or the goalpost. We need more research on the causes, implications, and prevention of concussions in soccer (See also Abstract 1–29.)

E.R. Eichner, M.D.

Chronic Traumatic Brain Injury in Professional Soccer Players
Matser JT, Kessels AGH, Jordan BD, et al (St Anna Hosp Geldrop, The Netherlands; Univ of Maastricht, The Netherlands; Charles R Drew Univ of Medicine & Science, Los Angeles; et al)
Neurology 51:791-796, 1998   1–29

Background.—Chronic traumatic brain injury is the long-term, cumulative neurologic consequence of concussive and subconcussive blows to the head. Such blows occur in soccer. The presence of chronic traumatic brain injury among professional soccer players was reported.

Methods.—Fifty-three active soccer players from several professional Dutch soccer clubs were studied along with 27 elite athletes in noncontact sports. All participants were examined neuropsychologically.

Findings.—Compared with the control group, the soccer players had impaired performances in memory, planning, and visuoperceptual processing. Among the soccer players, performances on memory, planning, and visuoperceptual tasks were correlated inversely with the number of concussions sustained during play and with the frequency of "heading" the ball. Performance on neuropsychological assessment also depended on field position, with forward and defensive players showing greater impairment.

Conclusions.—Participation in professional soccer may be associated with neurocognitive impairment. Impairments in the neuropsychologic functions of memory, planning, and visuoperceptual processing were documented in the current group of soccer players.

▶ This article adds to the controversy about brain injury in soccer. Depending on how well matched the control group and the soccer players were, these soccer players showed more cognitive impairment than swimmers and runners. That is, soccer players performed more poorly on verbal and visual memory, planning, and visuoperceptual processing tasks. The differences between groups seem subtle, but the authors build their case by correlating cognitive performance inversely with the number of concussions incurred in soccer and with the frequency of "heading" the ball. Yet surely there are inherent differences—differences that may influence cognition or test-taking—between athletes who choose to play soccer and those who choose to swim or run. In any case, concussions in ice hockey are on the rise,[1] with 60 to 70 per year now in the National Hockey League, second only to the 100 to 120 per year in the National Football League. It seems that concussions are also a risk in soccer.

E.R. Eichner, M.D.

Reference

1. Tegner Y, Lorentzon R: Concussion among Swedish elite ice hockey players. *Br J Sports Med* 30:251-255, 1996. (1997 YEAR BOOK OF SPORTS MEDICINE, pp 30-31.)

Concussion History in Elite Male and Female Soccer Players
Barnes BC, Cooper L, Kirkendall DT, et al (Duke Univ, Durham, NC; Univ of Los Angeles)
Am J Sports Med 26:433-438, 1998   1–30

Background.—In soccer, the head is used for controlling, passing, and shooting a soccer ball. There is concern about the cumulative effects of "heading" on soccer players. Neurophysiologic and neuropsychological changes have been reported in active and retired soccer players, and heading has often been cited as the cause of these changes. Concussive episodes can affect brain function, and a player's history of concussive episodes can greatly affect neurophysiologic and neuropsychological findings. An impact to an individual who had a previous concussion from the same type of impact can cause a more severe concussion. There is conflicting information about the effects of repeated heading in soccer players.

Methods.—All male and female soccer players who competed in the US Olympic Sports Festival in 1993 were interviewed. There were 137 players, and the mean age was 20.5. The mechanisms of injuries, frequency of injuries, and outcomes were determined.

Results.—In men, there were 74 concussions in 39 players; 50 of the injuries were grade I. In women, there were 28 concussions in 23 players; 19 of the injuries were grade I. In men, 48 of the 74 concussions were from collisions with another player. In women, 20 of the 28 concussions were from collisions with another player. The most common symptoms after these injuries were headache, a dazed feeling, and dizziness. On the basis of concussion history, the odds that a soccer player would sustain a concussion within a 10-year period were 50% for a man and 22% for a woman.

Discussion.—These findings indicate that concussion from player-to-player contact in soccer is a common hazard. None of the players in this study sustained a concussive episode from properly executed heading. More studies of the risk of sports-related head injuries and possible neurologic complications are needed.

► The major problem in dealing with concussion is to define exactly what you are talking about. In this study, the Colorado Medical Society Guidelines were used, with data being acquired by follow-up telephone interviews. The authors state that the athletes do not include the recollection of having been "dazed" after heading a ball as a specific head injury. Also, it is not clear how other factors, such as post-heading headaches, dizziness, and blurred vision, were or should be considered. Also questioned are the electroencephalogram abnormalities reported in the literature as necessarily being associated with repeated headache. Perhaps the best study design would be to follow a group of soccer players who were previously without symptoms to determine the occurrence and relationship of symptoms with the activity.

J.S. Torg, M.D.

Mild Brain Trauma in Sports: Diagnosis and Treatment Guidelines
Sturmi JE, Smith C, Lombardo JA (Ohio State Univ, Columbus)
Sports Med 25:351-358, 1998   1–31

Background.—Numerous guidelines for the diagnosis of mild brain trauma in sports have been published, but much confusion remains. The pathophysiology, diagnosis, and management of head injuries in athletes is reviewed.

Mechanisms of Head Injury.—Brain trauma is not uncommon in athletes; in any given year, about 20% of American high school football players experience a sports-related brain concussion. Other sports associated with high rates of head injury are boxing, ice hockey, rugby, motor racing, equestrian sports, martial arts, wrestling, gymnastics, soccer, cycling, alpine skiing, and diving. During these activities, a blow to the head—either direct or indirect—can cause brain injury. Given the brain's protective anatomy, most direct compressive forces are tolerated with little injury; the exception is a blow that causes fracture or hematoma. However, injuries due to acceleration or deceleration cause the brain's surrounding attachments to shear away, and these injuries are often serious. Additionally, a sharp blow to the athlete's torso or pelvis can cause a concussion. Forces can be dissipated by the athlete's equipment, a strong neck, and his or her ability to tense the neck muscles, thus lessening the severity of the injury. Fortunately, most head injuries are mild, and the athlete does not lose consciousness. Nonetheless, all athletes who sustain a head injury, regardless of whether they lose consciousness, should be evaluated for brain trauma.

Diagnosis of Brain Trauma.—Physicians must have a high index of suspicion regarding brain trauma in athletes. A careful history is important in assessment, including any symptoms of confusion, dizziness, headache, memory loss, fatigue, or nausea. Visual and other neurologic abnormalities must also be identified. Questions that test the athlete's orientation are important to detect posttraumatic amnesia. Knowing the athlete's personality and likelihood to downplay symptoms also helps in diagnosing brain trauma. Finally, tests should be repeated to ensure that cognitive or neurologic function is not deteriorating.

Management of the Athlete With Mild Head Injury.—At the very least, any athlete who sustains a concussion should be removed from play and examined. Similarly, loss of consciousness or amnesia also warrant withdrawal from competition. All symptoms must be completely resolved before the athlete is allowed to return to play. Furthermore, no matter how mild the injury seems, any evidence of functional deterioration requires immediate hospitalization, imaging, and neurosurgical consultation.

▶ This article brings into focus several interesting points. Ten "guidelines" have been published dealing with diagnosis and management of this condition in the athlete. The question is the concept of a "mild concussion." Importantly, regardless of the guideline used or the presumed degree of injury, there must be complete resolution of all symptoms before return to play.

J.S. Torg, M.D.

Emergency Removal of Football Equipment: A Cadaveric Cervical Spine Injury Model
Gastel JA, Palumbo MA, Hulstyn MJ, et al (Brown Univ, Providence, RI)
Ann Emerg Med 32:411-417, 1998   1–32

Purpose.—Proper early management of possible cervical spine injuries in football players is critical; yet there is no consensus regarding initial care. The situation is complicated by the presence of a football helmet and shoulder pads. Whereas EMTs are often trained to remove the helmet to avoid neck hyperflexion, sports medicine experts recommend against helmet removal in the field. A cadaver study was conducted to analyze the effects of a football helmet or shoulder pads on alignment of the unstable cervical spine.

Methods.—The study included 8 cadavers, average age 73. In each cadaver, a simulated bilateral facet dislocation was created at the C5-C6 motion segment. Before and after this injury, lateral cervical spine radiographs were obtained with the cadavers wearing no equipment, a helmet only, shoulder pads only, and a helmet and shoulder pads. The effects of the various equipment conditions on alignment of the unstable segment were analyzed.

Results.—Before the simulated injury was created, the neck was maintained in neutral alignment with helmet and shoulder pads in place. Lordosis was decreased by a mean of 9.6 degrees with the helmet only and increased by 13.6 degrees with the shoulder pads only. After destabilization of the cervical spine, C5-C6 forward angulation was increased by a mean of 16.5 degrees with the helmet only. At the same time, posterior disk space height was increased by 3.8 mm and dorsal element distraction by 8.3 mm. In the other 3 conditions, there were no significant differences from before to after destabilization.

Conclusions.—In football players with possible cervical spine injury, the cervical spine cannot be splinted in neutral position if the athlete is wearing a helmet without shoulder pads. The results suggest that the helmet and shoulder pads should be left in place until the patient reaches the emergency room, unless removal is needed for CPR. Alternatively, both the helmet and the pads may be removed, but one should not be left in place without the other.

Helmet and Shoulder Pad Removal From a Player With Suspected Cervical Spine Injury: A Cadaveric Model

Donaldson WF III, Lauerman WC, Heil B, et al (Univ of Pittsburgh, Pa)

Spine 23:1729-1733, 1998   1–33

Objective.—Cervical spine injuries can result in quadriplegia. The problem of removing the helmet and shoulder pads of an injured football player is not well understood. The issue of how much motion occurs with 2 types of cervical spine injuries when helmet and shoulder pads are removed was investigated in a cadaver model.

Methods.—Unstable C1-C2 segments were created by transoral osteotomy at the waist of the odontoid process in 3 cadavers, and at C5-C6 by sectioning the interspinous ligaments, facet capsules, posterior longitudinal ligaments, and posterior one third of the disk in 3 additional cadavers. Under fluoroscopic visualization, 4 people removed the helmets by first removing the face mask, then the chin strap, and then the ear pieces. With the neck stabilized, the helmet was removed. With the head stabilized, the shoulder pads were removed. Maximum displacements were recorded and analyzed.

Results.—Instability at C2 resulted in a change in angulation of 5.47 degrees, distraction of 2.98 mm, and a change in the space available for the cord of 3.91 mm when the helmet was removed. When shoulder pads were removed, the change in angulation was 2.9 degrees, distraction was 1.76 mm, and the change in the space available for the cord was 2.64 mm.

Conclusion.—A significant amount of movement can occur in an unstable cervical spine when helmet and shoulder pads are removed. The dangers of removal vary with the site of injury. Helmet removal tends to increase the flexion angle, whereas shoulder pad removal tends to increase extension. Posterior translation of 1 vertebral body on another during shoulder pad removal tends to reduce the anterior forces on the cadaveric spine.

▶ An appreciation of these 2 articles (Abstracts 1–32 and 1–33) requires insight into the controversy that has existed between emergency medicine physicians and technicians on 1 hand and team physicians and athletic trainers on the other. Existing emergency medical services guidelines mandate removal of protective headgear prior to transport of an individual suspected of having a cervical spine injury. These guidelines were implemented with motorcycle helmets in mind, so as to facilitate both airway accessibility and application of cervical spine-immobilizing devices. Clearly, such a procedure contradicts the longstanding principle, adhered to by team physicians and athletic trainers, of leaving the helmet in place, when a football player is suspected of having cervical spine injury, until the athlete is transported to a definitive medical facility.

It must be emphasized that this particular problem is of more than academic interest. Specifically, there have been occasions where emergency medical technicians, under the direction of emergency room physicians unfamiliar with the nuances of the relationship among helmet, shoulder pads, and the injured cervical spine, have precipitated an on-site turf battle by refusing to move the injured player before helmet removal. Again, such episodes represent more than an honest difference of opinion. They are clearly detrimental to the health and well-being of the injured player. It is the view of this observer that removal of the football helmet and shoulder pads on-site exposes the potentially injured spine to both unnecessary and awkward manipulation, as well as disrupting the immobilizing capacity of the helmet and shoulder pads. Also, removal of the helmet alone subjects a potentially unstable spine to a hyperlordotic deformity.

J.S. Torg, M.D.

Occurrence of Cervical Spine Injuries During the Rugby Scrum
Wetzler MJ, Akpata T, Laughlin W, et al (American Orthopaedic Rugby Football Assoc, Washington Crossing, Pa; South Jersey Orthopedic Associates, Voorhees, NJ; Rugby Magazine, New York; et al)
Am J Sports Med 26:177-180, 1998   1–34

Objective.—The scrum is responsible for almost 60% of cervical spine injuries occurring in rugby matches in the United States. The occurrence, cause, and reduction of cervical spine injuries during the rugby scrum were studied retrospectively.

Methods.—Injury data on 62 injured players were compiled from oral and written reports of coaches and officials, from medical records, and from conversations with injured players and their families.

Results.—Between 1970 and 1996, 36 (58%) of the players sustaining a cervical spine injury during a rugby game were injured during the scrum, with 23 (64%) of the injuries occurring during the engagement and 13 during the collapse of the scrum. Players injured during engagement were hookers (56%) and props (8%). Players injured during the collapse were hookers (22%), props (11%), and a second-row player (3%). There were 21 (58%) senior-level players and 15 (42%) junior-level players injured. Nine (25%) injuries occurred as a result of a mismatch in experience. Significantly more injuries occurred during the engagement than during the collapse. Hookers were significantly more likely than props to be injured. Junior players were significantly more likely than senior players to be injured.

Conclusion.—Cervical spine injuries to rugby players occur more frequently during the engagement phase of the scrum, to hookers, and to lower level players.

Spinal Injuries in New Zealand Rugby and Rugby League - A Twenty Year Survey

Armour KS, Clatworthy BJ, Bean AR, et al (Christchurch School of Medicine; Univ of Otago; Burwood Hosp, Christchurch)
N Z Med J 110:462-465, 1997   1-35

Background.—Some authors have reported a decrease in the frequency of serious spinal cord injuries in New Zealand rugby, whereas others have questioned such reports. Trends in the frequency of serious spinal cord injuries in rugby and rugby league during 20 years were investigated.

Methods and Findings.—Between 1976 and 1995, 119 rugby and 22 rugby league players were admitted to spinal injury units in New Zealand with serious spinal injuries. Forty-seven of these players were confined permanently to wheelchairs after injury. Frequency of injury increased steadily throughout the study period. Eighty-three percent of the injuries occurred in forwards and 17% in backs. Scrum produced the most injuries in rugby, and the tackle caused the most injuries in rugby league. The most spinal injuries occurred in April, early in the season. Since intense compulsory educational programs on safety were initiated 18 months ago, no serious spinal cord injuries have resulted from rugby scrums.

Conclusions.—Contrary to belief, spinal cord injuries in rugby have not declined since the rule changes in the mid 1980s. The current data can be used as an effective educational platform to increase the safety of rugby and rugby league.

Severe Cervical Spinal Cord Injuries Related to Rugby Union and League Football in New South Wales, 1984-1996

Rotem TR, Lawson JS, Wilson SF, et al (Univ of NSW, Sydney; Royal North Shore Hosp, Sydney, NSW; Prince Henry Hosp, Sydney, NSW)
Med J Aust 168:379-381, 1998   1-36

Background.—In the 1970s and early 1980s, the incidence of cervical spinal cord injuries sustained during rugby union or league football increased about 2-fold. Between 1984 and 1996, new rules were introduced, existing rules were enforced more strictly, and safety programs were offered, including exercises for strengthening players' neck muscles and preventing players with long thin necks from playing dangerous positions. The frequency and circumstances of serious cervical cord injuries associated with rugby union and league football in New South Wales between 1984 and 1996 were reported.

Methods and Findings.—During the review period, 115 rugby players were admitted to spinal units because of cervical spinal cord injuries. Permanent neurologic deficits resulted in 26 rugby union and 23 rugby league players. Two players died from injury sequelae within 2 weeks of hospitalization. No significant change in the rate of rugby-related spinal unit admissions was evident, although there was a small decrease in the number and incidence of patients with tetraplegia associated with rugby union, which was statistically significant when tested as a trend over time. Cervical spinal cord injuries resulting in complete tetraplegia were primarily associated with scrumlike plays in union and with tackles in league play.

Conclusions.—Serious cervical spinal injuries continue to be a problem in rugby union and league football. This sport is still inherently dangerous.

▶ Taylor et al. clearly identified spinal cord injuries resulting from Australian football as a major problem.[1] Despite such strategies as "new rules," "more strict enforcement of existing rules," "safety programs," "exercise for strengthening players' neck muscles," and "the banning of players with long thin necks from taking dangerous positions," cervical spine injuries remain a major problem. Some insight into the reason for this can be discerned in these 3 articles (Abstracts 1–34 through 1–36). Specifically, no mention is made of the classic mechanism of axial loading of the cervical spine that causes most of these injuries in collision sports. If you don't recognize or know the mechanism, how can you prevent the injury?

J.S. Torg, M.D.

Reference

1. Taylor TK, Coolican MR: Spinal cord injuries in Australian footballers, *Med J Aust* 147:112-118, 1987.

The Effects of Padded Surfaces on the Risk for Cervical Spine Injury
Nightingale RW, Richardson WJ, Myers BS (Duke Univ, Durham, NC)
Spine 22:2380-2387, 1997   1–37

Background.—Energy-absorbing equipment that protects the head from injury is assumed to decrease the risk for neck injury, also. However, research studies suggest this may not be true. The current *in vitro* study compared cervical spine injuries resulting from rigid head impacts and from padded head impacts.

Methods.—Eighteen cadaveric spines were used to test 6 combinations of impact angle and impact surface padding. The impact surface was oriented at −15, 0, or +15 degrees. The impact surfaces consisted of a 3-mm sheet of lubricated Teflon or 5 cm of polyurethane foam.

Findings.—Padded surface impacts resulted in significantly greater neck impulses and a significantly higher frequency of cervical spine injuries compared with rigid impacts. The angle of impact was also associated with the risk of injury.

Conclusions.—Highly deformable, padded contact surfaces should be used carefully when there is a risk for cervical spine injury. The orientation of the head, neck, and torso relative to the impact surface is at least as important in the risk of neck injury.

▶ The potential relevance of these observations regarding the risk for cervical spine injury with padded head impact pertains to the use of the currently available polyurethane helmet cover, which is being marketed with the presumption that it reduces recurrent cerebral concussive episodes. It is important to point out that it is not clear whether such padding is useful in reducing head injuries or that its use increases the risk of neck injury. I would certainly agree that "to ensure that measures designed to protect the head do not increase the risk for neck injuries, the effective padding should be rigorously tested." However, the test design should certainly simulate the clinical condition, thus placing the padding on the helmet side of the equation. Perhaps the most important observation is that "the surface padding used in this study was able significantly to reduce the magnitude of the measured head impact force and therefore the risk for head injury."

J.S. Torg, M.D.

Minimally Invasive Techniques in Spinal Surgery: Current Practice
Kambin P, Gennarelli T, Hermantin F (Allegheny Univ, Philadelphia)
Neurosurg Focus 4:1-10, 1998   1–38

Introduction.—Arthroscopic or endoscopic techniques of minimally invasive spinal surgery offer a useful and reliable alternative for the treatment of various spinal disorders. The authors review the current state of the art in minimally invasive spinal surgery, focusing on operations for herniated lumbar disk.

Arthroscopic Microdiskectomy.—Arthroscopic microdiskectomy is performed through the "triangular working zone" on the posterolateral cor-

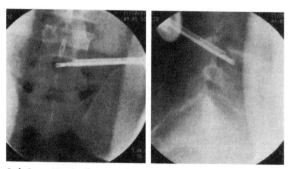

FIGURE 4.—**Left,** Intraoperative fluoroscopic examination after full insertion of forceps (extending 2 cm behind the tip of the cannula) demonstrating the posterior positioning of the instrument adjacent to the spinal canal. (In the anteroposterior projection, the tip of the inserted forceps is at the level of the spinal processes of the adjacent segments.) **Right,** Lateral fluoroscopic examination showing the tip of the instrument seen in the posterior one fourth of the anteroposterior diameter of the intravertebral disk. (Courtesy of Kambin P, Gennarelli T, Hermantin F: Minimally invasive techniques in spinal surgery: Current practice. *Neurosurg Focus* 4:1-10, 1998.)

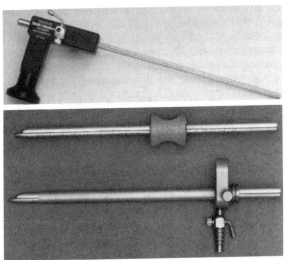

FIGURE 7.—**Upper**, photograph showing the working channel scope that is used in conjunction with a 5-mm ID access cannula. **Center**, a cannulated obturator and auxiliary obturator are passed through the oval bore of the jig. Note the beveled distal end of the auxiliary obturator that has a tendency to push the exiting root aside as it enters the annular fenestration. **Lower**, the jig is removed and the oval cannula is introduced over the two obturators. (Courtesy of Kambin P, Gennarelli T, Hermantin F: Minimally invasive techniques in spinal surgery: Current practice. *Neurosurg Focus* 4:1-10, 1998.)

ner of the disk. This zone is bounded by the exiting root on the antero-lateral boundary, the traversing root and dural sac on the medial side, and the proximal plate of the distal segment inferiorly. Careful attention to instrument positioning avoids neural injury, with the procedure performed through a subligamentous approach. The inclusion criteria are similar to those for open laminotomy and diskectomy. Arthroscopic disk surgery is not indicated for patients whose low back pain is caused by a degenerative process. To reach the herniated disk arthroscopically, the surgeon may use a uniportal or biportal approach. With use of the oval cannula, most paramedial, foraminal, or extraforaminal herniations can be addressed from a uniportal approach.

The needle is positioned in the triangular working zone under C-arm fluoroscopic guidance. The needle is replaced by a guidewire, then by a cannulated obturator, and then by the universal access cannula. Careful positioning of instruments in the disk is necessary for subligamentous removal of disk fragments (Fig 4). Annulotomy may be performed with direct vision through a working channel scope. Replacing the universal access cannula with an oval cannula allows broader access, further dorsal angulation of the forceps, and simultaneous introduction of an arthro-scope and forceps. This cannula is placed by means of a specially designed jig with an oval-shaped bore (Fig 7). If the bilateral portal approach is used, 2 working cannulas must be placed from right and left paramedial approaches.

Outcomes.—In their experience with 100 consecutive patients treated with arthroscopic minidiskectomy, the authors have achieved an 85% rate of successful outcomes at 2 years' follow-up. Other series have shown comparable results. Complications have included skin hypersensitivity and pseudocausalgic pain but no neurovascular complications.

Discussion.—For patients with herniated lumbar disks, arthroscopic minidiskectomy is a minimally invasive procedure that provides direct decompression of neural elements while protecting the contents of the spinal canal. The technique can be learned by any trained orthopedic surgeon or neurosurgeon. In properly selected patients, the outcomes are comparable to those of open laminotomy. The authors also review the technique of arthroscopic stabilization of lumbar motion segments by means of interbody arthrodesis.

▶ In those patients meeting the strict criteria and in the hands of these experienced and superb technicians, the results reported in this article can be achieved. Being personally familiar with the senior authors, I can attest to both their objectivity and technical prowess. The article vividly describes anatomical and radiographic considerations, inclusion and exclusion criteria, and surgical technique. It is certainly recommended reading for the interested surgeon. However, performance of the technique is not for the uninitiated.

J.S. Torg, M.D.

2 Injuries of Upper Limbs

A Dynamic Analysis of Glenohumeral Motion After Simulated Capsulolabral Injury: A Cavader Model
Apreleva M, Hasselman CT, Debski RE, et al (Univ of Pittsburgh, Pa)
J Bone Joint Surg Am 80-A:474-480, 1998
2–1

Objective.—Stability of the glenohumeral joint is not inherent, but rather provided by static and dynamic restraints. There is ongoing debate regarding the best operative approach to stabilizing the glenohumeral joint after capsulolabral injury. This cadaver study examined the effects of capsulolabral injury of varying severity on the kinematics of the glenohumeral joint.

Methods.—Nine fresh-frozen cadaver upper extremities were mounted for testing in a dynamic shoulder-testing apparatus. Increasing degrees of capsulolabral injury were created, from the labrum, to the capsule, to the anterior aspect of the glenoid rim. The effects of these injuries on glenohumeral joint kinematics during abduction in the scapular plane and external rotation were recorded using a 6-degrees-of-freedom magnetic tracking device. The study hypothesized that the dynamic restraint provided by the rotator cuff muscles would be sufficient to maintain glenohumeral "ball-and-socket" kinematics, even with a simulated Bankart lesion.

Findings.—The glenohumeral joint did not become dislocated in the presence of a large Bankart lesion, or even after the anterior aspect of the joint capsule. When both the anterior and posterior aspects of the joint capsule were divided, there was a significant increase in posterior translation during abduction in the scapular plane. Division of the entire joint capsule led to posterior dislocation in 2 of the 9 shoulders. Anterior and posterior translation were not increased by external rotation of the abducted arm.

Conclusions.—This biomechanical study shows that the rotator cuff muscles can maintain dynamic stability of the glenohumeral joint, even when static restraints—including the anterior aspect of the capsule and the anterior portion of the labrum—are disrupted. Anterior glenohumeral instability apparently involves a combination of muscle imbalance and

43

capsulolabral injury. The active stabilizers of the glenohumeral joint—ie, the rotator cuff muscles—warrant consideration during surgical reconstruction of capsulolabral injuries and defects, and during the design of rehabilitation protocols.

▶ This is an interesting study from the standpoint of design. However, the conclusions regarding the roles of the capsulolabral structures and rotator cuff muscles appear to be at variance with what occurs in the in vivo clinical state.

J.S. Torg, M.D.

The Active Compression Test: A New and Effective Test for Diagnosing Labral Tears and Acromioclavicular Joint Abnormality
O'Brien SJ, Pagnani MJ, Fealy S, et al (Hosp for Special Surgery, New York)
Am J Sports Med 26:610-613, 1998   2–2

Objective.—Superior labral tears are difficult to diagnose. Results of a prospective study evaluating a new diagnostic test for detection of labral abnormality and acromioclavicular joint abnormality were presented.

> *Technique.*—With the physician standing behind the patient, the patient flexes the affected arm forward at 90 degrees with the elbow at full extension, adducts the arm 10 to 15 degrees medial to the sagittal plane of the body and rotates it internally until the thumb points downward. The physician applies downward pressure on the arm. The maneuver is repeated with the palm fully supinated. The test is positive if there is pain with the first maneuver that is reduced or eliminated with the second maneuver. Pain on top of the shoulder or in the acromioclavicular joint is indicative of acromioclavicular joint abnormality whereas pain or painful clicking is diagnosed as labral abnormality.

Methods.—The specificity, sensitivity, and positive and negative predictive values of the new test were prospectively evaluated in 318 patients by an examiner who was blinded to the results of radiographic examination.

Results.—Of the 56 patients who had positive active compression tests, 53 were found to have labral tears at surgery. The 3 patients with false positive results had a reverse Hills-Sachs lesion, a hypermobile biceps tendon with multidirectional laxity and biceps tendinitis, and an anterior instability without a discrete labral tear. The sensitivity of the active compression test for labral abnormality was 100% (53/53), the specificity was 98.5% (200/203), the positive predictive value was 94.5% (53/56), and the negative predictive value was 100% (200/200). The sensitivity of the active compression test for acromioclavicular joint abnormality was 100% (55/55), the specificity was 96.6% (200/207), the positive predictive value was 88.7% (55/62), and the negative predictive value was 100% (200/200).

Conclusion.—The active compression test is a sensitive and specific technique for diagnosing acromioclavicular joint abnormality and labral abnormality.

▶ Presented is a clinical examination that is noninvasive, inexpensive, and has a sensitivity of 100% and a specificity of 97%. What more can one ask for?

J.S. Torg, M.D.

Posterior Labral Injury in Contact Athletes
Mair SD, Zarzour R, Speer KP (Duke Univ, Durham, NC)
Am J Sports Med 26:753-758, 1998

2–3

Background.—The National Collegiate Athletic Association rules allow blocking with arms fully extended and hands open. However, when a lineman blocks in this position, he may be at risk for posterior labral injury. Posterior labral injury in 9 contact athletes was described.

Methods and Findings.—Seven football offensive linemen, 1 defensive lineman, and 1 lacrosse player were found at arthroscopy to have posterior labral detachment from the glenoid. All had pain with bench pressing and during sports participation, compromising their ability to play effectively. Conservative measures did not alleviate the patients' symptoms. On examination with the patients under anesthesia, bilateral symmetric glenohumeral translation with no evidence of posterior instability was noted. The patients were treated with glenoid rim abradement and posterior labral repair with a bioabsorbable tack. All were able to complete at least 1 full season of contact sports and weightlifting without pain, with a follow-up of 2 or more years.

Conclusion.—When contact athletes ready their shoulder muscles in anticipation of impact with opponents, a compressive force at the glenohumeral joint results. Combined with a posteriorly directed force on impact, the resultant vector is a shearing force to the posterior labrum and articular surface. Repeated exposure results in posterior labral detachment without capsular injury. Consistently good outcomes result from posterior labral reattachment.

▶ The authors note that the diagnosis of posterior labral detachment is difficult because clinical symptoms are not specific. However, as reported, pain with bench pressing and participating in contact activities in which the opponent is engaged with arms in front of the body should certainly raise an index of suspicion. My own experience with both anterior and posterior labral detachments has been that attempted passive anterior or posterior subluxation frequently produces a palpable click. Report of a good outcome with posterior labral reattachment using bioabsorbable tacks is encouraging.

J.S. Torg, M.D.

Arthroscopic Management of Rotator Cuff Disease
Gartsman GM (Univ of Texas, Houston)
J Am Acad Orthop Surg 6:259-266, 1998   2–4

Objective.—A summary was presented of the 4 stages of rotator cuff disease and of the state of knowledge of arthroscopic surgical management.

Indications, Findings, Treatment.—The indications for arthroscopic treatment are the same as those for surgery and include pain and weakness that interferes with daily activities and does not respond to conservative methods. Arthroscopy is useful in the diagnosis of stage 2 impingement syndrome and conditions that may mimic it, such as glenohumeral instability, articular-surface partial rotator cuff tears, labrum tears, small areas of degenerative arthritis, posterior glenoid-cuff impingement, and lesions of the rotator interval.

Arthroscopy permits complete visual inspection of the glenohumeral joint. It is particularly valuable in diagnosing partial-thickness tears of the rotator cuff by allowing visualization of the articular surface. The technique can determine the presence and size of a tear in patients with false negative arthrography imaging studies and can reveal whether débridement, decompression, and/or repair is the best course of treatment. The value of arthroscopy in repair of complete tears is controversial, with some clinicians advocating complete arthroscopic repair and others preferring open surgery. Most surgeons prefer open procedures for release of adhesions. Arthroscopic débridement is the treatment of choice for irreparable tears.

Conclusion.—Whether arthroscopy or open procedures are best for managing rotator cuff disease remains controversial. Prospective, controlled clinical studies are needed to evaluate techniques and outcomes in a large patient population.

Arthroscopic Repair of Full-Thickness Tears of the Rotator Cuff
Gartsman GM, Khan M, Hammerman SM (Texas Orthopedic Hosp, Houston)
J Bone Joint Surg Am 80-A:832-840, 1998   2–5

Background.—Advances in operative technique have enabled the use of full-thickness tears of the rotator cuff to be repaired arthroscopically. One experience with arthroscopic repair was reported.

Methods.—Seventy-three patients, a mean 60.7 years at surgery, were followed up for 2 years or more. Eleven tears were less than 1 cm; 45 were 1 to 3 cm; 11 were 3 to 5 cm; and 6 were more than 5 cm. Sixty-nine tendons were repaired anatomically. Four were repaired a mean 3 mm medial to the anatomical insertion of the tendon. Repair necessitated a mean of 2.3 suture anchors. Sixty-three glenohumeral joints were normal. Ten had an intra-articular lesion. In 7 patients, the acromioclavicular joint was resected concomitantly.

Outcomes.—Active and passive range of motion was significantly improved postoperatively. The strength of resisted elevation increased from 7.5 to 14 pounds. The mean total University of California at Los Angeles score improved from 12.4 to 31.1 points. Mean total American Shoulder and Elbow Surgeons shoulder index score rose from 30.7 to 87.6 points. The mean absolute Constant and Murley score increased from 41.7 to 83.6 points. Pain scores also improved, with 78% of the patients rating pain relief as good or excellent. Ninety percent of the patients rated their satisfaction as good or excellent at the most recent examination. Eighty-four percent of the shoulders were rated as good or excellent after surgery, compared with none before surgery.

Conclusions.—Arthroscopic repair of full-thickness tears of the rotator cuff yields satisfactory results according to both traditional orthopedic and patient-assessed criteria. The advantages of the arthroscopic technique include smaller incisions, access to the glenohumeral joint for inspection and treatment of intra-articular lesions, no need to detach the deltoid, and less soft tissue dissection. However, this method is technically difficult.

▶ It appears in order to repeat Gartsman et al's word of caution regarding arthroscopic repair of rotator cuff tears. Specifically, they state that "these techniques can be recommended only for use by experienced orthopaedic surgeons ... An orthopaedic surgeon who performs open repairs infrequently should not attempt the arthroscopic procedure. The open operation is relatively simple and has a documented history of success. In contrast, the arthroscopic technique is technically demanding and is still in the developmental stage." A word to the wise is sufficient.

J.S. Torg, M.D.

Analysis of Collagen and Elastic Fibers in Shoulder Capsule in Patients With Shoulder Instability

Rodeo SA, Suzuki K, Yamauchi M, et al (Cornell Univ, New York; Univ of North Carolina, Chapel Hill)
Am J Sports Med 26:634-643, 1998   2–6

Objective.—Although surgery is necessary for shoulder instability that does not respond to conservative management, failure rates are higher for multidirectional than for unidirectional instability, suggesting underlying connective tissue abnormality. Collagen cross-links, collagen fibril diameter and density, amino acid composition, and elastic fibers in the shoulder capsule and skin were evaluated in 4 patient groups and in normal controls.

Methods.—Tissue samples were collected from 8 patients (1 woman), aged 18 to 28 years, with unidirectional anterior instability; 6 patients (2 men), aged 15 to 34 years, with multidirectional instability/primary surgery; 6 patients (2 men), aged 17 to 30 years, with multidirectional instability/revision surgery; and capsules from 5 shoulders of 3 normal controls harvested within 24 hours of death. The cause of instability and the degree of generalized joint laxity were determined, and a glenohumeral laxity score was calculated for the patients.

Results.—Compared with normal capsules, there were significantly more stable and reducible collagen cross-links in capsules from the patient groups. The average diameter of collagen fibrils was significantly larger in patient group capsules than in normal capsules. Patient group capsules contained significantly more cysteine and showed a significantly higher density of elastin staining than did normal capsules. There was a significant correlation between glenohumeral laxity and mean collagen fibril diameter and between an increasing number of dehydrohydroxylysinonorleucine reducible cross-links and decreasing collagen fibril diameter. Ligament laxity scores were significantly and negatively correlated with mean skin collagen fibril diameter. Mean skin collagen fibril diameter was significantly and negatively correlated with glenohumeral laxity. Group 1 (the unidirectional anterior instability group) and 2 (the multidirectional instability/primary surgery group) did not differ significantly in any parameter measured except for skin collagen diameter, which was significantly smaller in group 2 than in group 1.

Conclusion.—The decrease in skin collagen fibril diameter in group 2 compared with group 1 suggests a connective tissue abnormality in patients with multidirectional shoulder instability. Skin biopsies may be used to predict those patients likely to fail shoulder stabilization surgery.

▶ The authors have attempted to determine whether there are biochemical and morphological alterations in the extracellular matrix of the shoulder capsule and skin in patients with shoulder instability. However, they do point out that the distinction between glenohumeral laxity and glenohumeral instability is caused by variables other than just the biochemical and morphological composition. As seen, the strength of the capsule may not be different between patients with primary unidirectional anterior instability and those with multidirectional instability. Although suggested, the inference that skin biopsies be used to predict patients at high risk of recurrent instability after shoulder stabilization surgery is not supported by the data.

J.S. Torg, M.D.

Arthroscopic Transglenoid Stabilization Versus Open Anchor Suturing in Traumatic Anterior Instability of the Shoulder

Steinbeck J, Jerosch J (Westphalian Wilhelms Univ, Muenster, Germany)
Am J Sports Med 26:373-378, 1998   2–7

Introduction.—A stable inferior glenohumeral ligament-labral complex is necessary to maintain stability of the shoulder through a wide range of motion. The open Bankart repair is the current standard treatment for traumatic anterior instability of the shoulder. By reattaching the labrum and capsule directly to the glenoid rim, normal anatomy is restored. Techniques for arthroscopic stabilization of the shoulder have been developed during the last decades with success rates varying from 56% to 100%. The results of arthroscopic and open Bankart repair of traumatic anterior instability of the shoulder have not been prospectively studied. In 2 similar populations with traumatic unidirectional anterior glenohumeral instability, the results of arthroscopic and open Bankart repair were studied for a minimum follow-up of 2 years.

Methods.—Sixty-two consecutive patients with recurrent traumatic anterior instability of the shoulder were included in the study. Arthroscopic stability was performed on 30 patients and open Bankart repair was performed on 32 patients. The arthroscopic group was followed up for a mean of 36 months and the open Bankart repair group was followed up for a mean of 40 months. The arthroscopic technique used transglenoid sutures to reattach the labrum, whereas the open technique used bone anchors.

Results.—In the open repair group, redislocation occurred in 2 patients (6%), whereas in the arthroscopic repair group, redislocation occurred in 5 patients (17%). In the arthroscopic repair group, 3 of the 5 patients with redislocations had a reoperation. Good-to-excellent results were observed in 29 patients (90.6%) who had the open repair and in 24 patients (80%) who had arthroscopic repair. Postoperatively, the open repair group averaged 90.6 points by the Rowe scoring method while the arthroscopic repair group averaged 83.1 points. In 30 patients in the open repair group (94%) and in 25 patients in the arthroscopic repair group (93%), little or no limitations in postoperative sports activities were reported.

Conclusion.—The results of arthroscopic shoulder stabilization are inferior to those of the classic open Bankart procedure, despite similar patient populations and similar arthroscopic examinations to select the type of repair.

▶ The authors' observation that "the results of arthroscopic shoulder stabilization are inferior to those of the classic open Bankart procedure" is in keeping with my own experience.

J.S. Torg, M.D.

Complications in Arthroscopic Shoulder Surgery

Berjano P, González BG, Olmedo JF, et al (Cirugía Ortopédica y Rehabilitación ASEPEYO, Madrid)
Arthroscopy 14:785-788, 1998   2–8

Background.—Although arthroscopic surgery of the shoulder is considered safe, a variety of complications have been associated with this surgery. Few published studies have reported the incidence of these complications. The rate and types of observed complications occurring after shoulder arthroscopic surgery were analyzed.

Methods and Findings.—One hundred seventy-nine consecutive procedures performed by 1 surgeon were reviewed retrospectively. One hundred forty-one were arthroscopic alone, and 38 were arthroscopic plus open procedures. Overall, 9.5% of the procedures were associated with complications. The combined procedures had a complication rate of 5.3%; arthroscopy alone had a complication rate of 10.6%. However, few of the recorded complications compromised the clinical outcome of the patients.

Conclusion.—In this series, shoulder arthroscopic techniques had a complication rate of 9.5%. However, because few of the complications adversely affected clinical outcomes, arthroscopic techniques are still considered safe.

▶ Complications included respiratory distress, capsular tear, hematoma, excessive bleeding, infection, severe postoperative edema, and ulnar nerve neurapraxia. Not included were shoulder stiffness, recurrent instability, or persistent preoperative symptoms. Although a 9.5% complication rate is reported, it is concluded that the procedure is safe because clinical outcomes were not adversely affected—a conclusion that perhaps is to be questioned.

J.S. Torg, M.D.

Long-term Results of the Latarjet Procedure for the Treatment of Anterior Instability of the Shoulder

Allain J, Goutallier D, Glorion C (Hôpital Henri Mondor, Creteil, France)
J Bone Joint Surg Am 80-A:841-852, 1998   2–9

Background.—Few studies have analyzed the prevalence of glenohumeral osteoarthrosis after surgical stabilization of the shoulder. This prevalence and the factors leading to glenohumeral osteoarthrosis after the coracoid bone-block transfer procedure initially described by Latarjet were investigated.

Methods.—Ninety-five consecutive Latarjet procedures were performed because of recurrent anterior instability of the shoulder between 1969 and 1983. In 1993, data for review were available for 56 patients with 58 affected shoulders. Mean follow-up time was 14.3 years.

Findings.—At the most recent follow-up, none of the patients had recurrent dislocation. Six had apprehension with regard to possible dislocation, and 1 had occasional subluxation. Results were excellent or good in 88% of the patients, fair in 9%, and poor in 3%. No glenohumeral osteoarthrosis was noted in 22 shoulders. Thirty-four shoulders had centered glenohumeral osteoarthrosis: grade 1 in 25 shoulders, grade 2 in 4, grade 3 in 3, and grade 4 in 2. Two shoulders had grade 4 eccentric glenohumeral osteoarthrosis, with the humeral head more proximal than normal in relation to the center of the glenoid cavity. In contrast to the higher grades, grade 1 glenohumeral osteoarthrosis had no effect on shoulder function.

Conclusions.—In the patients available for follow-up in this series, the Latarjet procedure resulted in symptomatic glenohumeral osteoarthrosis only in shoulders with a preoperative tear of the rotator cuff or an intraoperative or postoperative complication. Shoulders should be assessed for a tear of the rotator cuff preoperatively, and the coracoid graft should be placed with care to avoid excessively lateral placement.

▶ As the saying goes, "A rose by any other name would smell as sweet." What I see here, on the basis of the authors' description of the procedure, is a modification of the Bristow procedure, a procedure that has fallen into disfavor in the United States. Although early results of the Bristow procedure have been reported as favorable, clearly it has not withstood the test of time, with instability, both in the form of subluxation and in dislocation, reoccurring, presumably because of eventual atrophy and weakness of the coracobrachialis/subscapularis muscular sling. Also, there have been reports of complications due to the coracoid screw, and of technical difficulties in salvaging the failures. In this study, 58% of the patients developed glenohumeral osteoarthritis, albeit most were grade I and 20% were determined to have had the condition preoperatively.

J.S. Torg, M.D.

Open Capsulorrhaphy With Suture Anchors for Recurrent Anterior Dislocation of the Shoulder
Ferretti A, De Carli A, Calderaro M, et al (Univ of Rome "La Sapienza")
Am J Sports Med 26:625-629, 1998   2–10

Background.—Various surgical procedures, including staple capsulorrhaphy, have been advocated to treat anterior dislocation of the shoulder. Because serious or potentially serious complications have been associated with staple use, the current authors began using nonabsorbable suture anchors in patients with recurrent anterior shoulder dislocation. The 2- to 4-year outcomes of open capsulorrhaphy with suture anchors are reported.

Methods.—Data on 40 of 42 consecutive open capsulorrhaphies with suture anchors were reviewed after a minimum of 2 years of follow-up.

The rating systems of Rowe and the Society of American Shoulder and Elbow Surgeons were used to assess outcomes.

Findings.—Ninety-five percent of the patients had satisfactory surgical outcomes. Eighteen of 22 patients involved in competitive overhead or collision sports before surgery were able to resume their preoperative playing levels. Of the 2 patients whose operations were unsuccessful, 1 had recurrent dislocation and 1 had a deep infection occurring as a complication of the surgical technique. In the latter patient, the deep infection healed after suture anchor removal.

Conclusions.—The results of open capsulorrhaphy with suture anchors are encouraging. This technique avoids the risks associated with the use of screws and staples. Longer-term follow-up is necessary to better define the role of this procedure in patients with recurrent anterior shoulder dislocation.

▶ The observations and conclusions of the authors with regard to the use of suture anchors during open capsulorrhaphy for recurrent anterior dislocation of the glenohumeral joint are in keeping with my own clinical experience.

J.S. Torg, M.D.

Continuous Passive Motion After Repair of the Rotator Cuff: A Prospective Outcome Study

Lastayo PC, Wright T, Jaffe R, et al (Univ of Florida, Gainesville)
J Bone Joint Surg Am 80-A:1002-1011, 1998   2–11

Objective.—Although continuous passive range-of-motion exercises after soft-tissue or joint replacement procedures are beneficial for maximizing full functional recovery after rotator cuff repair their effect on outcome has not been studied. The functional outcome of continuous passive motion exercises after rotator cuff repair was prospectively compared in a randomized study with that of manual passive range-of-motion exercises.

Methods.—After open repair of 32 rotator cuff tears (5 small, 18 medium, and 9 large), 31 patients (14 men), aged 30 to 80 years, were randomly allocated to receive continuous passive motion (17 patients) or manual passive range-of-motion exercises (15 patients) for 4 weeks. Thereafter, both groups practiced passive external rotation exercises and assisted passive elevation exercises. Patients were operated on by 1 surgeon and followed up for an average of 22 months. Outcome measures were pain, impairment, and disability.

Results.—Shoulder Pain and Disability Index scores were excellent for 27 (84%) shoulders, good for 2 (6%), fair for 2 (7%), and poor for 1 (3%). No significant differences were observed between groups with respect to pain, range-of-motion, or isometric strength. Manual passive range-of-motion exercises required fewer visits and were therefore more cost-effective than the usual 3 physical therapy visits per week.

Conclusion.—After rotator cuff repair, both continuous passive motion and manual passive range-of-motion exercises provide similar favorable outcomes.

▶ The authors report this to be a randomized study because 1 group received postoperative continuous passive motion and the other group received manual range of motion. However, it seems important that in the study design there should have been a third group in which neither was implemented. Also, there was no formal documentation of the compliance of patients or of modifications to the program after the first 4 weeks.

J.S. Torg, M.D.

Symptomatic Scapulothoracic Crepitus and Bursitis
Kuhn JE, Plancher KD, Hawkins RJ (Univ of Michigan, Ann Arbor; Albert Einstein College of Medicine, New York; Univ of Colorado, Denver)
J Am Acad Orthop Surg 6:267-273, 1998   2–12

Objective.—The 2 types of scapulothoracic crepitus—the painful "snapping scapula" caused by an osseous lesion in the scapulothoracic space and the less intense symptomatic scapulothoracic crepitus probably arising from a soft-tissue disorder—are related to, but different from, scapulothoracic bursitis. A discussion of the differences between these 2 disorders was presented.

Scapulothoracic Bursitis.—The anatomy of the subscapular region is described in Figure 1. The condition may occur with or without scapular crepitus, generally results from trauma or overuse, and is characterized by pain on use. Its symptoms are similar to those of elastofibroma. Initial treatment includes rest, analgesics, and nonsteroidal anti-inflammatory drugs. Corticosteroid injections, ice, heat, US, and periscapular muscle-strengthening exercises may be helpful. When symptoms do not resolve, arthroscopic or surgical resection of the bursa may be required.

Scapulothoracic Crepitus.—About 30% of patients with this condition have no pain. Scapular noises arise from anatomical changes in the tissue between the scapula and the chest wall or an incongruent scapulothoracic articulation. Underlying bone lesions include osteochondroma, hooked superomedial angle, Luschka's tubercle, or reactive bone spurs. Abnormalities in articulation can lead to scoliosis and thoracic kyphosis.

Diagnosis.—A history of repetitive overhead activity, examination, tangential radiographic views, and MRI can be useful in diagnosis.

Treatment.—Whereas conservative treatment is initially recommended, lesions usually must be resected to alleviate symptoms. Postural strengthening exercises, anti-inflammatory drugs, heat, massage, phonophoresis, US, and application of ethyl chloride can also help to eliminate pain.

Conclusion.—Conservative treatment of soft lesions is usually sufficient to resolve symptoms. For bony lesions or failure of conservation treatment, surgery or arthroscopy is necessary.

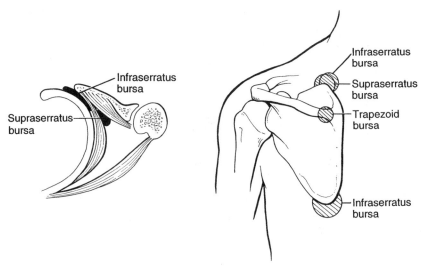

FIGURE 1.—Anatomical and adventitial bursae of the scapulothoracic articulation. **Left,** The infraserratus bursa is found between the serratus and the chest wall. Its borders are the origin of the serratus laterally and the rhomboid muscles medially. The supraserratus bursa is found between the serratus anterior and the subscapularis, with the lateral border extending to the axilla and the medial border extending to the insertion of the serratus. **Right,** sites where symptomatic bursitis may occur and the bursae that are affected. (From the American Academy of Orthopaedic Surgeons, copyright 1998. Reprinted from the *Journal of the American Academy of Orthopaedic Surgeons,* courtesy of Kuhn JE, Plancher KD, Hawkins RJ: Symptomatic scapulothoracic crepitus and bursitis. *J Am Acad Orthop Surg* 6:267-273, 1998, with permission. Courtesy of Kuhn JE, Hawkins RJ: Evaluation and treatment of scapular disorders, in Warner JJP, Iannotti JP, Gerber C (eds): *Complex and Revision Problems in Shoulder Surgery.* Philadelphia, Lippincott-Raven, 1997, pp 357-375.)

▶ The early literature describes a partial scapulectomy for the snapping of the scapula. It has been my experience that subscapular bursitis can be effectively managed with local steroid injections. Although there have been more recent reports alluding to arthroscopic treatment of this problem, I am not aware that this approach is commonly utilized. The rarely occurring scapular exostosis does require surgical removal.

J.S. Torg, M.D.

The Treatment of Symptomatic Os Acromiale
Warner JJP, Beim GM, Higgins L (Univ of Pittsburgh, Pa)
J Bone Joint Surg Am 80-A:1320-1326, 1998   2–13

Background.—Os acromiale is typically not associated with shoulder pain. Surgical management of symptomatic os acromiale is reported.

Methods.—The subjects were 14 patients (7 men, 7 women; mean age, 57) who had pain in the shoulder (15 shoulders) associated with os acromiale. All the patients had pain when the acromion in the affected region was palpated. Furthermore, no patient could actively flex the shoulder to more than 120 degrees even though only 8 patients had an associated rotator cuff tear. Radiography, MRI, or bone scan was used to confirm the os acromiale, located in the preacromion in 1 shoulder, the mesoacromion in 11 shoulders, and the metaacromion in 3 shoulders. In all cases, the anterior aspect of the acromion was discovered to be unstable at surgery. Three patients (3 shoulders) underwent excision of the unstable os acromiale. The remaining 11 patients (12 shoulders) underwent open reduction of the os acromiale and insertion of an autogenous iliac crest bone graft. In 4 of these patients (5 shoulders), internal fixation was provided by a tension band procedure involving pins and wires (group 1). In the other 7 patients (7 shoulders), internal fixation was provided by a tension band procedure involving cannulated screws with wires placed through them in a figure 8 configuration over the corticocancellous bone graft (group 2). After surgery, the shoulder was immobilized for 1 week, limited active motion was allowed after 6 weeks, and full active motion was allowed after 12 weeks.

Findings.—Of the 4 patients (5 shoulders) in group 1, fixation with pins and wires failed in 4 shoulders, causing nonunion and continued shoulder weakness and mild to moderate pain at rest. A solid osseous union occurred in 1 shoulder, and this patient could flex the shoulder to at least 140 degrees with no pain. Of the 7 patients (7 shoulders) in group 2, the screw and wire fixation failed in 1 shoulder, causing nonunion and continued limited shoulder movement and mild pain at rest. A solid osseous union occurred in 6 shoulders, with good results in 5 patients (shoulder flexion to at least 140 degrees with no pain) and poor results in 1 patient (shoulder flexion to 100 degrees, pain, and shoulder weakness because of a repeat rotator cuff tear). In the 7 shoulders in which union of the os acromiale occurred, hardware had to be removed in 5 because of discomfort or prominent hardware at the top of the shoulder. Union was confirmed when the hardware was removed, and the average time to union was 9 weeks.

Conclusions.—In patients with symptomatic os acromiale, autogenous bone grafting and rigid internal fixation with cannulated screws and wires placed through them in a figure 8 configuration generally results in union of the os acromiale and resolution of pain. The presence of a rotator cuff tear did not affect the outcome.

▶ Apparently, the key to successful operative management is to obtain rigid fixation across the site of nonunion. When only the tension band method was used, the failure rate was 80%. The authors believe that modifying their technique by using cannulated screws with wires placed through the screws and tightened in a figure 8 configuration resulted in a more rigid construct and kept the bone graft securely fixed over the top of the acromion.

J.S. Torg, M.D.

Injury of the Suprascapular Nerve at the Spinoglenoid Notch: The Natural History of Infraspinatus Atrophy in Volleyball Players

Ferretti A, De Carli A, Fontana M (Univ of Rome, La Sapienza)
Am J Sports Med 26:759-763, 1998   2–14

Background.—Suprascapular nerve injury at the spinoglenoid notch results in paralysis of the terminal branch of the nerve, with isolated atrophy of the infraspinatus muscle, loss of strength in external rotation, and inconstant pain. This injury occurs most often in volleyball players. One experience with the diagnosis and treatment of suprascapular nerve injury at the spinoglenoid notch in volleyball players was reviewed.

Patients and Findings.—Thirty-eight patients with isolated atrophy of the infraspinatus muscle were treated between 1985 and 1996. All were competitive volleyball players. The patients were 20 men and 18 women, aged 15 to 27 years. Thirty-five patients had no pain at the first examination and were treated with exercises to strengthen the external rotators. The other 3 patients had pain at the posterior aspect of the shoulder and underwent surgery. Sixteen of the 35 patients treated nonsurgically were reassessed at a mean of 5.5 years. Thirteen patients still played volleyball

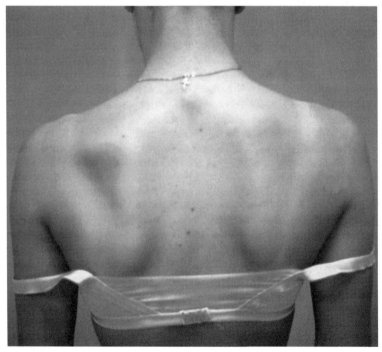

FIGURE 1.—**A,** Suprascapular nerve entrapment at the spinoglenoid notch in a 15-year-old female volleyball player with severe atrophy of the infraspinatus muscle. **B,** significant improvement of infraspinatus hypotrophy 2 years after surgical treatment. (Courtesy of Ferretti A, De Carli A, Fontana M: Injury of the suprascapular nerve at the spinoglenoid notch: The natural history of infraspinatus atrophy in volleyball players. *Am J Sports Med* 26:759-763, 1998.)

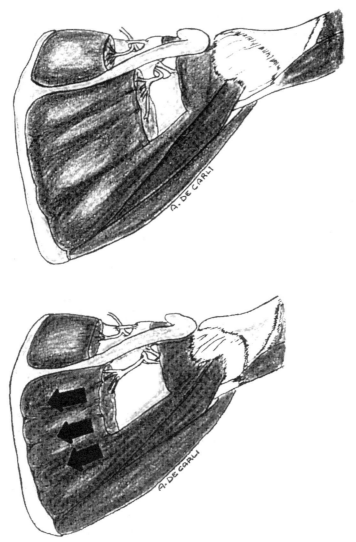

FIGURE 2.—Mechanism of suprascapular nerve impingement at the base of the scapular spine, caused by contraction of the infraspinatus muscle. (Courtesy of Ferretti A, De Carli A, Fontana M: Injury of the suprascapular nerve at the spinoglenoid notch: The natural history of infraspinatus atrophy in volleyball players. *Am J Sports Med* 26:759-763, 1998.)

and 3 had retired, symptom free. Infraspinatus muscle atrophy was unchanged in all patients on physical examination. Surgically treated patients were reassessed at a mean of 2 years' follow-up. All were able to play volleyball at pre-injury levels, though 1 patient had pain at the anterior aspect of the shoulder after strenuous activity. On physical examination, atrophy was notably reduced in 1 patient (Figs 1 and 2).

Conclusions.—Suprascapular nerve entrapment at the spinoglenoid notch, commonly seen in volleyball players, is usually a painless syndrome. In a carefully selected subgroup of patients with painful neuropathies, surgery is indicated.

▶ The interesting conclusion derived from this study is that, despite considerable muscle atrophy and loss of strength in external rotation, the effect on the athletes' performance was very limited. Also, long-term follow-up did not reveal progressive shoulder dysfunction or an increased incidence of impingement syndrome.

J.S. Torg, M.D.

Throwing Fracture of the Humeral Shaft: An Analysis of 90 Patients
Ogawa K, Yoshida A (Keio Univ, Tokyo)
Am J Sports Med 26:242-246, 1998   2–15

Objective.—Throwing fractures of the humeral shaft occur most frequently during pitching. The causes are not known. The characteristics of humeral shaft fractures sustained while pitching or throwing a ball and the causes of this type of fracture were retrospectively investigated.

Methods.—The physical status, history of athletic participation, and details of throwing at the time were reviewed for injury of 90 amateur athletes (1 woman), aged 12 to 43 years, who had sustained throwing fractures of the humeral shaft over the previous 18 years. The review used records and interviews. Most patients were in their 20s.

Results.—Sixty percent of patients were pitchers. Most fractures (91%) occurred during overhand or three-quarter overhand throwing. Little evidence of previously existing stress fracture was found. Most fractures were spiral, and most occurred immediately below the insertion of the deltoid muscle, at the junction of the middle and lower thirds of the humerus, or along the radial groove. The main fracture force appears to be an external rotation, with the fracture occurring during the acceleration phase of the throw in the middle to lower third of the humerus. Patients who practiced irregularly were at greatest risk.

Conclusion.—Patients who practice infrequently are more likely to have a throwing fracture of the humeral shaft. Fractures are the result of external rotation and occur during the acceleration phase of the throw in the middle to lower third of the humerus.

▶ This is perhaps the largest published series regarding this entity. All fractures were closed, external rotation spiral fractures that did not exhibit comminution, nor did they appear to be the result of fatigue. To be noted: 14 patients had associated radial nerve palsy, all of whom completely recovered.

J.S. Torg, M.D.

Stress Fractures of the Upper Limb

Brukner P (Olympic Park Sports Medicine Centre, Melbourne, Australia)
Sports Med 26:415-424, 1998   2–16

Objective.—Stress fractures of the arm are rarer than those of the leg. They occur in upper limb–dominated sports. Bony pain of gradual onset and bony tenderness in any athlete should alert the physician to the possibility of stress fracture of the arm.

Clavicle.—Two patients with clavicular stress fracture, a javelin thrower and a springboard diver, had maximal pain on abduction. Plain radiographs showed periosteal reaction. Fracture was confirmed with isotope scan in 1 case and plain tomography in the other.

Scapula.—Stress fractures can be related to occupation or sports activities. Axillary radiographs or bone scans have revealed the cause of shoulder pain that increased with resistance against adduction and flexion of the shoulder.

Humerus.—Most humeral fractures occur during sports played by adolescents with a recent increase in activity. Patients have swelling, ecchymosis, and extreme pain with active and passive motion of the arm. Radiographs, bone scans, and CT were diagnostic.

Olecranon.—Resulting from overuse and characterized by a gradual onset of pain over a period of weeks, olecranon fractures can be classified as stress fractures of the growth plate or of the olecranon itself (usually treated conservatively) or stress fracture of the tip of the olecranon (usually treated by surgical excision).

Ulna.—Stress fractures of the ulna, usually the result of overrotation, are characterized by tenderness and pain with movement and are confirmed by a bone scan.

Radius.—Stress fractures of the radius are characterized by forearm pain that may be bilateral and may be exacerbated by hyperextension of the wrist. Radiographs and bone scans are diagnostic.

Metacarpal.—Of 8 reported cases, 3 were occupational and 5 were sports related and resulted from extrinsic pressure from a solid object exerting a force on the bone. Increasing training intensity or changing technique increases the risk of metacarpal stress fractures.

Conclusion.—The majority of patients recover after a few weeks of rest and rehabilitation and are eventually able to return to full activity. Athletes may need to address problems of technique or overtraining.

▶ The value of this article is, if for no other reason, that it calls attention to the fact that stress fractures may involve the upper limbs. Certainly, stress fracture should be considered in the differential diagnosis of upper limb involvement where there is ill-defined pain in a physically active individual.

J.S. Torg, M.D.

Clinical, Functional, and Radiographic Assessments of the Conventional and Modified Boyd-Anderson Surgical Procedures for Repair of Distal Biceps Tendon Ruptures

D'Arco P, Sitler M, Kelly J, et al (Temple Univ, Philadelphia)
Am J Sports Med 26:254-261, 1998   2–17

Background.—The conventional Boyd-Anderson procedure (CBAP), which became the standard for surgical repair of distal biceps tendon ruptures after its inception in 1961, was associated with several complications. Since that time, several modifications of the CBAP have been developed. The clinical, functional, and radiographic outcomes of the conventional and modified Boyd-Anderson procedures for repair of distal biceps tendon ruptures were reported.

Methods and Findings.—Of 18 men undergoing surgical repair for unilateral distal biceps tendon ruptures, 13 participated in the study. Five had undergone CBAP, and 8 had undergone modified procedures. Return to premorbid activity levels, patient satisfaction with outcomes, and overall clinical results were generally favorable. Arms that had and had not been operated on did not differ significantly in elbow flexion, forearm supination, or upper extremity functional concentric peak torque and range of motion, after adjustment for dominance as a confounding variable. Radiographic findings showed no clinically remarkable signs of heterotopic ossification or proximal radioulnar synostosis.

Conclusions.—Conventional and modified Boyd-Anderson procedures for repair of distal biceps tendon ruptures are effective clinically, functionally, and radiographically. In general, these patients were very well satisfied with the results of their surgery.

▶ To avoid complications associated with the conventional Boyd-Anderson procedure—which included proximal radioulnar synostosis attributed to aggressive elevation of the anconeus muscle from the proximal ulna—the authors developed a modified Boyd-Anderson procedure. Rather than stripping the anconeus, a hemostat and subsequently the tendon itself is passed through the empty tunnel and into the space between the radius and the ulna. The tip of the hemostat is palpated on the dorsal surface of the forearm, and a 4-cm muscle splitting incision is made and developed down to the radial tuberosity. The arm is then placed in maximal pronation and the tendon is pulled through the passage and fixed through drill holes with nonabsorbable sutures. We have had experience with this technique and agree with the conclusions of the authors as to its efficacy.

J.S. Torg, M.D.

Early Detection of Osteochondritis Dissecans of the Capitellum in Young Baseball Players: Report of Three Cases
Takahara M, Shundo M, Kondo M, et al (Hokkaido Univ, Sapporo City, Japan)
J Bone Joint Surg Am 80-A:892-897, 1998   2–18

Introduction.—Repetitive throwing, as required in baseball, is thought to be an important etiological factor of osteochondritis dissecans. Little is known, however, about the primary changes leading to this disorder. A study of 44 young baseball players sought to detect these changes by examining their elbows with MRI and US.

Methods.—The boys ranged in age from 10 to 12 years. None had undergone a previous examination of the elbow. MRI was performed with a 1.5-tesla magnet, obtaining coronal and sagittal T2-weighted gradient-echo images. A real-time linear-array scanner equipped with a 7.5 MHz transducer (Fig 1) obtained anterior and posterior longitudinal ultrasonograms of the capitellum. Three boys were found to have an abnormality of the capitellum.

Results.—In all 3 cases, the T1-weighted images showed low signal intensity in the superficial aspect of the capitellum (Fig 2). In contrast, T2-weighted images revealed no abnormalities, and US demonstrated localized flattening of the subchondral bone and a normal outline of the articular cartilage. All 3 boys were advised to stop pitching, and the elbows healed spontaneously when followed this advice. One of the boys, how-

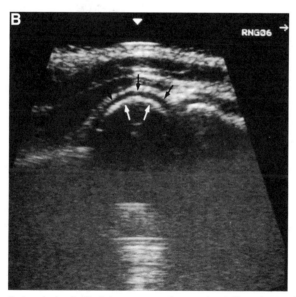

FIGURE 1.—**B,** Anterior longitudinal ultrasonogram of a normal capitellum, showing the subchondral bone of the capitellum as a high-signal-intensity round area (*white arrows*) and the articular cartilage as a low-signal-intensity round area (*black arrows*) over the subchondral bone. (Courtesy of Takahara M, Shundo M, Kondo M, et al: Early detection of osteochondritis dissecans of the capitellum in young baseball players: Report of three cases. *J Bone Joint Surg Am* 80-A, 892-897, 1998.)

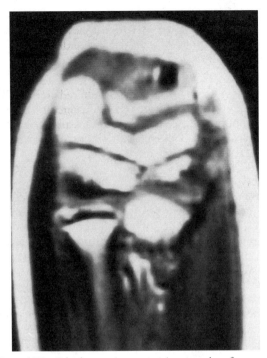

FIGURE 2.—Coronal T1-weighted magnetic resonance image, made at first examination, showing a low-signal-intensity in the superficial aspect of the capitellum. (Courtesy of Takahara M, Shundo M, Kondo M, et al: Early detection of osteochondritis dissecans of the capitellum in young baseball players: Report of three cases. *J Bone Joint Surg Am* 80-A, 892-897, 1998.)

ever, continued to pitch and was subsequently found to have typical osteochondritis dissecans.

Discussion.—Osteochondritis dissecans can develop as the result of a variety of conditions. Although numerous articles have discussed the etiology of the disease, little is known about the early changes that can occur. The identification of capitellar abnormalities by MRI and US suggest that these are early changes leading to osteochondritis dissecans. Early detection and treatment are important, because the lesion can become unstable or the bone fragment detached with delay.

▶ The ability of MRI to demonstrate what the authors believe to be the early changes of osteochondritis dissecans of the capitellum is interesting. However, whether or not the process is reversible by altering one's activities (i.e., pitching) remains to be seen.

J.S. Torg, M.D.

Snapping of the Medial Head of the Triceps and Recurrent Dislocation of the Ulnar Nerve: Anatomical and Dynamic Factors

Spinner RJ, Goldner RD (Duke Univ, Durham, NC)
J Bone Joint Surg Am 80-A:239-247, 1998

2–19

Introduction.—Few have reported snapping of the medial head of the triceps, and this entity may often go unrecognized. A failure to realize that the ulnar nerve and the medial head of the triceps can dislocate concurrently can lead to persistent symptoms after an otherwise successful transposition of the ulnar nerve. The 17 patients (22 limbs) described here had snapping (dislocation) of both the ulnar nerve and the medial head of the triceps over the medial epicondyle.

Methods.—The 15 male and 2 female patients had an average age of 25. In all but 3 cases, diagnosis of snapping of the medial head of the triceps and recurrent dislocation of the ulnar nerve was suspected clinically (Fig 1) and confirmed with MRI, CT, or both. Operative findings were confirmatory in the remaining 3 cases. Two patients were seen for painless snapping, 4 had snapping and pain in the medial aspect of the elbow, 3 had symptoms related to the ulnar nerve only, and 6 had snapping and symptoms related to the ulnar nerve. Four patients were asymptomatic and had snapping that was identified incidentally.

Results.—Six patients (7 limbs) were sufficiently symptomatic to be managed operatively. Five of these patients (6 limbs) had symptoms related to the ulnar nerve, and they underwent lateral transposition or excision of the dislocating medial head of the triceps in addition to decompression and transposition of the ulnar nerve. All 6 patients had an excellent result at an average of 4.5 years postoperatively. Specifically, all had a full range of

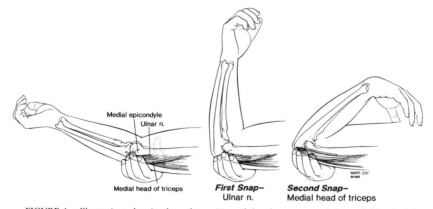

FIGURE 1.—Illustrations showing how the position of the ulnar nerve and the medial head of the triceps can be determined relative to the medial epicondyle as the elbow is flexed and extended actively or passively. In a patient who has snapping of the medial head of the triceps and dislocation of the ulnar nerve, the ulnar nerve dislocates at 90 degrees and the medial head of the triceps dislocates at approximately 110 degrees. (Printed by permission of the Mayo Foundation.) (Courtesy of Spinner RJ, Goldner RD: Snapping of the medial head of the triceps and recurrent dislocation of the ulnar nerve: Anatomical and dynamic factors. *J Bone Joint Surg Am* 80-A:239-247, 1998.)

motion, with no snapping and no symptoms related to the ulnar nerve. Among patients managed conservatively, control of symptoms related to the ulnar nerve was achieved in 4 limbs and control of pain from the snapping in 4 limbs.

Discussion.—Snapping of the medial head of the triceps may have a spectrum of clinical presentations. Not all dislocating triceps snap, and snapping may be painless. Patients may have pain in the medial aspect of the elbow, snapping, ulnar neuropathy, or a combination of the three. Treatment of snapping of the triceps can be nonoperative in many cases if symptoms are mild, intermittent, or positional.

▶ The clinical relevance of this article is clear. Persistent snapping after an otherwise successful transposition of the ulnar nerve can result from failure to recognize concurrent dislocation of the nerve and medial head of the triceps.

J.S. Torg, M.D.

Medial Elbow Joint Laxity in Professional Baseball Pitchers: A Bilateral Comparison Using Stress Radiography
Ellenbecker TS, Mattalino AJ, Elam EA, et al (Scottsdale Sports Clinic, Ariz; Clinical Diagnostic Radiology Ltd, Phoenix, Ariz; Milwaukee Brewers Baseball Club, Milwaukee, Wis)
Am J Sports Med 26:420-424, 1998   2–20

Purpose.—Baseball pitchers and other throwing athletes place large, repetitive valgus stress on the elbow during the cocking and acceleration phases. This can lead to injuries of the ulnar collateral ligament (UCL), found at the medial aspect of the ulnahumeral joint. Evaluation of the UCL is an essential part of injury prevention and management in throwing athletes. This study compared medial elbow laxity in the throwing and nonthrowing arms of professional baseball pitchers.

Methods.—The study included 40 uninjured professional baseball pitchers. All underwent measurement of active range of motion for elbow and wrist extension and flexion, followed by bilateral stress radiography using the Telos GA-IIE stress device to apply valgus stress to the elbow. Medial joint laxity in both elbows was calculated by measuring the joint space width between the humeral trochlea and the ulnar coronoid process on anteroposterior radiographs with a 15-daN valgus stress versus no stress.

Results.—Under stress, mean medial joint space opening was 1.20 mm in the dominant arm versus 0.88 in the nondominant arm. Thus, the dominant extremity showed 0.32 mm greater medial joint width opening on application of valgus stress. Range of motion measurements showed that elbow extension was significantly reduced in the dominant arm compared with the nondominant arm. Elbow flexion and wrist extension range of motion were also significantly reduced in the dominant arm.

Conclusions.—Uninjured professional baseball pitchers show increased medial elbow laxity in the throwing arm, compared with the opposite arm. More study is needed to define patterns of medial elbow laxity in other upper extremity athletes, and the relationship between stress radiography and UCL injury. Stress radiography is apparently a reliable test for medial elbow laxity in throwing athletes.

Elbow Valgus Stress Radiography in an Uninjured Population
Lee GA, Katz SD, Lazarus MD (Albert Einstein Med Ctr, Philadelphia)
Am J Sports Med 26:425-427, 1998   2–21

Background.—The diagnosis of valgus instability of the elbow is based on history and physical examination. Nonetheless, some authors have used gravity valgus stress radiography to aid the diagnosis by measuring the medial ulnahumeral distance before and after stress. The amount of ulnahumeral gapping that occurs in normal elbows was measured with stress valgus radiographs.

Methods.—The subjects were 20 men and 20 women (mean age, 27) with no history or physical examination findings of elbow pain or trauma. Both elbows were radiographed with the elbow positioned in extension and again with the elbow in 30 degrees of flexion. Medial ulnahumeral distance was measured in 3 conditions: no stress, valgus stress by gravity, and applied valgus stress of 25 N (about 5 pounds).

Findings.—Results did not differ based on the subject's gender, hand dominance, or side. Ulnahumeral distances increased significantly with increasing stress: Ulnahumeral distances in extension and 30 degrees of flexion during no stress were 3.3 ± 0.4 and 3.5 ± 0.5 mm, respectively. During valgus stress by gravity, the ulnahumeral distances were significantly greater, 3.7 ± 0.5 and 4.0 ± 0.7 mm. During applied valgus stress, the ulnahumeral distances were again significantly greater than in the other 2 conditions, 4.4 ± 0.5 and 4.7 ± 0.6 mm.

Conclusions.—Valgus stress causes a significant increase in ulnahumeral distances in normal elbows. This fact can be used in the diagnosis of valgus instability of the elbow by comparing valgus stress radiographs of the injured elbow with those of the uninjured contralateral elbow. However, valgus stress radiography of only the injured elbow should not be used to diagnose valgus instability of the elbow because even normal elbows show increased ulnahumeral gapping; thus, without a comparison with the contralateral elbow, false-positive results could become common.

▶ The significance of these 2 articles (Abstracts 2–20 and 2–21) relates to the idea that reconstruction of the ulnar collateral ligament complex is indicated in symptomatic individuals with laxity demonstrated by valgus stress radiography. Lee et al observed that there was no significant difference in medial ulnahumeral gapping when comparing contralateral elbows in normal volunteers. Ellenbecker, on the other hand, studying "uninjured" professional baseball pitchers demonstrated a 0.32 mm difference between elbows. It should be noted that in the second group "a significant decrease in elbow extension was measured on the dominant arm compared with the nondominant extremity". We may ask what was the relationship between the flexion contracture and the observed minuscule valgus gapping. Clearly, the role of stress radiography as a determinant for surgery remains somewhat unclear.

J.S. Torg, M.D.

Acute Skier's Thumb Repaired With a Proximal Phalanx Suture Anchor
Zeman C, Hunter RE, Freeman JR, et al (Orthopaedic Associates of Asper, Colo; Aspen Found for Sports Medicine, Education and Research, Colo)
Am J Sports Med 26:644-650, 1998   2–22

Background.—Various fixation methods are used in the direct repair of acutely avulsed ulnar collateral ligament (UCL) of the thumb. The use of

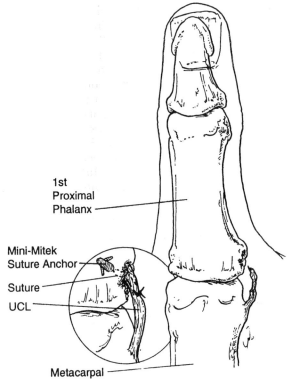

1st
Proximal
Phalanx

Mini-Mitek
Suture Anchor

Suture

UCL

Metacarpal

FIGURE 6.—Technique for suturing the distal end of the ulnar collateral ligament to the proximal phalanx with a Mitek suture anchor. (From Zeman C, Hunter RE, Freeman JR, et al: Acute skier's thumb repaired with a proximal phalanx suture anchor. *Am J Sports Med* 26:644-650, 1998. Courtesy of Bovard R, et al: Grade III avulsion fracture repair on the UCL of the proximal joint of the thumb. *Orthop Rev* 23:167-169. Copyright, 1994 by Quadrant Healthcom Inc.)

a Mitek Mini Anchor in fixing the distal end of the UCL of the thumb to the base of the proximal phalanx has been described recently (Fig 6).

Methods.—Fifty-eight patients with grade III sprains of the UCL underwent early repair using a suture anchor for fixation. Forty-five patients were available for an interview at least 12 months after the procedure. A 14-point questionnaire was administered to determine functional outcomes.

Findings.—Ninety-eight percent of the patients interviewed said they had a stable repair, felt satisfied with the surgery, and would have it again if needed. Ninety-eight percent reported a functional range of motion and no hindrance in their daily activities. Seventeen percent reported mild discomfort, but only 7% experienced pain with activities. Mean time to return to skiing was 1.7 days.

Conclusions.—Early surgery using a suture anchor can provide a strong, stable repair in patients with acute UCL rupture. The high success rate may be attributed to accurate diagnosis as well as prompt treatment with a minimally traumatizing technique.

▶ Acute rupture of the ulnar collateral ligament is a common injury in skiers. In view of the fact that 78% of the patients in this series had "some type of a Stener lesion," the authors' observation that surgery was indicated is sound. However, the results determined on the basis of the patient's self examination and a questionnaire response can be questioned. More importantly, there was no control group with which to compare the efficacy of the suture anchor technique.

J.S. Torg, M.D.

3 Injuries of Lower Limbs

Tennis After Total Hip Arthroplasty
Mont MA, LaPorte DM, Mullick T, et al (Johns Hopkins Univ, Baltimore, Md)
Am J Sports Med 27:60-64, 1999   3–1

Background.—Many active persons undergoing hip arthroplasty wish to continue playing tennis after surgery. One group of patients who continued to play tennis after hip arthroplasty was surveyed regarding their functional abilities and degree of satisfaction.

Methods.—A questionnaire was mailed to all US Tennis Association member associations in 3 states to identify players who had had hip arthroplasty. Fifty men and 8 women, aged 47 to 89, were identified.

Findings.—Only 14% of these patients' surgeons had approved of their playing tennis. Thity-four percent of the surgeons recommended only doubles. After a mean of 8 years, 3 patients needed revision surgery. One year after arthroplasty, the patients played both singles and doubles about 3 times a week. All were very satisfied with their hip arthroplasties and their increased ability to play tennis.

Conclusion.—Physicians should advise caution in tennis activities after hip arthroplasty. Such patients wishing to play tennis should be followed up annually to determine whether osteolysis is occurring prematurely. Further research on the general effects of playing tennis on total hip arthroplasty is needed.

▶ Encouraging is the fact that not only did these tennis players improve markedly from their symptomatic to their postarthroplastic states, but it appears that their level of play was restored to that of their presymptomatic state. The results of this study suggest that revision rates in tennis players with total hip arthroplasty were no worse that those of individuals who were less active. However, the authors acknowledge a "selection bias" in the study and draw no conclusions regarding revision rates.

J.S. Torg, M.D.

Hamstring Strains in Athletes: Diagnosis and Treatment

Clanton TO, Coupe KJ (Univ of Texas, Houston)
J Am Acad Orthop Surg 6:237-248, 1998   3–2

Objective.—Hamstring injuries are common, well-defined athletic injuries. The diagnosis and treatment of hamstring strains in athletes are discussed.

Basic Science.—The contractile nature of the musculotendinous unit consists of type I (slow-twitch) and type II (fast-twitch) fibers. The hamstring muscle group, made up of the biceps femoris, the semitendinosus, and the semimembranosus, functions during the early-stance phase of gait for knee support, during the late-stance phase for propulsion, and during midswing to control leg momentum. Injury occurs at the musculotendinous junction where forces are concentrated and, typically, results from hamstring strength imbalances and lack of adequate flexibility.

Clinical Findings.—Most hamstring injuries are acute. A physical examination should include palpation of the entire length of the muscle. Strains should be classified into direct and indirect injuries and categorized as mild (pulled), moderate (partial tear), or severe (complete rupture). CT, US, and MRI are diagnostic, with MRI being the most definitive and the most expensive. Acute strains are treated with usually less than 1 week of immobilization; rest; ice; compression; and elevation to control hemorrhage, pain, and edema. Administration of nonsteroidal anti-inflammatory drugs is controversial. Muscle strength quickly returns as long as there is no reinjury. Careful mobilization, with pain-free stretching and strengthening exercises, gradually helps the athlete to regain flexibility and endurance, reduce inflammation, and prevent reinjury. Isokinetic measurements may be useful for determining the extent of healing and strength balance. Progress in functional activities is the best indication of healing. Surgical repair is usually necessary only for complete rupture at the origin or insertion.

Conclusion.—Hamstring strain injuries in athletes are generally self-limiting and rarely require surgical repair. Conservative management and careful mobilization are usually all the treatment required.

▶ This is an excellent and comprehensive review of the subject. The original article is recommended reading for all those involved in primary care of the athlete.

J.S. Torg, M.D.

Rectus Femoris Muscle Tear Appearing as a Pseudotumor

Temple HT, Kuklo TR, Sweet DE, et al (Walter Reed Army Med Ctr, Washington, DC)
Am J Sports Med 26:544-548, 1998   3–3

Background.—Quadriceps muscle strains are common sports injuries. However, sometimes a rectus femoris muscle tear can appear as a soft tissue mass of the anterior thigh, with or without a significant trauma history. One experience was reported.

Patients and Findings.—Seven patients with an unexplained soft tissue mass of the thigh were seen at a military medical center between 1992 and 1996. All were male, aged 15 to 73 years. Three patients were active-duty soldiers; 3, military dependents; and 1, a retired serviceman. In all patients, clinical examination revealed a palpable, mildly tender mass. Laboratory and plain radiographic findings were normal. On MR images, lesions were seen as an obvious but often ill-defined mass at the musculotendinous junction of the rectus femoris muscle. Tissue biopsy was performed in 4 patients to exclude soft tissue sarcoma. Histologic examination demonstrated fibrosis, degeneration of muscle fibers, and chronic inflammatory cells with no evidence of malignancy.

Conclusions.—A chronic rectus femoris muscle tear can mimic a soft tissue tumor or sarcoma, which need to be ruled out in the differential diagnosis of such injuries. These injuries may occur acutely or may indicate overuse caused by repeated microtrauma. Clinicians can confirm the diagnosis of muscle tear by careful history, physical examination, and selective radiographic studies. The patient's full functional recovery can be expected.

▶ The lesion reported presents as a well-defined nontender mass at the musculotendinous junction on the rectus femoris muscle. It is characteristically associated with a palpable defect. To this observer, the location and defect are in and of themselves diagnostic. As this article points out, "Only rarely, if ever, should a biopsy be undertaken."

J.S. Torg, M.D.

Patellar Tendon Defect During the First Year After Anterior Cruciate Ligament Reconstruction: Appearance on Serial Magnetic Resonance Imaging

Bernicker JP, Haddad JL, Lintner DM, et al (Baylor College of Medicine, Houston)
Arthroscopy 14:804-809, 1998   3–4

Objective.—Reconstruction of the anterior cruciate ligament (ACL) is most commonly performed using the central third of the patellar tendon. Although the defect heals with time, no one had chronicled this healing process. MRI was used to evaluate prospectively the healing of the patellar tendon defect in the first year after ACL reconstruction.

Methods.—MRI scanning, using a 1.5-Tesla superconducting magnet, was performed on 12 consecutive patients (6 males), aged 15 to 48 years, who underwent arthroscopic ACL repair at 3 weeks, 3 months, 6 months, and 1 year after surgery. After surgery, the tendon defect was not closed, and the peritenon was closed with sutures. The tendon gap and the patellar bone harvest site were evaluated for healing.

Results.—The defect decreased significantly but did not disappear completely over the study period. The overall tendon width decrease was 6%. The ratio of defect to tendon widths decreased significantly by 58%, and the overall length decreased 4%. The increase in cross-sectional area was only 9%. By 6 months, the patellar bone graft was integrated into the patella in 10 of 12 patients. At 1 year, there was no significant soft-tissue formation in 3 patients, 5 had a thin layer (less than 50% of the adjacent normal tissue), and 4 had reformed tissue of equal thickness and appearance to overlying tissue.

Conclusion.—Although the patellar tendon defect had decreased by an average of 62% at 1 year after surgery, only 2 patients had healed completely, and some had not healed at all. Tendon width and length decreased. The greatest change occurred between 3 and 6 months after surgery. Thereafter, healing slows.

▶ Surprise, surprise. The patella tendon is not a tadpole. Even more interesting would be correlation of postoperative defect appearance and clinical symptoms. Indirectly, this study appears to support the concept of using the medial or lateral third of the patella tendon as a source of ACL graft.

J.S. Torg, M.D.

Which Factors Predict the Long-term Outcome in Chronic Patellofemoral Pain Syndrome? A 7-Yr Prospective Follow-up Study

Natri A, Kannus P, Järvinen M (UKK Inst, Tampere, Finland; Univ of Tampere, Finland; Univ of Vermont, Burlington)
Med Sci Sports Exerc 30:1572-1577, 1998   3–5

Objective.—Patellofemoral pain syndrome (PFPS) is a common sports injury that often becomes chronic. Although a variety of conservative and operative managements are available, no long term prospective studies have demonstrated the benefit of treatment. The factors that predict long-term outcome after conservative treatment of chronic PFPS were prospectively investigated.

Methods.—The effects of 19 variables—including age, sex, body composition, athletic activity, duration of symptoms, follow-up time, and radiologic and clinical evaluations of the knee joint—were studied 7 years after 6 weeks of conservative treatment for chronic PFPS in 49 consecutive patients (22 men) with an average age of 27 years. There were 45 patients

(20 men) with an average age of 34 years available at follow-up. Ten patients had surgery during the follow-up. The outcome assessment included Visual Analogue Scale pain score and Lysholm and Tegner functional knee scores.

Results.—Muscle strength was significantly and negatively correlated with Lysholm and Tegner scores. Patients with bilateral symptoms during the follow-up had poorer Tegner and Lysholm scores than did patients who did not have symptoms in the other knee. The patella apprehension test was significantly correlated with the Lysholm and Tegner scores at baseline and with the Tegner score at follow-up. Baseline patellar crepitation scores were significantly correlated with follow-up Lysholm score and were nonsignificantly correlated with Visual Analogue Score pain and Tegner score. Age and height were significant predictors of outcome, accounting for 60% of the variation of Lysholm score and 52% of the variation in Tegner score. Radiologic imaging studies were not predictive of outcome.

Conclusion.—Systematic rehabilitation of the quadriceps muscle with a period of restriction is the treatment of choice for chronic PFPS.

▶ When considering factors that affect chronic PFPS, there are some that can be controlled—such as amount of activity, weight, and quadriceps strength—and some on which we have no control, such as height and age. The authors have concluded that a period of limiting activities that cause pain, increasing quadriceps strength, and weight reduction are factors that can improve the long-term outcome of chronic PFPS.

F.J. George, A.T.C., P.T.

The Plica Syndrome: Diagnostic Value of MRI With Arthroscopic Correlation

Jee W-H, Choe B-Y, Kim J-M, et al (Catholic Univ, Seoul, Korea)

J Comput Assist Tomogr 22:814-818, 1998   3–6

Background.—Alhough MRI has been used extensively for assessing internal derangement of the knee, few investigators have reported use of MRI of the medial plicae. The value and efficacy of MRI in diagnosing plica syndrome were studied, along with MR criteria for pathologic medial plicae.

Methods.—The MR images of 55 patients with arthroscopically confirmed pathologic mediopatellar plicae were compared with those of 100 patients without plicae. Axial multiplanar gradient-recalled (MPGR), axial T1-weighted, and sagittal T2-weighted MR images were obtained and assessed for all medial plicae width and length.

Findings.—The sensitivity and specificity of axial MPGR images for diagnosing plica syndrome were 73% and 78%, respectively; for sagittal T2-weighted imaged, they were 71% and 83%, respectively; and for the combination of these images, they were 95% and 72%, respectively. With

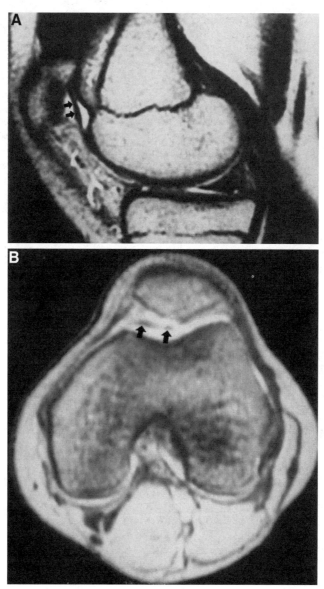

FIGURE 5.—Pathologic medial plica of Sakakibara type D in a 19-year-old man. **A,** sagittal T2-weighted (2,000/75) MR image of the knee shows a hypointense band (*arrows*) anterior to the medial condyle of the femur. **B,** axial multiplanar gradient-recalled (550/15, 20 degree flip angle) MR image of the knee demonstrates a thick low-intensity band (*arrows*) with a width of 4+, above the medial condyle of the femur extending beyond the trochlear groove of the femur (*arrows*). (Courtesy of Jee W-H, Choe B-Y, Kim J-M, et al: The plica syndrome: Diagnostic value of MRI with arthroscopic correlation. *J Comput Assist Tomogr* 22:814-818, 1998.)

the criterion of extension beyond the medial end of the patella on axial MPGR images, the incidence of pathologic medial plica increased (Fig 5).

Conclusion.—MRI is a useful noninvasive screening tool for diagnosing plica syndrome before arthroscopy. This modality may be an efficient alternative to invasive arthrography or CT arthrography for detecting pathologic medial plicae.

▶ This article nicely demonstrates the ability of MPGR imaging to demonstrate medial plicae. To be noted, however, is the fact that the authors were unable to correlate the severity of symptoms with the size or breadth of the synovial plica.

J.S. Torg, M.D.

Operative Treatment and Arthroscopic Findings in Chronic Patellar Tendinitis
Griffiths GP, Selesnick FH (Miami Sports Medicine Fellowship, Coral Gables, Fla)
Arthroscopy 14:836-839, 1998   3–7

Background.—Although patellar tendinitis usually responds well to conservative treatment, some patients continue to have symptoms. The outcomes of 1 group of patients with chronic patellar tendinitis treated surgically after the failure of extensive conservative therapy were reported.

Methods.—Seven patients, age 20 to 45 years, with a total of 8 affected knees underwent surgery. Five patients were professional or collegiate athletes. The mean symptom duration was 1.4 years before surgery was performed. Operative treatment consisted of knee arthroscopy and open repair with excision of degenerated tissue and stimulation of a healing response of the patellar tendon abnormality. The mean follow-up was 3.6 years.

Findings.—Marked fibrotendinous degeneration was consistently found during surgery and on pathologic study. Outcomes—as determined subjectively with SF36, objectively with Biodex testing, and by return to previous level of competition—were judged to be excellent in 86% of the patients and fair in 14%.

Conclusion.—Patients with chronic patellar tendinitis that does not improve with well-supervised, comprehensive conservative treatment should undergo operative repair. If surgery is performed, concomitant arthroscopy should be considered, as there appears to be a strong correlation with associated intra-articular pathology.

▶ The observations of the authors are in keeping with my own clinical experience. Performing the procedure with local infiltrative anesthesia facilitates identifying the area of tendon involvement in that point pressure will elicit pain. Then, of course, the procedure involves "cutting out the pain."

J.S. Torg, M.D.

The Effect of Knee Bracing After Anterior Cruciate Ligament Reconstruction: A Prospective, Randomized Study With Two Year's Follow-up

Risberg MA, Holm I, Steen H, et al (Univ of Oslo, Norway; Martina Hansens Hosp, Baerum, Norway)
Am J Sports Med 27:76-83, 1999   3–8

Background.—For many years, rehabilitation after anterior cruciate ligament (ACL) reconstruction has included knee braces. The effects of knee bracing after ACL reconstruction on knee joint laxity, lower limb function, the cross-sectional area of the thigh, and the incidence of further intra-articular injury were investigated.

Methods.—Sixty patients were assigned randomly to rehabilitative braces for 2 weeks, followed by function braces for 10 weeks (group 1), or to no braces (group 2). Data were recorded before and at 6 weeks, 3 and 6 months, and 1 and 2 years after surgery. Assessment included KT-1000 arthrometry, the Cincinnati knee score, goniometry for range of motion, CT to determine thigh atrophy, Cybex 6000 isokinetic testing to determine muscle strength, 3 functional knee tests, and a visual analogue pain assessment scale.

Findings.—At all follow-up assessments, the 2 groups did not differ in knee joint laxity, range of motion, muscle strength, functional knee tests, or pain. However, knee function was significantly improved in group 1 compared with group 2 at 3 months, even though the braced group had significantly increased thigh atrophy compared with the nonbraced group at that assessment.

Conclusion.—Knee bracing after ACL reconstruction appears to have no effect on knee joint laxity, range of motion, muscle strength, functional knee tests, patient satisfaction, or pain. However, the Cincinnati knee score improved significantly with bracing at 3 months postoperatively, although thigh atrophy was increased. Prolonged bracing significantly reduced quadriceps muscle strength compared with bracing for a shorter time. Bracing did not appear to decrease the risk of further injury to the meniscus or cartilage in the tibiofemoral joint.

▶ The observations and conclusions of the authors regarding the general lack of effectiveness of bracing after ACL reconstruction is in keeping with my own clinical experience.

J.S. Torg, M.D.

Septic Arthritis of the Knee Following Anterior Cruciate Ligament Reconstruction: Results of a Survey of Sports Medicine Fellowship Directors

Matava MJ, Evans TA, Wright RW, et al (Washington Univ, St Louis; Slippery Rock Univ, Pa)
Arthroscopy 14:717-725, 1998   3–9

Objective.—Septic arthritis is an uncommon complication after reconstruction of the anterior cruciate ligament (ACL). There is little information about treatment of septic arthritis. The literature was reviewed to determine whether septic arthritis after ACL reconstruction is as rare as has been thought and whether there exists a standard of care among experts regarding prevention and treatment of this complication.

Methods.—A questionnaire was mailed to 74 surgeons listed in the Sports Medicine Fellowship Program in the 1995 *Postgraduate Orthopaedic Fellowship Directory* of the American Academy of Orthopaedic Surgeons to assess their experience and practices in performing ACL surgery, number of years in practice, number of ACL reconstruction performed annually, graft choice, surgical technique, use of postoperative drains, use and duration of prophylactic antibiotics, and the number of postoperative infections treated in the past 2 and 5 years.

Results.—The 61 responders (82%) had been in practice for an average of 17.3 years and performed an average of 98 ACL reconstructions annually. Most (77%) chose the patellar tendon graft, followed by the hamstring graft (23%). Endoscopic reconstruction was the method of choice for 72% of responders 75% of the time, whereas 16% used arthroscopically assisted surgery 75% of the time. Preoperative prophylactic antibiotics were prescribed by 98% of surgeons 75% of the time or more, and 77% prescribed postoperative prophylactic antibiotics 75% of the time or more. Slightly more than half (51%) used a drain. Thirty percent had treated an ACL infection within the past 2 years, and 26% had treated an ACL infection within the past 5 years. Culture-specific IV antibiotics and surgical irrigation of the joint were the treatments chosen by 85% of responders.

For an infected allograft, 64% of the responders used IV antibiotics and surgical irrigation of the joint for the initial treatment, and 93% used them as part of the treatment regimen. IV antibiotics with surgical irrigation and graft retention was the most common treatment (39%) for resistant infection. Graft removal was chosen by 31%. Revision after graft removal for infection was performed in 6 to 9 months by 49% of responders.

Conclusion.—There was general agreement that septic arthritis after ACL reconstruction was rare and that treatment should have included culture–specific IV antibiotics and joint irrigation with graft retention, with graft removal reserved for graft infection or resistant infection.

▶ It is to be noted that antibiotic prophylaxis reduces the risk of infection 4-fold in clean surgical cases, whereas the use of a drain has been shown to increase the rate of infection. However, this study indicates that there is no significant difference in the number of infections based on the surgeons' case load, graft choice, or method of reconstruction. The important point made is that both graft excision and hardware removal are considered only for those infections resistant to initial treatment and for the infected allograft.

J.S. Torg, M.D.

The Effect of Exercise and Rehabilitation on Anterior-Posterior Knee Displacements After Anterior Cruciate Ligament Autograft Reconstruction

Barber-Westin SD, Noyes FR, Heckmann TP, et al (Deaconess Hosp, Cincinnati, Ohio; HealthSouth Rehabilitation Corp, Cincinnati, Ohio)
Am J Sports Med 27:84-93, 1999   3–10

Background.—Current trends in rehabilitation after anterior cruciate ligament (ACL) reconstruction focus on aggressive or accelerated exercise protocols that permit immediate full weightbearing and a return to high levels of athletic activity as early as 3 to 4 months after surgery. The effect of rehabilitation strength training and return to activities on anterior-

TABLE 4.—Timing and Details of Abnormal Anterior-Posterior Displacements in 21 Patients

First Abnormal Displacement (weeks)	Displacement (mm)	Rehabilitation Phase When Detected	Latest Arthrometer Measurement*	Last Follow-up (Months)	Type of ACL Rupture
6	3.0	Early strength training	4.5	35	Chronic
8	4.5	Early strength training	3.0	26	Chronic
8	5.5	Early strength training	5.5	23	Chronic
10	4.5	Early strength training	6.0	27	Chronic
12	4.0	Early strength training	4.0	24	Chronic
16	3.5	Early strength training	3.0	25	Acute
16	6.5	Intensive strength training	8.0	26	Chronic
20	3.0	Intensive strength training	3.5	24	Chronic
20	3.0	Intensive strength training	10.0	27	Chronic
20	4.0	Intensive strength training	3.5	30	Acute
24	10.5	Early strength training†	10.5	(revised)	Chronic
24	5.0	Return to sports activities	9.0	(revised)	Acute
28	4.0	Intensive strength training	5.0	30	Chronic
35	3.5	Return to sports activities	3.5	27	Chronic
52	3.5	Return to sports activities	7.0	24	Acute
52	4.5	Intensive strength training	4.0	24	Acute
104	4.0	Early strength training†	4.0	25	Chronic
104	4.0	Return to sports activities	4.0	24	Chronic
104	7.0	Return to sports activities	7.0	24	Acute
104	3.5	Return to sports activities	3.5	30	Acute
208	4.0	Return to sports activities	4.0	24	Acute

*Involved minus noninvolved side at 134 newtons of force.
†Patient never completed rehabilitation program, never performed strenous strength training, or returned to sports.
(Courtesy of Barber-Westin SD, Noyes FR, Heckmann TP, et al: The effect of exercise and rehabilitation on anterior-posterior knee displacements after anterior cruciate ligament autograft reconstruction. *Am J Sports Med* 27:84-93, 1999.)

posterior knee displacements after patellar tendon autogenous ACL reconstruction was investigated.

Methods.—Nine hundred thirty-eight measures were collected sequentially for 142 patients with the KT-2000 arthrometer. Rehabilitation consisted of immediate knee motion and early weightbearing, light participation in sports at 6 months, and competitive sports at 8 months or later.

Findings.—At 2 or more years after surgery, 85% of the patients had normal displacements—less than 3 mm of increase at 134 newtons; 10% had 3 to 5.5 mm of increase, and 5% had more than 5.5 mm of increase and were considered failures. The initial onset of abnormal displacements was unassociated with the length of time after surgery or the rehabilitation program. Of the 7 grafts that failed, 6 did so in the first year after surgery (Table 4).

Conclusions.—Individualized, evaluation-based rehabilitation is needed after ACL reconstruction. The use of instrumented arthrometer testing to determine AP displacements is recommended before progression to the more strenuous phases of rehabilitation.

▶ The authors stress the need for individualized, evaluation-based rehabilitation programs after ACL surgery. They recommend using arthrometer testing as the evaluation tool, before progressing to more strenuous levels of rehabilitation. They state that the arthrometer cannot be used to determine functional status and that there are a number of variables that contribute to overall knee foundation.

F.J. George, A.T.C., P.T.

Home-based Rehabilitation for Anterior Cruciate Ligament Reconstruction

Fischer DA, Tewes DP, Boyd JL, et al (Minneapolis Sports Medicine Ctr)
Clin Orthop 347:194-199, 1998   3–11

Objective.—Rehabilitation after anterior cruciate ligament (ACL) reconstruction is important for maximizing functional outcome. There is only 1 study comparing home-based and clinic-based rehabilitation programs. The results of a postoperative, home-based rehabilitation program after ACL reconstruction were compared with results from a more traditional clinic-based rehabilitation program. The study used a randomized, prospective design.

Methods.—During a 2-year period, 54 patients (26 female), aged 15 to 44 years, were randomly assigned to a home-based rehabilitation program (n = 27; 11 female) or to a traditional clinic-based program (n = 27; 14 female). Patients had had no previous knee reconstruction, were not professional athletes, and had no complicating medical conditions. There was a minimum of 6 weeks between injury and reconstruction. Patients in the home-based group had supervised visits at 1, 2, 3, 4, 6, and 12 weeks. The clinic-based group had 24 physical therapy appointments in the first 6 months. Patients were followed for at least 6 months. Preoperative and postoperative Lysholm and health status questionnaire scores were recorded.

Results.—The clinic-based group was significantly younger than the home-based group (27 vs. 32 years). Lysholm scores; physical examination results; and hop test, KT-1000 test, and HSQ results were similar for the 2 groups.

Conclusion.—Home-based rehabilitation programs after ACL reconstruction provide good, cost-effective results for selected patients.

▶ I agree with the conclusion that home-based rehabilitation programs after ACL reconstruction provides good, cost-effective results for selected patients. Here, importantly are the key words "selected patients." In the young, well-motivated individual with a mentality likened to that of a Marine Corps recruit, the system works.

In our clinic, we have a trainer/therapist carefully instruct the postoperative patient in our exercise protocol, then have the patient perform the exercises in the health club of choice. It is important that progress be carefully monitored and that the patient understands the sequential parameters of motion-strength goals. The advantage of this modus operandi could obviate both the underaggressive and overaggressive approaches of many therapists, as well as the faking and baking modality schedules that invariably unnecessarily increase expense.

J.S. Torg, M.D.

Factors Contributing to Function of the Knee Joint After Injury or Reconstruction of the Anterior Cruciate Ligament

Dye SF, Wojtys EM, Fu FH, et al (Univ of California, San Francisco; Univ of Michigan, Ann Arbor; Univ of Pittsburgh, Pa; et al)
J Bone Joint Surg Am 80-A:1380-1393, 1998   3–12

Objective.—The factors that govern restoration of knee function after injury or anterior cruciate ligament reconstruction are discussed in terms of musculoskeletal function.

Restoration of Knee Function.—No studies have compared outcomes of conservative versus operative treatment with respect to joint function. The concept of musculoskeletal joint function encompasses the capacity to generate, transmit, absorb, and dissipate loads and to maintain tissue homeostasis.

Envelope of Function.—The concept of envelope of function combines and connects the idea of load transference and tissue homeostasis to present a picture of the functional capacity of the knee using a load and frequency distribution to define a safe range of loading (the envelope of function).

Factors Contributing to Joint Function.—Several factors contribute to the functional capacity of any joint. These include anatomical factors, such as macromorphology and micromorphology, structural integrity, and bio-mechanical characteristics of knee components; kinematic factors, such as the pattern of sequential tightening of the fibers of the anterior cruciate ligament and the dynamic function of all of the complex neuromuscular control mechanisms; physiologic factors, such as the biochemical and metabolic processes that maintain and restore homeostasis in joints and musculoskeletal components; and nonoperative and operative treatments.

Indicators of Functional Restoration.—Indicators that a joint is being loaded within its capacity are absence of discomfort, of warmth, of swelling, and of functional instability.

Overview.—Restoration of knee function requires restoration of structural, biomechanical, kinematic, and physiologic factors that maximize the load transference capacity of the knee joint safely and predictably by using the envelope-of-function construct. Decreasing loading across a joint to a safe level compatible with maintenance of tissue homeostasis, while maintaining an active lifestyle, is likely to result in successful treatment.

▶ Starting with the premise that perfection (that is, full restoration of preinjury status) is often not achieved and that long-term results are often not completely satisfactory following reconstruction of the anterior cruciate ligament, the authors attempted to define factors involved in the maximization of the load-transference capacity of the knee joint. The article points out that continued presence of warmth, swelling, and mild discomfort with certain loading activities is caused by loss of joint homeostasis.

J.S. Torg, M.D.

Repeatability of Patellar Cartilage Thickness Patterns in the Living, Using a Fat-suppressed Magnetic Resonance Imaging Sequence With Short Acquisition Time and Three-Dimensional Data Processing

Tieschky M, Faber S, Haubner M, et al (Ludwig-Maximilians-Universität München, Germany; Klinikum Großhadern, Munich, Germany; Institut für Medizinische Informatik und Systemforschung, Neuherberg, Germany; et al)
J Orthop Res 15:808-813, 1997   3–13

Background.—MRI can directly delineate articular cartilage in vivo. However, artifacts at the bone-cartilage interface, poor contrast-to-noise ratios with adjacent tissues, and other shortcomings limit its utility in measuring cartilage thickness. The reproducibility of in vivo cartilage thickness measurements by fat-suppressed MRI with a short acquisition time, 3-dimensional (3-D) data reconstruction, and digital data processing was described.

Methods.—The subjects were 8 healthy volunteers 23 to 32 years old with normal knees. Their right knees were examined by transverse MRI with a T1-weighted, fat-suppressed, FLASH-3D (fast low angle shot) sequence; the entire transverse data set was acquired in 4 minutes 10 seconds. Data sets were acquired with the knees in 6 different positions to determine the replicability of cartilage thickness measurements. A minimal-distance algorithm was used to reconstruct the data 3-dimensionally for measurements of cartilage volume and thickness.

Findings.—Across all 48 data sets, the coefficients of variation for cartilage volume determinations ranged from 0.81% to 3.70%, with a mean of 1.35%. Cartilage volumes did not change significantly during repeated measurements. Across all 48 data sets, 250 randomly selected coordinate points were analyzed to determine how many of the pixels could be attributed to an identical cartilage thickness interval (0.5 mm). A mean of 75.1% ± 4.1% of the pixels could be attributed to the same interval, 14.8% ± 2.4% of the pixels deviated by 1 interval, 6.6% ± 1.5% of the pixels deviated by 2 intervals, and only 3.5% ± 1.8% of the pixels deviated by more than 2 intervals.

Conclusions.—A fat-suppressed, FLASH-3D MRI sequence with 3-dimensional reconstruction and digital data processing reliably determined the thickness of cartilage in the knee. The method is fast, reproducible, and noninvasive, and may provide a new method for measuring cartilage thickness clinically.

Magnetic Resonance Imaging of Articular Cartilage in the Knee: An Evaluation With Use of Fast-Spin-Echo Imaging

Potter HG, Linklater JM, Allen AA, et al (Hosp for Special Surgery, New York City)
J Bone Joint Surg Am 80-A:1276-1284, 1998   3–14

Background.—MRI is well suited for the evaluation of articular cartilage, although the best MRI sequence for detection of chondral abnormalities remains unclear. Fat-suppressed volumetric gradient-echo sequences have been suggested but have significant drawbacks. This study evaluated a specialized proton-density-weighted, high-resolution, fast-spin-echo sequence for evaluation of chondral lesions in the knee.

Methods.—The study included 88 patients who underwent MRI examination followed by knee arthroscopy during a 20-month period. Sagittal, axial, and coronal scans were performed using the specialized fast-spin-echo sequence, previously reported of value in assessing other structures within the knee. The scans were read in prospective fashion, with 2 independent readers using the 5-point Outerbridge classification to grade the patellar facets, trochlea, femoral condyles, and tibial plateaus. The same system was used at arthroscopy, usually performed within 2 months of MRI scanning.

Results.—Two hundred forty-eight arthroscopic lesions were identified in a total of 616 articular surfaces (Fig 3A). Chondral softening was detected in 82 surfaces; mild ulceration in 75; deep ulceration, fibrillation, or a flap without subchondral bone exposure in 53; and full-thickness wear in 38. The sensitivity of MRI scanning in detecting chondral lesions was estimated at 87%, with a specificity of 94%, accuracy of 92%,

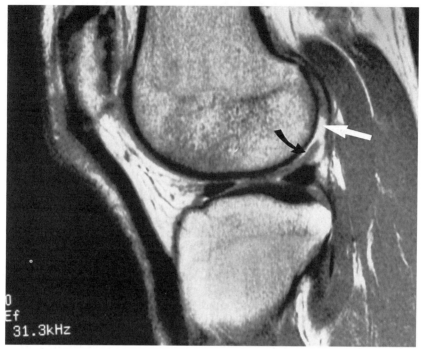

FIGURE 3.—Man, 34 years, had symptoms suggestive of a meniscal tear, including intermittent locking of the knee. A, sagittal fast-spin-echo magnetic resonance image demonstrating a discrete full-thickness chondral defect (*white arrow*) over the posterior margin of the lateral femoral condyle, with an adjacent chondral flap (*black arrow*). (Courtesy of Potter HG, Linklater JM, Allen AA, et al: Magnetic resonance imaging of articular cartilage in the knee: An evaluation with use of fast-spin-echo imaging. *J Bone Joint Surg Am* 80-A:1276-1284, 1998.)

positive predictive value of 85%, and negative predictive value of 95%. Interobserver agreement was near perfect.

Conclusions.—With the fast-spin-echo sequence used in this study, MRI provides a valuable approach for evaluation of the articular cartilage of the knee. This imaging approach offers high accuracy with low interobserver variability. It will be useful in identifying chondral lesions amenable to arthroscopic treatment, as well as for post-treatment evaluation.

Accuracy of Cartilage Volume and Thickness Measurements With Magnetic Resonance Imaging

Eckstein F, Schnier M, Haubner M, et al (Ludwig-Maximilians-Universität München, Munich, Germany; GSF Research Ctr Neuherberg, Oberschleiß-heim, Germany; Klinikum Großhadern, Munich, Germany)
Clin Orthop 352:137-148, 1998   3–15

Background.—Currently there is no established noninvasive method to measure cartilage volume and thickness in the osteoarthritic knee. The accuracy of MRI with 3-dimensional (3-D) data reconstruction in measuring cartilage volume and thickness of the knee was explored.

Methods.—Eight normal knee joints were harvested from cadavers (mean age at death, 50.6 years) within 48 hours of death. Specimens were examined by sagittal MRI with a fat-suppressed gradient echo sequence. A contrast agent was then injected and a sagittal CT arthrogram was obtained with the knee in extremity. The knee was repositioned, then 15 minutes later another sagittal CT arthrogram was obtained. A minimal-distance algorithm was used to reconstruct the data 3-dimensionally for measurements of cartilage volume and thickness. Additionally, a 32-year-old patient with anterior knee pain and recurrent patellar dislocation was examined by MRI with 3-D reconstruction and by arthroscopy to determine whether the MRI method could be used clinically to measure cartilage volume and thickness.

Findings.—The results of MRI and CT arthrography correlated extremely well (r = 0.998). Across all 32 joint surfaces examined, the total cartilage volumes based on MRI were 2.6% higher than those based on CT arthrography (P = .027). Most of this difference was accounted for by different measurements in the patella. Across all 32 joint surfaces examined, the mean absolute volume deviation between MRI and CT arthrography was 3.3%, which was not significantly different than that between the 2 CT arthrographic measurements (3.6%). MRI and CT arthrography also correlated closely in determining cartilage thickness in 48 joint regions. There was exact agreement in 28 regions; MRI was higher in 8 regions; and CT arthrography was higher in 12 regions (mean difference, −0.2 thickness intervals of 0.5 mm each). Across all 48 joint regions examined, the mean absolute thickness deviation between MRI and CT arthrography was 0.6 intervals, which was not significantly different than that between the 2 CT arthrographic measurements (0.5 intervals). MRI in the patient identified a focal cartilage defect in the lateral facet of the patella, which was verified by arthroscopy.

Conclusions.—3-D MRI can accurately assess cartilage volume and thickness in all 4 joint surfaces of the human knee. This noninvasive method may prove useful in assessing patients with osteoarthritis of the knee.

▶ Although MRI has assumed a major role in the diagnosis of interarticular knee pathology, current techniques have not been able to delineate full thickness cartilage defects clearly without enhancement. In view of a recent interest in surgical management of articular cartilage defects, the relevance of these 3 articles (Abstracts 3–13 through 3–15) become apparent. With regard to the technique of Tieschky et al., it is important to note that their "results are valid for healthy cartilage and the conclusions should not be directly transferred to the situation of an osteoarthritic joint".

J.S. Torg, M.D.

Clinical Results of Meniscus Repair in Patients 40 Years and Older

Barrett GR, Field MH, Treacy SH, et al (Mississippi Sports Medicine and Orthopaedic Ctr, Jackson)

Arthroscopy 14:824-829, 1998   3–16

Objective.—Some clinicians have reported that meniscus repair in older patients is less successful than in younger patients. The clinical outcome of meniscal repair in the older population was prospectively investigated in all patients aged 40 years or older who underwent meniscal repair between September 1989 and March 1995.

Methods.—After workers' compensation patients had been excluded, 37 patients (11 women), aged 42 to 50 years, who underwent the standard inside-out technique with posterior incision (N = 31) or the T-fix suture anchor repair (N = 6) performed by the same surgeon, were followed for a minimum of 2 years. There were 19 left knees and 18 right knees repaired, and 28 were repaired acutely. Anterior cruciate ligament (ACL) tears were simultaneously repaired in 22 patients.

Results.—Five patients (13.5%) continued to have symptoms at last follow-up and had joint line tenderness, and 2 had a positive McMurray test. Three patients were reoperated. Patients with acute tears had a lower failure rate than did patients with older tears (11% vs. 22%). Four patients had medial meniscus tears and 1 had a failed lateral meniscus repair. Patients with tears greater than 2 cm had a higher failure rate than did patients with tears less than 2 cm (10 vs. 18%). The failure rate was 50% for complex tears, 20% for bucket handle tears, and 0% for vertical tears. Only 1 patient (4.5%) with ACL reconstruction failed, but 4 patients (27%) without reconstruction failed. Of 5 patients who underwent sec-ond-look arthroscopy, 3 had no evidence of healing.

Conclusion.—The overall success rate for meniscus repair in older pa-tients was 86.5%. Patients who had concurrent ACL repair had a higher success rate.

▶ As the authors point out, only 6% of meniscal tears in their older patient population underwent repair. More accurate is the statement that "most meniscal tears in older patients are of a degenerative nature and not ame-nable to repair."

J.S. Torg, M.D.

The Chondrogenic Potential of Human Bone-Marrow-derived Mesen-chymal Progenitor Cells

Yoo JU, Barthel TS, Nishimura K, et al (Case Western Reserve Univ, Cleve-land, Ohio)

J Bone Joint Surg Am 80-A:1745-1757, 1998   3–17

Background.—Mesenchymal progenitor cells can be used in the repair of musculoskeletal tissue. However, in vitro models are needed to investigate the mechanisms of progenitor cell differentiation. The induction of in vitro chondrogenesis with human bone-marrow–derived osteochondral progenitor cells in a reliable, reproducible culture system was reported.

Methods and Findings.—After the removal and fractionation of human bone marrow, adherent cell cultures were established and the cells passed into an aggregate culture system in a serum-free medium. The cell aggregates initially contained type I collagen, and neither type II nor type X collagen was identified. Typically, type II collagen was identified in the matrix by day 5, with the immunoreactivity localized in the area of metachromatic staining. By day 14, types II and X collagen were apparent throughout the cell aggregates, except for the outer region which consisted of flattened, perichondrial-like cells in a matrix rich in type I collagen. Aggrecan and link protein were found in extracts of the cell aggregates, suggesting that large aggregating proteoglycans of the type in cartilaginous tissues had been synthesized by the newly differentiating chondrocytic cells. The small proteoglycans, biglycan and decorin, were also found in extracts. Immunohistochemical staining with antibodies specific for chondroitin 4-sulfate and keratan sulfate showed a uniform proteoglycan distribution throughout the extracellular matrix of the cell aggregates. The bone-marrow–derived cell preparations were passed in monolayer culture up to 20 times, with the cells permitted to grow to confluence at each passage. After each passage, the chondrogenic potential of the cells was maintained.

Conclusion.—Progenitor cell chondrogenesis is the basis for the in vivo repair of fractures and damaged articular cartilage. This cellular differentiation may be studied in this model of in vitro chondrogenesis of human bone-marrow–derived osteochondral progenitor cells. The maintenance of chondrogenic potential after a more than billion-fold expansion suggests that these cells will be useful clinically in the repair of bone and cartilage.

▶ This is an interesting and important study (albeit in vitro) with potential application for repair of interarticular chondral defects. Clearly, the use of mesenchymal progenitor cells of bone for cartilaginous repair has the advantages of an extensive reserve of these cells, ease of removal, and expandability in culture. At this time, an understanding of their behavior in vivo is not well understood, but these in vitro studies appear to be most encouraging.

J.S. Torg, M.D.

Treatment of Articular Cartilage Defects of the Knee With Autologous Chondrocyte Implantation

Gillogly SD, Voight M, Blackburn T (Atlanta Knee and Shoulder Clinic, Ga; Belmont Univ, Nashville, Tenn; Tulane Inst of Sports Med, New Orleans, La)
J Orthop Sports Phys Ther 28:241-251, 1998   3–18

Background.—Treating focal full-thickness articular defects in the knee continues to be a challenge. Articular cartilage defects and treatment with autologous chondrocyte implantation were discussed.

Discussion.—Significant chondral defects frequently cause persistent joint line pain, swelling, and catching in the knee. Such defects can also lead to progressive onset of early osteoarthritis. Traditional treatment such as marrow stimulation, which gives access to the bone-blood supply by penetrating the subchondral bone to provide mesenchymal stem cells in the fibrin clot, have yielded mixed early outcomes and fair to poor long-term outcomes. Autologous chondrocyte implantation provides chondrocytes committed to forming type II cartilage. This treatment appears to provide hyaline-like repair tissue, with corresponding improvement in the histologic, biomechanical, and durability characteritics. Better clinical outcomes have been reported in as many as 90% of patients with femoral condyle defects, with a mean reported postoperative follow-up of 4 years and up to 10 years. We can expect further developments and refinements in this treatment approach, producing even better outcomes in patients with this difficult clinical condition (Fig 1).

▶ As this article states, "The treatment of focal full thickness articular defects in the knee has continued to present a challenge, with no traditional treatment method providing consistent acceptable long-term clinical results." Initial clinical studies have reported encouraging results with autologous chondrocyte implantation. Peterson[1] has reported on 219 consecutive patients with an average 4-year follow-up (range, 2-12 years). In addition to improved objective and subjective clinical results, follow-up biopsy specimens demonstrated hyaline-like tissue with type II collagen present. He has also reported on the clinical durability of the repaired tissue. The down-side to the procedure is that it is done in 2 stages; is expensive and is not covered by many insurance carriers; and, to some degree, the jury remains out with regard to a definitive assessment of its efficacy.

J.S. Torg, M.D.

Reference

1. Peterson L: Autologous chondrocyte transplantation. Articular cartilage repair, regeneration and transplantation symposium. Presented at the 65th annual meeting of the American Academy of Orthopaedic Surgeons, New Orleans, La, March, 1998.

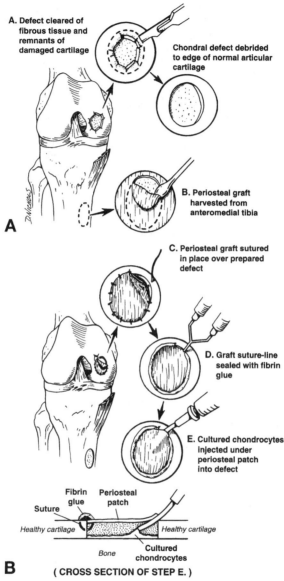

A. Defect cleared of fibrous tissue and remnants of damaged cartilage

Chondral defect debrided to edge of normal articular cartilage

B. Periosteal graft harvested from anteromedial tibia

A

C. Periosteal graft sutured in place over prepared defect

D. Graft suture-line sealed with fibrin glue

E. Cultured chondrocytes injected under periosteal patch into defect

Suture

Fibrin glue

Periosteal patch

Healthy cartilage   Healthy cartilage

Bone   Cultured chondrocytes

B   (CROSS SECTION OF STEP E.)

FIGURE 1.—A and B, Autologous chondrocyte implantation procedure. (Courtesy of Gillogly SD, Voight M, Blackburn T: Treatment of articular cartilage defects of the knee with autologous chrondrocyte implantation. *J Orthop Sports Phys Ther* 28:241-251, 1998.)

Isolated Arthroscopic Meniscal Repair: A Long-term Outcome Study (More Than 10 Years)

Johnson MJ, Lucas GL, Dusek JK, et al (Univ of Kansas, Wichita)
Am J Sports Med 27:44-49, 1999   3–19

Background.—Previous research suggests that meniscal repair has an advantage over meniscectomy in that it preserves meniscal tissue, which results in reduced pain and prevention of osteoarthritis in the knee joint. However, long-term outcome studies are needed to substantiate this claim. A 10-year follow-up of repaired isolated meniscal tears in patients with intact cruciate and collateral ligaments was reported.

Methods.—Forty-eight patients undergoing 50 arthroscopic repairs of meniscal tears were included in the retrospective analysis. All were operated on by 1 surgeon. None of the patients had concomitant ligament damage to the knee. The mean follow-up was 10 years 9 months. Clinical success was defined as a history of pain of grade 1 or less and the absence of locking, catching, or giving way; a physical examination showing no significant effusion and a painless and negative jump sign; and no subsequent operations on the repaired meniscus.

Findings.—Patient satisfaction was high. Clinical confirmation, possible in only 38 knees, demonstrated a 76% success rate. Bilateral standing radiographs of the 38 operated knees, assessed by Fairbank's classification, showed that 8% of the operated knees had minimal joint changes, compared with 3% in the contralateral, nonoperated knee.

Conclusion.—Arthroscopic meniscal repair in knees with isolated meniscal tears can be clinically and radiographically successful in the long term. The findings suggest that essentially all torn menisci should be repaired and that increasing rim width is associated with poorer outcomes.

▶ Repairs of the lateral meniscus had an 85% success rate as compared with a 72% success rate for medial meniscal tears. At variance with the literature was the observation that as the distance from the posterior horn to the start of the tear increases, the rate of clinical success decreases. The conclusion that the data support the advisability of repairing all meniscal tears is questioned by the authors' statement that they "cannot say with certainty which type of tear responds best to repair."

J.S. Torg, M.D.

Natural History of Anterior Knee Pain: A 14- to 20-Year Follow-up of Nonoperative Management

Nimon G, Murray D, Sandow M, et al (Nuffield Orthopaedic Centre, Oxford, England)
J Pediatr Orthop 18:118-122, 1998   3–20

Background.—The results of the various surgical procedures used to treat anterior knee pain (AKP) syndrome have seldom been compared with the natural outcome of the condition. The long-term follow-up of 1 group of girls with idiopathic AKP that was not treated surgically was reported.

Methods and Findings.—Sixty-three patients, aged 10-19 years, were enrolled in the study. Follow-up ranged from 14 to 10 years, with a mean of 16 years. At the last follow-up assessment, 22% of the patients reported no pain. Seventy-one percent of patients said their symptoms seemed better than at the initial assessment. Eighty-eight percent rarely or never needed analgesics, and 90% continued to participate in sports regularly. However, about 1 in 4 patients continued to have significant symptoms. No predictors of persistent symptoms could be identified.

Conclusions.—Seventy-three percent of adolescents with AKP, in whom clinical examination and standard radiographs exclude serious pathology, will improve with no treatment. Surgical treatment is not justified until a procedure can be shown to yield a better outcome or until the subset of patients who will not improve spontaneously can be identified.

▶ Surgeon, spare the knife! A needed study on the natural history of anterior knee pain in adolescent girls (63 girls, mean age 15.5 years at outset) is described in this article. All patients complained of pain going up and down stairs, on squatting, and after prolonged sitting. Most had retropatellar tenderness and crepitus but otherwise normal knees. Radiographs were normal. Sure enough, after a mean follow-up of 16 years—without surgery—most of the participants were getting along fine and 90% were still active in sports. Granted, 1 in 4 of the participants still had pain, but their knees still seemed normal.

E.R. Eichner, M.D.

Discoid Lateral Meniscus in Children: Long-term Follow-up After Total Meniscectomy
Räber DA, Friederich NF, Hefti F (Children's Hosp, Basel, Switzerland)
J Bone Joint Surg Am 80-A:1579-1586, 1998   3–21

Objective.—Whereas short-term results of total or partial meniscectomy in children showed favorable results, long-term follow-up has revealed a high prevalence of osteoarthrotic changes. The prevalence of osteoarthritis after total diskectomy in children was retrospectively reviewed.

Methods.—Of 28 children, aged 3 to 14 years, who underwent total diskectomy between 1961 and 1991, 14 patients (3 boys), with 17 surgically treated knees, were available for follow-up. Demographic information, preoperative history, alignment of the knee, intraoperative findings, and current status of the menisci, along with the patient's subjective assessment of the knee, symptoms, range of motion, stability of the ligaments, compartmental findings, evidence of pathologic change at the donor site, radiographic findings, and results of functional testing, were reviewed.

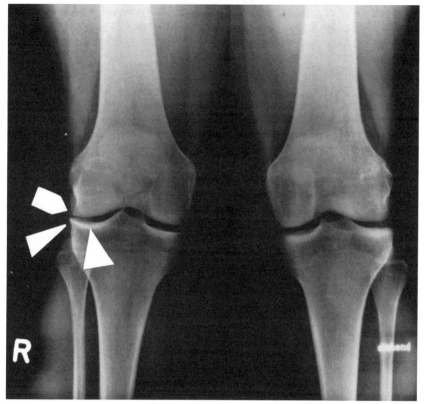

FIGURE 1.—Case 2. Anteroposterior radiograph, made 20 years after a meniscectomy, showing the formation of a ridge along the margin of the lateral femoral condyle as well as spurring and sclerosis of the tibial plateau (*arrows*) in the right knee. The latest overall grade was B, according to the system of the International Knee Documentation Committee. (Courtesy of Räber DA, Friederich NF, Hefti F: Discoid lateral meniscus in children: Long-term follow-up after total meniscectomy. *J Bone Joint Surg Am* 80-A:1579-1586, 1998.)

Results.—At latest follow-up, according to the International Knee Documentation Committee rating system, 12 knees were asymptomatic (grade A), 4 were moderately painful with swelling and a history of giving way (grade B), and 1 was severely painful during participation in sports (grade C). Four patients had had a second operation. Ten knees showed evidence of osteoarthritis (Fig 1).

Conclusion.—Total diskectomy in children should be avoided.

▶ The conclusion that "total meniscectomy for the treatment of discoid meniscus in children should be avoided whenever possible" is well known. Unfortunately, the authors did not deal with how to approach the problem. Other possibilities to consider could include partial meniscectomy, meniscal repair, or doing nothing.

J.S. Torg, M.D.

Evaluation of the Anatomy of the Common Peroneal Nerve: Defining Nerve-at-Risk in Arthroscopically Assisted Lateral Meniscus Repair
Deutsch A, Wyzykowski RJ, Victoroff BN (Case Western Reserve Univ, Cleveland, Ohio)
Am J Sports Med 27:10-15, 1999   3–22

Background.—The factors that contribute to the prevalence of peroneal nerve injury include errors in arthroscopic technique, not using a posterior incision and deflecting retractor, and anatomical variability. This 2-part study documented the relevant regional anatomy and potential risk for nerve injury during repair of lateral meniscus tears.

Methods and Findings.—In part 1 of the study, 70 cadaver legs were dissected to assess the relevant anatomy of the common peroneal nerve. Ten percent showed division of the common peroneal nerve into deep and superficial branches proximal to the knee joint. In 30% of the legs, a previously unreported cutaneous branch emanated from the common peroneal trunk. In part 2 of the study, 10 cadaver knees were subjected to arthroscopically assisted inside-out lateral meniscus repair. As the suture position was sequentially posterior, divergence between suture groups increased. When posterior retraction was not used, nerve branch capture occurred in 20% of the knees. Retractor use eliminated nerve involvement. Significant anatomical variability was observed in the course and branching pattern of the common peroneal nerve at the level of the lateral joint line. During meniscus repair, the risk of injury to the peroneal nerve was associated with suture position because of the proximity of anatomical structures and the tendency for suture divergence with soft tissue tethering (Fig 1).

Conclusion.—The course and branching pattern of the common peroneal nerve at the level of the lateral joint line shows significant anatomical variability. Attention to meticulous technique and comprehensive knowledge of anatomical variation will help protect the peroneal nerve during arthroscopic lateral meniscus repair.

▶ The purpose of this study was, in the words of the authors, to "define the anatomical course of the common peroneal nerve and improve existing anatomic understanding and arthroscopic technique to help surgeons avoid peroneal nerve injury during arthroscopic lateral meniscus repair." The authors have clearly accomplished this goal.

J.S. Torg, M.D.

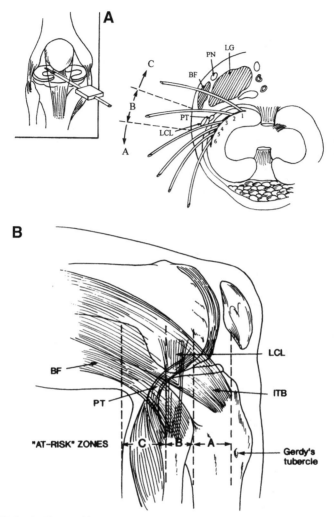

FIGURE 1.—A, Zone-specific meniscus repair cannulas were used to sequentially pass 6 vertical mattress sutures along the lateral meniscus. The suture needles were placed from the contralateral medial portal across a surgically created longitudinal tear in the peripheral portion of the posterior two thirds of the lateral meniscus *(inset).* The suture needle positions were numbered 1 through 6 from posterior to anterior. The lateral aspect of the knee was divided into 3 specific zones (A, B, and C) based on bony and soft-tissue landmarks. **B,** Demarcation of zones. *Abbreviations: LG,* lateral gastrocnemius muscle; *PN,* peroneal nerve; *BF,* biceps femoris muscle; *PT,* popliteus tendon; *LCL,* lateral collateral ligament; *ITB,* iliotibial band. (Courtesy of Deutsch A, Wyzykowski RJ, Victoroff BN: Evaluation of the anatomy of the common peroneal nerve: Defining nerve-at-risk in arthroscopically assisted lateral meniscus repair. *Am J Sports Med* 27:10-15, 1999.)

Treatment of Articular Cartilage Defects in Athletes: An Analysis of Functional Outcome and Lesion Appearance

Blevins FT, Steadman JR, Rodrigo JJ, et al (Univ of New Mexico, Albuquerque; Steadman Hawkins Clinic, Vail, Colo; Univ of California, Sacramento; et al)
Orthopedics 21:761-768, 1998   3–23

Introduction.—Two groups of athletes, 1 high-level competitive and the other recreational, were reviewed for the results of microfracture treatment of full-thickness chronic and acute chondral defects. Such chondral lesions can progress, causing pain, dysfunction, and osteoarthritis.

Methods.—Group A included 48 patients engaged in professional or high-level competitive sports at the time of their injury. The 188 patients in group B were involved in recreational sports at various levels on a regular basis. All were asked to complete a questionnaire at study entry and on an annual basis postoperatively. Symptoms were graded on a scale of 1 (none) to 4 (severe), function on a scale of 1 (no limitation) to 5 (unable to perform specified activities), and activity levels on a scale of 1 (lowest) to 10 (highest). Chondral lesions were graded on a scale of 1 (normal-appearing articular cartilage) to 4 (full-thickness cartilage loss with exposed subchondral bone). All patients underwent a microfracture procedure and a postoperative rehabilitation program that employed a continuous passive motion machine.

Results.—The 2 patient groups were similar, except that those in group B were older (average 38 vs. 26 years) and were treated at a longer interval after the injury (median 94 vs. 20.5 weeks). Average follow-up was 3.7 years for group A and 4 years for group B. In both groups, functional evaluation forms showed significant improvements from the time of microfracture to final follow-up. Both groups experienced the greatest improvement during the first postoperative year. In group B, pain scores deteriorated slightly between postoperative years 3 and 4. Second-look arthroscopy tapes, available for 26 group A and 54 group B athletes, showed average improvements in grade of 1.6 and 1.4, respectively. Among the 31 group A athletes who completed the sports outcome questionnaire, 77% returned to competition at a mean of 9.3 months posttreatment.

Discussion.—Numerous techniques have been employed for the purpose of resurfacing articular cartilage lesions, but many have limitations or are invasive and expensive. Outcomes in both the high-level and recreational athletes suggest a low-risk, simple, and inexpensive arthroscopic procedure such as microfracture can play an important role as an initial attempt at biologic resurfacing.

▶ Apparently, this was not a randomized study with regard to treatment modalities, in that the authors "could not justify establishing a control group consisting of patients with untreated chondral lesions." The study also leaves several questions unanswered. What are the biochemical composition and durability of the repaired tissue? Most importantly, is this technique superior to simply débriding loose cartilage tissue and subchondral plate back to bleeding bone?

J.S. Torg, M.D.

Rehabilitation Following Surgical Procedures to Address Articular Cartilage Lesions in the Knee
Irrgang JJ, Pezzullo D (Univ of Pittsburgh, Pa)
J Orthop Sports Phys Ther 28:232-240, 1998   3–24

Background.—Effective rehabilitation after surgery for articular cartilage lesions of the knee requires an understanding of the structure and function of articular cartilage. These authors review the structure of articular cartilage and related research on the effects of use and disuse on both normal and injured articular cartilage.

Discussion.—Articular cartilage is avascular. Its nutrition is derived mainly from synovial fluid, resulting in a limited potential for regeneration. Basic science studies have shown that compressive loading may positively affect articular cartilage healing. However, excessive shear loading may be detrimental. Controlled range-of-motion exercises should be a part of rehabilitation after surgery for articular cartilage lesions. Exercises to enhance muscle function should minimize shear loading or the joint surfaces in the area of the lesion. A period of protected weight bearing is often indicated, followed by progressive loading of the joint (Table 2).

Conclusions.—Rehabilitation after surgery for articular cartilage lesions should include range-of-motion exercises to regain motion and stimulate cartilage healing, exercises to enhance muscle function, exercises in progressive weight bearing, and low impact aerobic exercises. Excessive immobilization and shear loading with the joint under compression must be avoided. Exercises should progress systematically, and goals for return to activity must be realistic.

▶ A comprehensive treatment and rehabilitation program for articular cartilage lesions is described in this article. The authors emphasize the importance of compressive forces and shear loading. The rehabilitation program they recommend should not jeopardize the healing lesion. Realistic goals should be established to avoid progessive degeneration of the knee. Please read Abstract 4-16.

F.J. George, A.T.C., P.T.

TABLE.—Summary of Rehabilitation Considerations After Surgical Procedures for Articular Cartilage Lesions of the Knee

Procedure	Range of Motion Considerations	Considerations for Enhancing Muscle Function	Weight-Bearing Considerations
Arthroscopic lavage and débridement	Passive and unloaded active range of motion exercises with no restrictions on range of motion	Isometric and limited arc resisted open and closed chain exercises as tolerated	Partial weight bearing or weight bearing as tolerated gait Discontinue assistive devices when: Full passive knee extension At least 100° of flexion No knee extensor lag Able to ambulate without symptoms or gait deviations
Abrasion arthroplasty subchondral drilling and microfracture procedures	Unloaded passive range of motion exercises in range as tolerated	Isometric exercises at angles which do not engage the articular cartilage lesion Limited arc resisted open and closed chain exercises after 4 to 6 weeks	Non-weight bearing or touch down gait for 6 weeks Progress to weight bearing at tolerated gait after 6 weeks Discontinue assistive devices when conditions for arthroscopic lavage and débridement met
Osteochondral grafts	Unloaded passive range of motion exercises in range as tolerated May need to restrict motion dependent on fixation of graft	Isometric exercises at angles which do not engage the articular cartilage lesion Limited arc resisted open and closed chain exercises after 4 to 6 weeks	Non-weight bearing or touch down gait for 6 weeks Progress to weight bearing at tolerated gait after 6 weeks Discontinue assistive devices when conditions for arthroscopic lavage and débridement met
Osteotomy	Unloaded passive range of motion exercises in range as tolerated	Isometric quadriceps exercises with no loading across osteotomy site for 4-6 weeks (ie., quad sets and unloaded straight leg raises until the osteotomy site has healed) Limited arc resisted open and closed chain exercises after 4 to 6 weeks	Partial weight bearing or weight bearing as tolerated with rehabilitation brace locked in full extension for 4-6 weeks Discontinue assistive devices when conditions for arthroscopic lavage and débridement met

(Courtesy of Irrgang JJ, Pezzullo D: Rehabilitation following surgical procedures to address articular lesions in the knee. *J Orthop Sports Phys Ther* 28:232-240, 1998.)

Bone Bruise of the Knee: Histology and Cryosections in 5 Cases

Rangger C, Kathrein A, Freund MC, et al (Universitätsklinik für Unfallchirurgie, Innsbruck, Australia)
Acta Orthop Scand 69:291-294, 1998   3–25

Background.—Bone bruise injuries have been reported in the knee, wrist, calcaneus, foot, ankle, and hip. However, there have been no reports on the histology of bone bruise lesions.

Patients and Findings.—The histopathologic and cryosectional appearance of bone bruise injuries of the knee, as detected on MRI, were studied in 5 patients. Histologic assessment of bone biopsies from 3 patients showed microfractures of cancellous bone, edema, and bleeding in the fatty marrow. Fragments of hyaline cartilage mixed with highly fragmented bone trabecules were detected between intact lamellar bone trabecules. In addition, postmortem specimens were obtained from 2 additional patients killed in motor vehicle accidents. In 1 knee, MRI showed bone bruise injuries of the lateral femoral condyle and the lateral tibial plateau. The other specimen showed anterior cruciate ligament disruption, a medial meniscus tear, and bone bruise injury of the tibial plateau and lateral femoral condyle. The specimens were embedded in physiologic saline solution and frozen, and 1 mm slices were removed from the surfaces by rotationcryotomy. Subchondral lesions and bleeding occurred, corresponding to the MR images (Fig 2).

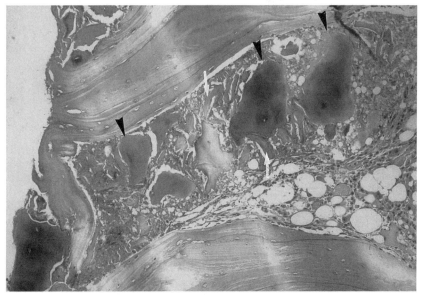

FIGURE 2.—Histologic evaluation demonstrates microfractures of cancellous bone (*light arrows*), fragments of hyaline cartilage (*black arrows*) between intact lamellar bone trabecules, and new bone formation. (Courtesy of Rangger C, Kathrein A, Freund MC, et al: Bone bruise of the knee: Histology and cryosections in 5 cases. *Acta Orthop Scand* 69:291-294, 1998.)

Conclusions.—Histologic and cryosectional analysis of bone bruise of the knee showed microfractures of cancellous bone, bleeding, and edema, in the absence of damage to the articular surface at arthroscopy. In addition, fragments of hyaline cartilage were found between intact lamellar trabecules of the subchondral bone, indicating involvement of the deep layers of articular cartilage.

▶ The value of this article is that it substantiates the contention of the radiologist that "bone edema" and "bone bruise" do, in fact, represent discernible pathology.

J.S. Torg, M.D.

Meniscal Repair in the Young Athlete
Mintzer CM, Richmond JC, Taylor J (Tufts Univ, Boston)
Am J Sports Med 26:630-633, 1998   3–26

Background.—Partial meniscectomy and meniscal repair are now performed instead of meniscectomy because it is recognized that the menisci have a crucial role in the normal functioning of the knee joint. Although the incidence of reported intra-articular knee injuries in young athletes is increasing, there is little information on the long-term outcome and success rate of meniscal repair in adolescents.

Methods.—Twenty-six patients age 17 years or younger had 29 meniscal repairs. All meniscal repairs were performed with the use of using arthroscopic techniques. Patients underwent follow-up reviews and examinations. The SF-36 Health Status Survey and the International Knee Documentation Committee evaluation form were administered. The follow-up time was 2 to 13½ years.

Results.—Follow-up data were available for all 26 patients. Each patient had a full range of motion with no effusion, joint line tenderness, or McMurray sign. No patient had symptoms of locking. Repeat surgery for nonhealed meniscal repair was not needed in any patient. SF-36 data indicated an average physical functioning score of 91 and an average role physical score of 91. Lysholm scores averaged 90. International Knee Documentation Committee evaluations indicated that 85% of the patients were performing level I activities.

Discussion.—These long-term results indicate that excellent healing rates after meniscal repair are possible in adolescent patients. The healing rates obtained are often higher than the healing rates in the adult population. Even longer follow-up is needed to determine whether successful repair can also decrease the incidence of early degenerative joint changes.

▶ The observations of the authors regarding the propensity of peripheral meniscal tears to heal are in keeping with my own clinical experience. Of note, 13 of the 17 knees had tears of the lateral meniscus with associated anterior cruciate ligament disruptions. Clearly, the moral of this story is, in the young athlete, "fix them and they will heal."

J.S. Torg, M.D.

Open Meniscal Repair: Clinical and Magnetic Resonance Imaging Findings After Twelve Years
Muellner T, Egkher A, Nikolic A, et al (Univ of Vienna)
Am J Sports Med 27:16-20, 1999   3–27

Background.—The prognosis for patients after meniscal repair has improved because of better understanding of meniscal tears and the meniscal blood supply and because of the development of better methods of treating such tears. Meniscal repair was performed by open surgery before the advent of arthroscopic techniques. There is little information on the long-term healing rates of open meniscal repair.

Methods.—The results of open meniscal repair after at least 11 years were determined in 22 patients who had 23 open meniscal repairs. Clinical outcomes were compared with results of MRI and radiographic evaluations. Patient history, physical examination findings, KT-1000 arthrometer testing, the Orthopaedische Arbeitsgemeinschaft Knie evaluation scheme, Tegner activity score, weight-bearing radiographs, and MRI provided follow-up data.

Results.—Of the 22 patients, 2 had retears, which occurred in unstable knees. Radiographs showed no degenerative changes in 17 of 23 compartments. More than 50% of the repaired menisci had grade III and IV signal alterations on MRI scans.

Discussion.—In these patients, the long-term survival rate of repaired menisci was 91%. MRI is unsuitable for observing the healing process of repaired menisci, although it remains ideal for diagnosing meniscal tears.

▶ This article makes several interesting points. First, 22 of the 23 repairs were performed on acute tears. This perhaps accounts for the higher retear rate reported by other investigators who attempted to repair chronic meniscal tears. Importantly, it is pointed out that the MRI has limited use in the evaluation of tear healing.

J.S. Torg, M.D.

Arthroscopic Partial Meniscectomy: A 12-Year Follow-up and Two-Step Evaluation of the Long-term Course

Schimmer RC, Brülhart KB, Duff C, et al (Univ Hosp of Zurich, Switzerland; Joint and Sports Traumatology, Zurich, Switzerland)
Arthroscopy 14:136-142, 1998   3–28

Introduction.—The first arthroscopic meniscectomy was performed at the University Hospital of Zurich in 1978. Long-term results of arthroscopic partial meniscectomy at this hospital are presented.

Methods.—Arthroscopic partial meniscectomy was performed on 200 patients. A questionnaire was used to interview patients 4 years and 12 years after surgery. The questionnaire assessed knee status according to the criteria of Tapper and Hoover and according to Lysholm's score.

Results.—Follow-up information was available for 119 patients. Four years after surgery, 91.7% of patients rated their results as excellent or good; 12 years after surgery, 78.1% of patients rated their results as excellent or good. The vast majority of patients were able to return to work and their previous sports activity level. Early results of patients with isolated meniscal lesions were representative and did not change significantly throughout the study. Damage to articular cartilage had the greatest effect on long-term results. Such damage did not affect knee function several years after surgery, but after 5 years patients became more symptomatic. Only 62% of patients with additional cartilage damage rated their results as excellent or good 12 years after surgery, whereas 94.8% of patients with isolated meniscal tears rated their results as excellent or good 12 years after surgery. Results after untreated rupture of the anterior cruciate ligament were similar.

Discussion.—Arthroscopic partial meniscectomy appears to be the definitive treatment for isolated meniscal lesions of the knee joint. Rapid recovery and excellent early results are typical. A stable long-term course without significant deterioration from the resected meniscal part is common.

▶ Long-term course outcome studies with consecutive evaluation points are exceptions to the rule. The downside of this particular study is that it was based on a questionnaire evaluation. However, other long-term results published after open meniscectomy also dispel the idea of its being "harmless surgery." As the authors state, "In contrast to this, the course of the isolated meniscal tear treated arthroscopically was impressively good after a mean follow-up of 12 years." The other noteworthy observation is that deterioration of long-term results was directly associated with pre-existing injury to the articular surface.

J.S. Torg, M.D.

Evaluation and Treatment of Posterior Cruciate Ligament Injuries

Harner CD, Höher J (Univ of Pittsburgh, Pa)
Am J Sports Med 26:471-482, 1998 3–29

Background.—Management of injuries involving the posterior cruciate ligament (PCL) remains controversial. The current approaches to the diagnosis and treatment of these injuries is reviewed.

Types of PCL Injuries and Their Evaluation.—The incidence of PCL injuries ranges from 3% in a general population to 37% of patients in an emergency department. The severity of PCL injuries also varies, with isolated injuries more frequent in athletes and combined injuries more common in the general and emergency department populations. Isolated PCL injuries are classified by the extent of tear: partial (grades I or II) or complete (grade III). Although it can be difficult to distinguish grade III isolated PCL tears from combined PCL injuries, making this distinction is crucial because with combined injuries, knee dislocation or vascular injuries must be suspected. Another aspect of the injury important to treatment is whether it is acute or chronic.

The evaluation of possible PCL injury begins with determining the mechanism of the injury. The posterior drawer test should be performed to identify and grade the injury; if pain or swelling prevents this test, magnetic resonance imaging should be performed. If the posterior tibial translation is more than 10 mm, involvement of the posterolateral corner must be ruled out by reducing the tibia to the neutral position and testing the posterolateral corner at 30 and 90 degrees of flexion. If a combined PCL injury is suspected, vascular (especially the pulses in the feet) and neurologic (especially the peroneal nerve) injuries should be ruled out. Radiographs are also needed to identify any avulsion fracture fragments.

Treatment of PCL Injuries.—For acute PCL injuries, patients with grades I or II isolated injuries can generally be managed with 4 to 6 weeks of relative rest followed by physical therapy. For those with isolated grade III injuries, 4 weeks of full extension with subsequent physical therapy is required to avoid posterior tibial subluxation. Furthermore, if the patient is a young athlete or has a femoral "peel-off" injury, surgery may be required. Acute PCL injury combined with lateral, medial, or anterior cruciate ligament injury requires prompt surgery, with reconstruction of the PCL and repair or reconstruction of the collateral ligaments followed by postoperative immobilization and rehabilitation. For chronic isolated PCL injuries, conservative treatment with quadriceps rehabilitation and modification of activity generally suffices. However, a grade III isolated injury associated with pain, instability, or a positive bone scan may require surgery. Chronic PCL injury combined with injury to the other collaterals requires reconstruction of the PCL and the involved collateral ligaments. Postoperatively, the knee should be immobilized for 2 to 4 weeks, then physical therapy begun. Surgery typically involves reconstruction of the anterolateral component of the PCL with a graft. Other techniques for reconstruction under investigation include fixing the graft directly to the tibia and a double-bundle reconstruction technique.

▶ Despite increases in understanding of knee mechanics, improved technology, and success in dealing with anterior cruciate ligament disruption, management of injury to the PCL remains somewhat problematic. With regard to surgical reconstruction, I agree with the authors that it is usually recommended for injuries to the PCL that occur in combination with injury to other structures.

J.S. Torg, M.D.

The Effects of a Popliteus Muscle Load on In Situ Forces in the Posterior Cruciate Ligament and on Knee Kinematics: A Human Cadaveric Study
Harner CD, Höher J, Vogrin TM, et al (Univ of Pittsburgh, Pa)
Am J Sports Med 26:669-673, 1998   3–30

Background.—Rupture of the posterior cruciate ligament (PCL) is often accompanied by injury to the structures of the posterolateral knee. The PCL and posterolateral structures have a close functional relationship and act together to restrain posterior tibial translation and tibial rotation.

Methods.—Ten human cadaveric knees (donor age, 58-89 years) were examined to study the effect of simulated contraction of the popliteus muscle on in situ forces in the PCL and on changes in knee kinematics. A

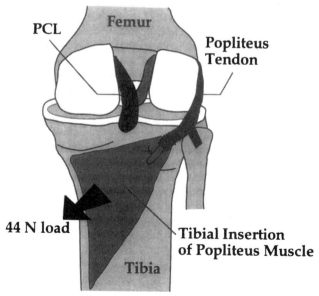

FIGURE 2.—Experimental setup of simulated popliteus muscle contraction. (Courtesy of Harner CD, Höher J, Vogrin TM, et al: The effects of a popliteus muscle load on in situ forces in the posterior cruciate ligament and on knee kinematics. *Am J Sports Med* 26:669-673, 1998.)

robotic manipulator/universal force moment sensor system was used. The kinematics of intact knees and in situ forces in the ligament were determined using a 110-N posterior tibial load (simulated posterior drawer test). A repeat test was performed using an additional 44-N load to the popliteus muscle (Fig 2). The PCL was then sectioned and the tests were repeated.

Results.—The additional load to the popliteus muscle significantly decreased the in situ forces in the ligament from 9% at 90 degrees of flexion to 36% at 30 degrees of flexion. There were no significant effects on posterior tibial translation in intact knees. In ligament-deficient knees, however, posterior tibial translation decreased by up to 36% of the translation caused by ligament transection. A coupled internal tibial rotation of 2 degrees to 4 degrees at 60 degrees to 90 degrees of knee flexion occurred in intact knees and ligament-deficient knees with the additional popliteus muscle load.

Discussion.—Both the popliteus muscle and the PCL work to resist posterior tibial loads. The popliteus muscle may be an important factor in protecting the PCL and intact knee and can contribute to knee stability when the ligament is absent or deficient. Popliteus muscle function should be restored when there is injury to the popliteus complex.

▶ This is an excellent article that elevates the popliteus muscle, which has been viewed as somewhat of a nonentity, to the status of major supporting structure of the knee joint. The study, although it is cadaveric, strongly suggests a functional interaction between the popliteus muscle and PCL. However, the data do not support the conclusion that the popliteus muscle "may play an important dynamic role in protecting the PCL in the intact knee and helping to stabilize the knee in case of PCL deficiency."

J.S. Torg, M.D.

Reconstruction of the Lateral Collateral Ligament of the Knee With Patellar Tendon Allograft: Report of a New Technique in Combined Ligament Injuries
Latimer HA, Tibone JE, ElAttrache NS, et al (Kerlan-Jobe Orthopaedic Clinic, Los Angeles; Univ of California, Orange)
Am J Sports Med 26:656-662, 1998   3–31

Background.—Compared with other knee ligament injuries, combined ligament injuries to the knee that include the posterolateral corner are not well documented. A new technique for reconstructing the lateral collateral ligament of the knee was described.

Methods and Findings.—Ten patients with combined cruciate ligament and posterolateral instability who underwent surgical reconstruction between 1991 and 1994 were studied. All knees had at least 20 degrees increased external rotation at 30 degrees of knee flexion. Varus instability ranged from 1+ to 3+. Five knees with posterior cruciate ligament rup-

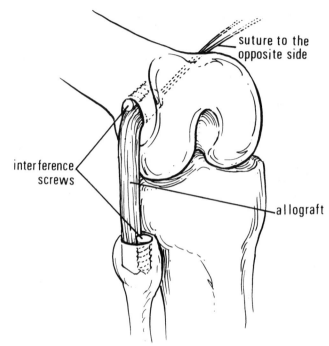

FIGURE 2.—The graft was advanced into the femoral tunnel and was secured with an interference screw. (Courtesy of Latimer HA, Tibone JE, ElAttrache NS, et al: Reconstruction of the lateral collateral ligament of the knee with patellar tendon allograft: Report of a new technique in combined ligament injuries. *Am J Sports Med* 26:656-662, 1998.)

tures had at least a 2+ Lachman test result. All lateral collateral ligaments were reconstructed with a bone-patellar tendon-bone allograft secured with interference screws. The surgeon placed fixation tunnels in the fibular head and at the isometric point on the femur (Fig 2). Autograft or allograft material was used to reconstruct the cruciate ligaments. Mean follow-up was 28 months.

Findings.—In all but 1 knee, the excessive external rotation at 30 degrees of flexion was corrected. Six patients had no varus laxity. In the remaining 4, varus laxity was 1+ at 30 degrees of flexion. The posterior drawer test result declined to a mean of 1+, and the Lachman test results declined to between 0 and 1+. Mean Tegner score was 4.6. Five patients resumed their preinjury activity level, and 4 returned to 1 level lower.

Conclusions.—Reconstructing the lateral collateral ligament with a patellar tendon allograft corrects not only the varus but also the external rotatory instability. This is a promising procedure for patients with instability resulting from lateral ligament injuries of the knee.

▶ The authors have presented a novel and innovative approach for management of varus or anterior cruciate ligament/posterior cruciate ligament instability. Clearly, this is a most difficult problem to manage in the chronic state. To be noted, the study group of 10 patients is small. Four of the 10 patients underwent subsequent surgical procedures, and the degree of the decrease in varus laxity was not determined quantatively. I would agree with the conclusion that "larger number of patients, more surgical experience, and longer follow-up are necessary before the status of this operation can be established in the treatment of lateral instability."

J.S. Torg, M.D.

Tibial Stress Injuries: An Aetiological Review for the Purposes of Guiding Management
Beck BR (Stanford Univ, Calif)
Sports Med 26:265-279, 1998   3–32

Background.—In the past 3 decades, few advances have been made in the management of tibial stress injuries, such as tibial stress fracture and medial tibial stress syndrome. An etiologic review of tibial stress injuries was undertaken to help guide future management.

Review.—Tibial overuse injuries result from chronic, intensive, weight-bearing training as commonly practiced by athletes and military recruits. In general, the most effective treatment is thought to be rest, often for prolonged periods, which can significantly disrupt a patient's lifestyle or career. However, knowledge of the nature of tibial stress injuries has increased substantially, suggesting alternative management strategies and ways to prevent such injury. Most recent studies indicate that tibial stress injuries result from the repetitive tibial strain created by loading during chronic weight-bearing activities. Evidence suggests an association between repeated tibial bending and stress injury as a function of strain-related modeling, in the case of medial tibial stress syndrome, and a strain-related positive feedback mechanism of remodeling, in the case of stress fracture.

Understanding the fundamental pathology and etiology of tibial stress injuries can help clinicians select effective management techniques. Recommendations for promoting recovery from tibial stress injury include rest from pain-provoking activities for 3 to 4 days at the first sign of injury and resumption of activity when free of pain again during running; maintenance of aerobic fitness by reduced weight-bearing exercise; a gradual return to training; and, if a particularly quick return to activity is necessary, the use of a pneumatic tibial brace to splint the tibia and reduce strain during weight-bearing. Persons with tibial stress injuries should not excessively stretch the gastrocnemius and soleus muscles, perform leg muscle strengthening exercises, engage in high-intensity activities, or train on unusually soft or uneven surfaces.

▶ This is an excellent review article with a bibliography of 179 citations. The original article is recommended reading for the interested clinician.

J.S. Torg, M.D.

Blood Supply of the Achilles Tendon

Ahmed IM, Lagopoulos M, McConnell P, et al (Univ of Leeds, England; Harrogate District Hosp, England)
J Orthop Res 16:591-596, 1998   3–33

Background.—The Achilles tendon is a common site of injury and rupture from overuse. The pathogenesis of rupture may involve the pattern of blood supply in the Achilles tendon. The Achilles tendon blood supply was investigated.

Methods and Findings.—Angiographic and histologic methods were used to study 12 human cadaveric specimens. Angiography confirmed the fact that the blood supply to the tendon is from 3 areas: the musculotendinous and osseotendinous junctions and the paratenon, with the posterior tibial artery being the major contributor. Qualitative and quantitative histologic examinations showed a poor blood supply through the length of the Achilles tendon. There were a small number of blood vessels per cross-sectional area, which generally did not significantly vary along the length of the tendon.

Conclusion.—Poor vascularity of the Achilles tendon may prevent adequate tissue repair after trauma, resulting in further tendon weakening.

▶ There is a dichotomy in the observations and conclusions of this article. The authors suggest that poor vascularity may prevent adequate tissue repair following trauma, leading to further weakening of the tendon. They conclude, on the other hand, that "The findings of this study suggest that the blood supply to the Achilles tendon may not be an important factor in tendon rupture, unless extensive microdamage exists."

J.S. Torg, M.D.

Achilles Tendon Injuries

Saltzman CL, Tearse DS (Univ of Iowa, Iowa City)
J Am Acad Orthop Surg 6:316-325, 1998   3–34

Objective.—The incidence of overuse Achilles tendon injuries is about 25%. The etiology, diagnosis, and treatment of Achilles tendon injuries are discussed.

Etiology.—Overuse injuries can result from a variety of causes including biomechanical, mechanical, and age, as well as training errors.

Classification.—The 3 stages of tendon inflammation and degeneration are paratenonitis, paratenonitis with tendinosis, and tendinosis, each with its own histologic findings and clinical signs and symptoms.

Diagnosis.—Physical examination should include comparison of calf girth on the affected and unaffected legs, and notation of any tenderness, crepitation, warmth, swelling, nodularity, and substance defects.

Imaging.—US and MRI are 2 helpful diagnostic modalities.

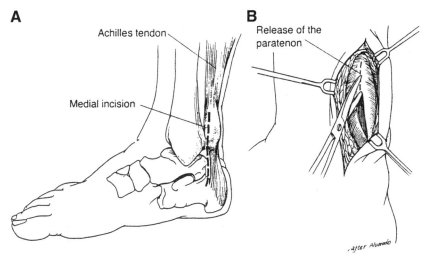

FIGURE 5.—A, The medial longitudinal incision minimizes risk to the sural nerve and short saphenous venous system. **B,** After creation of full-thickness flaps, the paratenon is released, and any thickened areas are excised. (Reprinted from the *Journal of the American Academy of Orthopaedic Surgeons* courtesy of Saltzman CL, Tearse DS: Achilles tendon injuries. *J Am Acad Orthop Surg* 6:316-325, copyright 1998, American Academy of Orthopaedic Surgeons, with permission.)

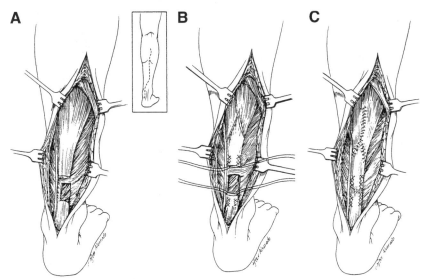

FIGURE 10.—Technique for V-Y lengthening of the triceps surae. **A,** A medial incision is extended proximally in a gently curving S (*inset*). The tendon ends are debrided, and the repair site is prepared by windowing the deep posterior fascia. **B,** a V cut is made in the triceps surae aponeurosis. **C,** After approximation of the tendon ends, the aponeurosis is closed. (Reprinted from the *Journal of the American Academy of Orthopaedic Surgeons* courtesy of Saltzman CL, Tearse DS: Achilles tendon injuries. *J Am Acad Orthop Surg* 6:316–325, copyright 1998, American Academy of Orthopaedic Surgeons, with permission.)

Treatment.—Paratenonitis is usually treated conservatively. Tendinosis is initially treated conservatively but may require surgical excision of the paratenon if symptoms are resistant (Fig 5). Whether acute rupture should be treated conservatively or surgically is controversial, although surgery is often preferred in younger, more athletic patients. Chronic rupture, particularly when there is a gap, can generally be treated successfully only by surgery (Fig 10).

Conclusion.—Overuse injuries of the Achilles tendon are usually successfully managed conservatively. Acute rupture may be managed surgically or conservatively. Chronic rupture may require reconstruction.

▶ This article is a comprehensive review of Achilles tendon injuries based on a histopathologic scheme for classification, a process that facilitates a logical approach to treatment. The original article is recommended reading for the interested practitioner.

J.S. Torg, M.D.

The Clinical Diagnosis of Subcutaneous Tear of the Achilles Tendon: A Prospective Study in 174 Patients

Maffulli N (Univ of Aberdeen, Scotland)
Am J Sports Med 26:266-270, 1998   3–35

Objective.—Diagnosis of a complete subcutaneous tear of the Achilles tendon is sometimes illusive. The clinical history may be deceptive. The sensitivity, specificity, and positive and negative predictive values of several clinical diagnostic tests of subcutaneous Achilles tendon rupture were reviewed.

Methods.—Between September 1983 and March 1996, 174 patients (25 women) underwent tests for a unilateral complete subcutaneous tear of the Achilles tendon. The tests used were palpation, calf squeeze, Matles, Copeland, and O'Brien. Times between injury and clinical visit were day of injury (N = 98), 1 to 3 days (N = 45), 4 to 7 days (N = 14), 8 to 14 days (N = 7), and 14 to 28 (N = 10). An additional 28 patients (7 women), initially given a misdiagnosis of Achilles tendon tear, took the same tests. All patients were tested by the same person who was blinded to the diagnoses.

Results.—Patients treated conservatively were significantly older than patients treated surgically. Time between injury and clinical visit did not have an effect on the sensitivity or predictive value of the tests. The respective awake and anesthesia sensitivities were 0.73 and 0.81 for the Gap test, 0.96 and 0.96 for the calf squeeze, 0.88 and 0.94 for the Mates test, 0.78 and 0.81 for the Copeland test, and not applicable and 0.80 for the O'Brien test. The corresponding awake and anesthesia positive predictive values were 0.82 and 0.85, 0.98 and 0.96, 0.92 and 0.97, 0.92 and 0.88, and not applicable and 0.85. At least 2 tests were positive for all patients with tears. For patients with no Achilles tendon tear, only the palpation, calf squeeze, and Matles tests were performed. Two patients had false positive results by the Matles test. The respective specificity and negative predictive values of the 3 tests were 0.89 and 1, 0.93 and 1, and 0.85 and 0.92.

Conclusion.—Tests for subcutaneous Achilles tendon tears were sensitive, specific, and accurate.

▶ As pointed out by the author, it is not unusual for nonspecialists to misdiagnose a complete rupture of the Achilles tendon. It has been my experience that the Thompson test (calf squeeze test) is uniformly positive, regardless of the length of time after injury. Not only is this test sensitive, specific, and accurate, it is also noninvasive and economical.

J.S. Torg, M.D.

Early Active Motion and Weightbearing After Cross-stitch Achilles Tendon Repair
Aoki M, Ogiwara N, Ohta T, et al (Sapporo Med Univ, Japan)
Am J Sports Med 26:794-800, 1998   3–36

Background.—Achilles tendon ruptures are becoming increasingly common. Such injury usually occurs in middle-aged persons engaging in strenuous exercise. The clinical outcomes of cross-stitch tendon repair and early rehabilitation were evaluated.

Methods.—Twenty-two patients with closed Achilles tendon ruptures sustained during sports underwent repair with Kirschmayer core suture and cross-stitch epitenon suture. Early active ankle motion with weightbearing was begun after surgery. Mean follow-up was 24.6 months.

Findings.—Ninety-one percent of the tendons healed without rupturing again. Nine percent partially ruptured again at 23 and 56 days after repair. At a mean of 9.7 days, active ankle extension ranged from a negative value to 0 degrees. Ankle motion recovered to normal at a mean of 6 weeks. Patients were able to bear weight fully without heel raising in a mean of 16.4 days. Heel raising with both legs became possible in a mean of 7.3 weeks. Full sports activity was resumed in 13.1 weeks. Mean time to the area of high-intensity signal at the tendon repair site on T2-weighted MR images was 6.9 weeks. The tendon repair site became low-intensity signal at an average of 12.6 weeks, indicating excellent tendon healing (Fig 1).

Background.—Strong, stable tendon repair and an early rehabilitation protocol appear to restore good muscle and joint function in patients with Achilles tendon rupture. The use of Kirschmayer core suture and cross-stitch epitenon suture may enable athletes to return to sports in a shorter time than has been previously reported.

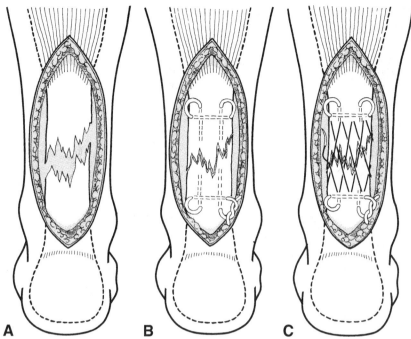

FIGURE 1.—The Kirschmayer core suture and cross-stitch epitenon suture repair technique is demonstrated. **A,** a 10 cm skin and fascial incision was performed over the Achilles tendon. **B,** paratenon over the Achilles tendon was spared on both tendon ends. The Kirschmayer core suture with Number 2 Tevdek was applied to connect proximal and distal tendon ends in an appropriate length. **C,** the cross-stitch epitenon suture with 2-0 Maxon was placed inside the tendon grasps of the Kirschmayer core suture. (Courtesy of Aoki M, Ogiwara N, Ohta T, et al: Early active motion and weightbearing after cross-stitch Achilles tendon repair. *Am J Sports Med* 26:794-800, 1998.)

Early Full Weightbearing and Functional Treatment After Surgical Repair of Acute Achilles Tendon Rupture

Speck M, Klaue K (Univ of Berne, Switzerland; Ospedale Regionale San Giovanni, Bellinzona, Switzerland)
Am J Sports Med 26:789-793, 1998   3–37

Background.—The best treatment of acute Achilles tendon rupture has not been established. The effects of limited immobilization and early motion with full weightbearing on the healing pattern after operative repair of acute Achilles tendon ruptures were studied.

Methods.—Twenty patients, aged 27 to 83 years, were treated by a prospective protocol. All underwent open repair, which included Kessler-type suture and simple apposition sutures (Fig 1). Postoperatively, the patients were treated with a plantigrade splint for 24 hours, with 6 weeks of early full weightbearing in a removable walker (Fig 2). Assessment at 3, 6, and 12 months postoperatively included clinical and US examination and a new 100-point scoring system.

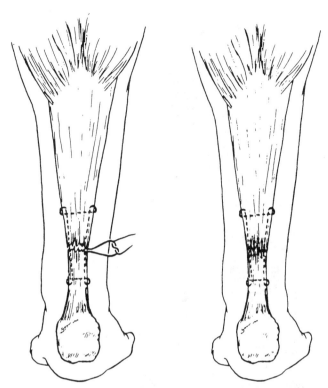

FIGURE 1.—In the Kessler suture repair technique, the ruptured ends of the tendon are approximated using a stitch through each stump, 2.5 cm from the rupture. The foot is then plantar flexed 10 degrees and the suture's ends are tied. (Courtesy of Speck M, Klaue K: Early full weightbearing and functional treatment after surgical repair of acute Achilles tendon. *Am J Sports Med* 26:789-793, 1998.)

Findings.—At 3 months, the mean score was 73 points; at 6 months, 86 points; and at 1 year, 94 points. All patients were able to resume sports activities at their preoperative levels. No significant differences were noted in ankle mobility and isokinetic strength. No ruptures occurred. One patient had a deep venous thrombosis 3 weeks after surgery after prematurely stopping thromboprophylaxis.

Conclusions.—Early careful ankle mobilization and full weightbearing in a removable walker after primary repair of the Achilles tendon do not appear to increase the risk of repeat rupture. An accelerated rehabilitation program improved early foot function, with excellent recovery of plantar flexion strength and amplitude.

▶ These 2 articles (Abstracts 3–36 and 3–37) by Aoki et al and Speck et al clearly demonstrate the efficacy of early active motion and weightbearing following open repair of Achilles tendon ruptures. To be noted, Speck used a number zero absorbable polydioxanone suture. Presumably, this would obviate any potential problems associated with a nonabsorbable suture. Impressive is the fact that early full weightbearing and unloaded ankle

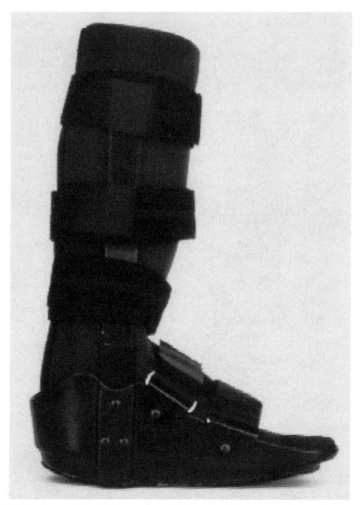

FIGURE 2.—Removable ankle-foot-orthosis (*AFP*) "walker" equipped with a rocking sole, which minimizes the lever effect of the foot onto the heel cord. The removable walker allows for full weight-bearing and passive range-of-motion exercises. (Courtesy of Speck M, Klaue K: Early full weightbearing and functional treatment after surgical repair of acute Achilles tendon. *Am J Sports Med* 26:789-793, 1998.)

motion did not increase risk of re-rupture, when the repair was protected by a removable walker with a roll ramp. Speck believes that the ramp is important because it avoids the lever effect provided by the foot. The article cites an experimental study in which absorbable sutures were used for repair of rabbit Achilles tendon lacerations with postoperative results comparable with those of nonabsorbable sutures. This observation in itself is an important contribution.

J.S. Torg, M.D.

Magnetic Resonance Imaging During Healing of Surgically Repaired Achilles Tendon Ruptures

Karjalainen PT, Aronen HJ, Pihlajamäki HK, et al (Helsinki Univ Central Hosp; Univ of Helsinki; Mount Sinai Med Ctr, Miami Beach, Fla)

Am J Sports Med 25:164-171, 1997   3–38

Background.—Imaging techniques may be useful for detecting complications after the surgical treatment of Achilles tendon ruptures. MRI features during the healing of surgically repaired Achilles tendon ruptures were reported.

Methods.—Twenty consecutive patients with 21 surgically repaired Achilles tendon ruptures were studied by MRI at 3 and 6 weeks and 3 and 6 months after repair. Clinical and functional assessments were also performed at the time of scanning.

Findings.—At 3 months after surgery, 19 Achilles tendons showed an intratendinous area of high-density signal on proton density-weighted and T2-weighted images. The 3 patients with the largest lesions had clinically poor outcomes at 3 months. Patients with smaller intratendinous lesions recovered normally. In addition, the 5 patients who walked abnormally at 3 months had significantly larger intratendinous lesions than those who walked normally. In all patients, the cross-sectional region of the rejoined Achilles tendon demonstrated the greatest increase after cast removal, occurring between 6 weeks and 3 months after surgery. The largest tendon area was measured at 3 months postoperatively in all cases (Figs 2 and 5).

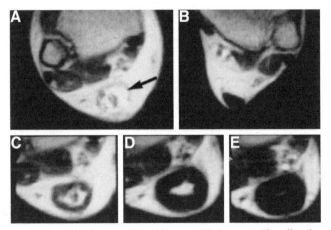

FIGURE 2.—**A,** T2-weighted images (TR, 2000 msec; TE, 80 msec). The affected tendon shows high-intensity signal (*arrow*) with a peripheral thin rim of low-intensity signal area and also low-intensity elements centrally. **B,** The unaffected side. **C,** At 6 weeks, the intratendinous lesion and the margin of the Achilles tendon are better visualized on T2-weighted images than on proton density-weighted images. **D,** At 3 months, the periphery of the healing tendon has returned to its normal low-intensity signal level. The intratendinous lesion inside the tendon is rather small. Note that the cross-sectional area of the healing tendon is 7 times as large as that on the unaffected side (**B**). **E,** At 6 months, the scar is barely seen and the edema around the tendon has decreased compared with previous follow-ups. (Courtesy of Karjalainen PT, Aronen HJ, Pihlajamäki HK, et al: Magnetic resonance imaging during healing of surgically repaired Achilles tendon ruptures. *Am J Sports Med* 25:164-171, 1997.)

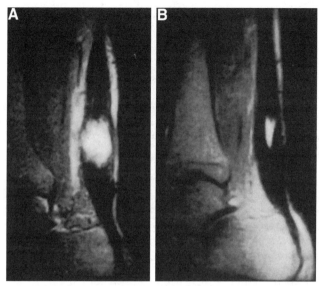

FIGURE 5.—Sagittal T2-weighted MR images (TR, 1500 msec; TE, 55 msec) of a patient with a poorly healed Achilles tendon rupture subsequently requiring a reoperation. **A,** at 3 months after initial injury the tendon has a large area of intratendinous lesion formation (incomplete healing). Note the large rounded and compact appearance of the central scar and thin peripheral low intensity fibers. The patient had consistent pain and an abnormal walk. He had a second surgery; the lesion was removed, and the tendon was augmented with a Lindholm plasty. **B,** at 6 months after reoperation the lesion had decreased significantly. (Courtesy of Karjalainen PT, Aronen HJ, Pihlajamäki HK, et al: Magnetic resonance imaging during healing of surgically repaired Achilles tendon ruptures. *Am J Sports Med* 25:164-171, 1997.)

Conclusions.—MRI is a valuable tool for assessing the internal structure of surgically repaired Achilles tendons during the reunion process. The long-term appearance of this process has yet to be determined.

▶ Certainly, rupture of the Achilles tendon, either acute or chronic, is a clinical diagnosis. However, this study very nicely depicts, in terms of both signal intensity and cross-sectional area, sequential changes that occur in healing. Of note, there is no correlation between MRI changes and activity participation.

J.S. Torg, M.D.

Acute Achilles Tendon Rupture in Badminton Players
Fahlström M, Björnstig U, Lorentzon R (Univ Hosp of Umeå, Sweden)
Am J Sports Med 26:467-470, 1998   3–39

Background.—Badminton is a popular sport in Sweden. The incidence, nature, and treatment of acute Achilles tendon ruptures in badminton players were reported.

Methods.—Thirty-one patients sustaining badminton-related acute Achilles tendon ruptures between 1990 and 1994 were followed up retrospectively by questionnaire. The patients were 27 men and 4 women, with a mean age of 36 years. Ninety-seven percent said they were recreational players or beginners.

Findings.—Ninety-four percent of the injuries occurred in the middle or at the end of the game. Sixteen percent of the patients had noticed previous local symptoms. In the long term, patients undergoing surgery had a significantly shorter sick leave than those treated conservatively. None of the surgically treated patients and 2 nonsurgically treated patients had reruptures. The surgically treated patients appeared to have fewer lingering symptoms and a greater level of sports activity after the injury.

Conclusions.—Specific treatment of minor injuries and adequate training of strength, endurance, and coordination are important for preventing badminton-related acute Achilles tendon rupture. Surgical treatment and careful postoperative rehabilitation are most effective in treating Achilles tendon ruptures in badminton players of any age and sports level.

▶ The data neither indicate nor contraindicate a connection between warming up and stretching habits and Achilles tendon rupture. Although the authors suggest that an important reason for acute Achilles tendon rupture is fatigue with impaired neuromuscular function and coordination of the triceps surae, this also is not supported by data. I do agree that surgical treatment is the recommended approach to dealing with this problem.

J.S. Torg, M.D.

Effect of Coordination Training on Proprioception of the Functionally Unstable Ankle
Bernier JN, Perrin DH (Univ of Virginia, Charlottesville)
J Orthop Sports Phys Ther 27:264-275, 1998   3–40

Background.—Exercises are advocated to improve joint proprioception and coordination of the functionally unstable ankle. However, there is little evidence that such exercises have any effect on proprioception and balance. The effect of coordination training on proprioception of the functionally unstable ankle was investigated.

Methods.—Forty-five patients with ankle instability were randomly assigned to a control (group 1), sham (group 2), or training (group 3) group. Patients in group 3 trained 3 days a week, 10 minutes each day, doing various balance and proprioception exercises. Postural sway and active and passive joint position sense were evaluated.

Findings.—Significant 4-way interactions were found for postural sway modified equilibrium score, for anterior and posterior sway as well as for medial and lateral sway. Group 3 performed significantly better on the posttests than groups 1 and 2 did. Joint position sense or postural sway index did not differ significantly among groups.

Conclusions.—Balance and coordination training apparently can improve some measures of postural sway. Whether joint position sense can be improved in the functionally unstable ankle remains unclear.

▶ Ankle rehabilitation programs must include coordination and proprioception exercises. Proprioceptive neuromuscular facilitation exercises, balance boards, and functional exercises will help to achieve total rehabilitation. If an athlete has sustained a severe ankle injury, a protective device such as a lace-up ankle brace is recommended for return to activity after rehabilitation goals are met. In many situations, adhesive tape is used, either alone or with an ankle brace, to prevent reinjury or to allow the athlete to return to activity.

F.J. George, A.T.C., P.T.

Prospective Evaluation of the Ottawa Ankle Rules in a University Sports Medicine Center: With a Modification to Increase Specificity for Identifying Malleolar Fractures
Leddy JJ, Smolinski RJ, Lawrence J, et al (State Univ of New York, Buffalo)
Am J Sports Med 26:158-165, 1998   3–41

Background.—The Ottawa Ankle Rules (OARs) are easy-to-use clinical decision guidelines for using radiography in patients with acute ankle injuries in an emergency department. The ability of the OARs for detecting clinically significant ankle and midfoot fractures and for reducing the need for radiography was evaluated prospectively at a sports medicine center. In

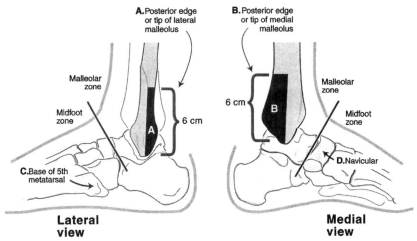

Lateral view   **Medial view**

FIGURE 1.—The Ottawa Ankle Rules are positive, and radiography is indicated, if there is bone tenderness at A or B (ankle series) or C or D (foot series) or if there is inability to bear weight both immediately after injury and during examination (4 steps, regardless of limping). The malleolar tenderness rule involves palpation along the posterior borders of the malleoli. (Adapted from Stiell et al) (Courtesy of Leddy JJ, Smolinski RJ, Lawrence J, et al: Prospective evaluation of the Ottawa ankle rules in a university sports medicine center: With a modification to increase specificity for identifying malleolar fractures. *Am J Sports Med* 26:158-165, 1998).

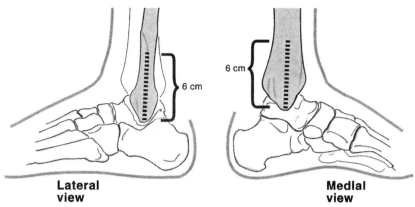

Lateral view   **Medial view**

FIGURE 2.—The Buffalo modification for malleolar tenderness moves the area of palpation to over the crests or midportions of the malleoli, away from the ligamentous attachments. The remainder of the OAR are otherwise the same. (Courtesy of Leddy JJ, Smolinski RJ, Lawrence J, et al: Prospective evaluation of the Ottawa ankle rules in a university sports medicine center: With a modification to increase specificity for identifying malleolar fractures. *Am J Sports Med* 26:158-165, 1998).

addition, a modification was developed to improve specificity for identifying malleolar fracture.

Methods.—Patients seen within 10 days of ankle injury were studied. The sensitivity, specificity, and potential decrease in radiography use were determined for the OARs in 132 patients. The new "Buffalo" rule was applied in a subset of 78 patients.

Findings.—Eleven clinically significant fractures were identified. The OARs would have decreased the need for radiography by 34% without resulting in missed fractures, for a sensitivity and specificity of 100% and 37%, respectively. Specificity for malleolar fracture for the new "Buffalo" rule was significantly higher than that of the OAR malleolar rule, at 59% and 42%, respectively. Sensitivity remained at 100%. The potential reduction in the need for radiography using the new rule was 54%, significantly greater than without the new rule (Figs 1 and 2).

Conclusions.—The OARs may significantly decrease the need for radiography in patients with acute ankle and midfoot injuries in a sports medicine center. Incorporating the Buffalo modification could enhance specificity for malleolar fractures without compromising sensitivity and could further significantly decrease the need for radiography.

▶ Rules are absolute; guidelines are relative. Whatever happened to the maxim, "Never say never, never say always"? Certainly, such problems as acute osteochondral fractures of the chondral dome, lis franc sprains, and tumors will be missed. But clearly the lawsuits won't.

J.S. Torg, M.D.

Long-term Results of Watson-Jones Tenodesis of the Ankle: Clinical and Radiographic Findings After Ten to Eighteen Years of Follow-up

Sugimoto K, Takakura Y, Akiyama K, et al (Nara Med Univ, Kashihara, Japan)
J Bone Joint Surg Am 80-A:1587-1595, 1998   3–42

Objective.—Tenodesis is the treatment of choice for chronic lateral ankle instability. Whereas short-term results with the Watson-Jones tenodesis are satisfactory, long-term studies have yielded controversial results. The clinical and radiographic changes in ankles and subtalar joints are reported 10 to 18 years after a Watson-Jones tenodesis.

Methods.—Between 1979 and 1989, a Watson-Jones tenodesis was performed on 37 unstable ankles in 36 patients, thirty-four ankles in 33 patients (9 male), aged 14 to 57 at time of surgery, were available for follow-up an average of 13 years 8 months later. Radiographic evaluation was performed on 25 patients (26 ankles) at follow-up, and the remaining 6 patients were interviewed by telephone.

Results.—Results were excellent for 19 ankles, good for 11, fair for 3, and poor for 1. The mean American Orthopaedic Foot and Ankle Society ankle-hindfoot score was 90 on a 100-point scale. The final score was negatively correlated with both age at surgery and age at follow-up. Six patients had postoperative complications. Radiographic results showed exostosis in 18 ankles. There was no narrowing of the joint space. There was no relationship between clinical results and radiographic osteoarthrotic changes.

Conclusion.—Long-term results after the Watson-Jones tenodesis are good.

▶ The authors conclude that "the results of the modified Watson-Jones tenodesis were good; did not deteriorate over time; and, although not ideal, were much better than we expected." One has to wonder what the authors expected.

J.S. Torg, M.D.

Reconstruction of the Lateral Ankle Ligaments Using a Split Peroneus Brevis Tendon Graft

Sammarco GJ, Idusuyi OB (Univ of Cincinnati, Ohio; Southern Illinois Univ, Springfield)
Foot Ankle Int 20:97-103, 1999   3–43

Objective.—The surgical treatment of chronic primary and recurrent ankle instability in patients with high demands or with failure of a primary surgical reconstruction was discussed in the context of modified use of a split peroneus brevis tendon graft in light of the newer surgical techniques and bone fixation devices.

Methods.—Between 1991 and 1995, lateral ankle reconstructions using a split peroneus brevis graft were performed on 31 chronically unstable

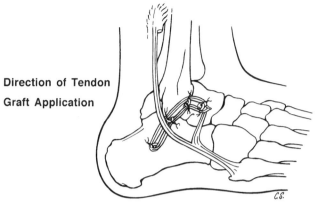

Direction of Tendon Graft Application

FIGURE 6.—The tendon graft was doubled back on itself and sutured back to each of the anchors in reverse, creating a double thickness tendon graft which is anatomical in position and stabilizes both the ankle and subtalar joints. (Courtesy of Sammarco GJ, Idusuyi OB: Reconstruction of the lateral ankle ligaments using a split peroneus brevis tendon graft. *Foot Ankle Int* 20(2):97-103, 1999.)

ankles in 30 patients (13 females), aged 12 to 47 years. The average time from injury to repair was 23 months.

> *Technique.*—A 4-cm incision was made from the lateral malleolus distally. Using a "pigtail" tendon stripper, 15 cm of one half of the peroneus brevis tendon was harvested and pulled distally into the wound. Bone anchors were inserted into the anterior border of the lateral facet of the talar dome, the anterior talofibular insertion, the insertion of the anterior talofibular ligament on the lateral malleolus, the insertion of the calcaneofibular ligament on the lateral malleolus, and the anterior border of the insertion of the calcaneofibular ligament on the calcaneus. The tendon graft was sutured to the anchors with the ankle in the neutral position. The tendon was then doubled back on itself and again sutured to the anchors to create a double thickness (Fig 6).

Results.—Patients were followed for an average of 44 months. Functional results were excellent in 20 ankles, good in 9, fair in 1, and poor in 1. Ankle stability did not deteriorate with time for 30 ankles. Complications included dysesthesia, hypoesthesia, or both, which resolved when bone anchors were removed. At follow-up, 3 patients had mild pain on the job or when participating in sports, 10 patients had some subtalar motion that did not affect activities of daily living or sports participation. Thirty of 31 patients believed the surgery had improved function.

Conclusion.—This technique is safe, effective, simple, and reliable for reconstruction ankles of patients with high demand, longstanding instability, or failed primary reconstruction.

▶ The authors present still another reconstructive procedure for lateral ankle ligament instability. They report the technique as being both simple and reliable. Innovative is the use of bone anchors to secure the graft as well as a slotted tendon stripper, allowing for a smaller surgical incision. Unfortunately, the study was not designed for comparison with another simple reliable procedure such as that described by Brostrom.[1,2]

J.S. Torg, M.D.

References

1. Brostrom L: Sprained ankles. V: Treatment and prognosis in recent ligament ruptures. *Acta Chir Scand* 132:537-550, 1966.
2. Brostrom L: Sprained ankles. VI: Surgical treatment of "chronic" ligament ruptures. *Acta Chir Scand* 132:551-565, 1966.

Ankle Orthoses Effect on Single-Limb Standing Balance in Athletes With Functional Ankle Instability

Baier M, Hopf T (Orthopädische Universitätsklinik Homburg/Saar, Germany)
Arch Phys Med Rehabil 79:939-944, 1998   3–44

Background.—Many athletes wear ankle orthoses to prevent recurrent ankle sprains during training and competition. Such orthoses may affect proprioception. The effect of a rigid or flexible ankle orthosis on postural sway in a single-limb stance was investigated by stabilometry.

Methods.—Twenty-two athletes with functional ankle instability and 22 healthy athletes participated in the study. Stabilometry in single-limb stance was performed on a force platform. Athletes were assessed while standing on each leg, with and without a rigid or flexible ankle orthosis.

Findings.—Both the rigid and flexible ankle orthoses decreased mediolateral sway velocity significantly. The flexible ankle orthosis also significantly changed the sway pattern by reducing the percentage of linear movements of fewer than 5 degrees per 0.01 seconds.

Conclusions.—Ankle orthoses decrease mediolateral sway velocity in athletes with functional ankle instability, possibly because the orthoses improves mediolateral proprioception. By stimulating cutaneous afferents, ankle orthoses provide additional data on joint position, which may result in more accurate correctional movements in single-limb stance and reduce mediolateral sway velocity. The greater decrease in mediolateral sway velocity in athletes with ankle instability, compared with the decrease in healthy athletes, supports this notion.

▶ The ankle orthoses that the authors describe as flexible are considered moderately rigid when compared to the lace-up braces that many athletes wear. The authors have concluded that the orthosis will improve proprioception in the functionally unstable ankle, providing a mechanical stabilizing effect as well. These orthoses are more expensive than traditional lace-up ankle braces, however.

F.J. George, A.T.C., P.T.

Ultrasonography in the Differential Diagnosis of Achilles Tendon Injuries and Related Disorders: A Comparison Between Pre-operative Ultrasonography and Surgical Findings

Paavola M, Paakkala T, Kannus P, et al (Tampere Univ Hosp, Finland; Tampere Univ, Finland; UKK Inst, Tampere, Finland)
Acta Radiol 39:612-619, 1998   3–45

Background.—Although clinical assessment with a careful history alone is usually sufficient for diagnosing complete Achilles tendon rupture, 20% to 30% of such injuries are not diagnosed correctly by primary care physicians. The value of US in the diagnosis of various Achilles tendon disorders was investigated.

Methods.—Seventy-nine patients with Achilles tendon symptoms were included in the analysis. Preoperative US findings were compared with surgical findings.

Findings.—Of the 26 surgically verified cases, US examination yielded only 1 false negative finding. In the diagnosis of retrocalcanear bursitis, 6 of 8 cases were identified by US, with no false positive findings.Ultrasonography yielded no false positive findings in patients with peritendinitis and tendinitis. However, there were 7 false negative US findings among the 40 surgically verified peritendinitis and tendinitis cases, indicating that a negative US result in a clinically suspected case of this disorder is not reliable. Also, US did not adequately differentiate partial tendon rupture from a focal tendon degeneration, though the occurrence and location of such a lesion were identified by US (Fig 3).

Conclusions.—US is reliable for locating Achilles tendon abnormalities, estimating their severity, and determining most conditions that require surgical intervention. However, US is not completely reliable for diagnosing peritendinitis or tendinitis and does not differentiate partial tendon ruptures from focal degenerative lesions.

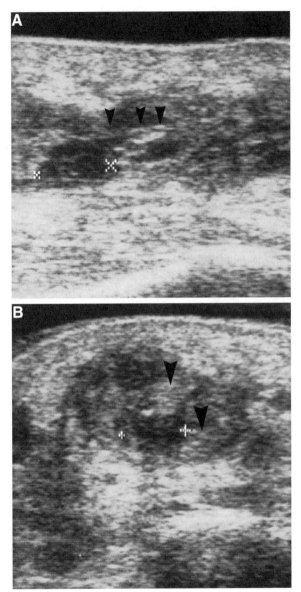

FIGURE 3.—**A**, Longitudinal and **B**, transverse US images of a complete Achilles tendon rupture with some intact fibers (*arrowhead*). The US finding was confirmed surgically. (Courtesy of Paavola M, Paakkala T, Kannus P, et al: Ultrasonography in the differential diagnosis of Achilles tendon injuries and related disorders: A comparison between preoperative ultrasonography and surgical findings. *Acta Radiol* 39:612-619, 1998.)

Use of Ultrasonography Versus Magnetic Resonance Imaging for Tendon Abnormalities Around the Ankle

Rockett MS, Waitches G, Sudakoff G, et al (Harris County Podiatric Surgical Residency, Houston; Univ of Washington, Seattle; Univ of Chicago)
Foot Ankle Int 19:604-612, 1998   3–46

Background.—Although US is being used increasingly for diagnosing musculoskeletal abnormalities in the shoulder, knee, and hand, its use in the assessment of ankle tendon disorders has been limited. The use of US in imaging pathologic conditions of ankle tendons was described.

Methods and Findings.—Twenty-eight patients undergoing surgery for tendon disorders around the ankle were studied prospectively. Before surgery, all patients had real-time, high-resolution US with a 7.5 or 10 mHz transducer. In addition, 20 patients underwent MRI of the ankle before surgery. Intraoperatively, 54 tendons were examined, revealing 24 intrasubstance or complete tendon tears. Surgical findings were compared with US and MRI findings. The sensitivity, specificity, and accuracy of US were 100%, 89.9%, and 94.4%, respectively. Findings on MRI had a sensitivity of 23.4%, a specificity of 100%, and an accuracy of 65.8%.

Conclusions.—High-resolution, real-time US should be the first-line diagnostic modality in patients suspected of having a specific tendon tear around the ankle. US is more sensitive and accurate than MRI for detecting such tears. Also, US is faster, less costly, more available, and more interactive than an MR examination, with minimal-to-no patient contraindications.

▶ It appears that US can be used for evaluating tendon abnormalities about the ankle. However, US is not completely reliable for diagnosing peritendinitis and tendinitis and cannot be used to differentiate focal degenerative lesions from tendon ruptures.

J.S. Torg, M.D.

Subtalar Arthroscopy: Indications, Technique, and Results

Williams MM, Ferkel RD (Univ of California, Los Angeles; Southern California Orthopedic Inst, Van Nuys)
Arthroscopy 14:373-381, 1998   3–47

Background.—Although numerous reports have addressed arthroscopic examination of the ankle, few have focused on arthroscopy of the subtalar joint. This study reviewed an experience with subtalar joint arthroscopy in 50 patients, including indications, technique, and results.

Patients.—Fifty consecutive patients undergoing subtalar arthroscopy were reviewed. Each patient had concomitant ankle arthroscopy to determine the exact source of pain. There were 26 men and 24 women, average age 34. Each patient had symptoms such as pain, swelling, stiffness, locking, or catching that had failed to respond to conservative measures.

Arthroscopy was performed with 2.7 and 1.9 mm arthroscopes using standard and accessory portals with joint distraction. In patients with subtalar pathology requiring operative arthroscopy, patient outcomes were independently assessed at an average follow-up of 48 months.

Outcomes.—Subtalar arthroscopy had no major complications. Twenty-one patients were treated for chronic lateral ankle pain after inversion injury. Arthroscopy revealed no abnormal findings in the subtalar joint, and no operative subtalar arthroscopy was performed. In the remaining 29 patients, subtalar joint arthroscopic diagnoses included synovitis in 7 patients, degenerative joint disease in 5, subtalar dysfunction in 5, chondromalacia in 4, nonunion of the os trigonum in 4, arthrofibrosis in 2, loose bodies in 1, and osteochondral talus lesions in 1. At follow-up, the results were scored as excellent in 76% of these patients, good in 10%, fair in 10%, and poor in 3%. Forty percent of patients with degenerative joint disease had fair or poor results. Other factors contributing to less favorable results were associated ankle pathology and patient activity level.

Conclusions.—Subtalar arthroscopy is a valuable diagnostic and therapeutic procedure. No subtalar pathology is found in patients with chronic ankle pain after inversion injury. In patients with various forms of subtalar pathology, long-term follow-up reveals a high rate of good to excellent results. Posterior subtalar joint arthroscopy is a difficult procedure that only surgeons with experience in small-joint arthroscopy should attempt.

▶ Notably, the authors point out that "posterior subtalar arthroscopy is a technically demanding and difficult procedure that should only be performed by arthroscopists experienced with small joint arthroscopy."

J.S. Torg, M.D.

Subtalar Instability Following Lateral Ligament Injuries of the Ankle
Yamamoto H, Yagishita K, Ogiuchi T, et al (Tokyo Med and Dental Univ)
Injury 29:265-268, 1998   3–48

Introduction.—Despite the large number of reports concerning the pathology, diagnosis, and treatment of ankle instability, there is little information on subtalar joint instability. Several techniques for stress radiography of the subtalar joint have been described for measurement of the subtalar tilt angle or displacement of the calcaneus on the talus. However, each of these methods has had inherent difficulties. The Telos equipment for stress radiography was used to examine the stability of the subtalar joint.

Methods.—The Telos equipment was used to apply 150 N of inversion stress to the calcaneus for stress radiography. The studies were performed with the x-ray beam directed onto the posterior subtalar joint at angles of 30 degrees lateromedially and 40 degrees caudocranially. The films were used to measure the subtalar tilt angle as an indicator of subtalar joint stability. Intraobserver and interobserver variability were assessed in 20

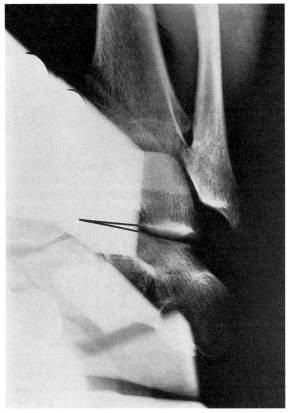

FIGURE 2.—The subtalar tilt angle in stress radiograph was the angle of the line of the posterior articular surface of the talus and the line of posterior articular surface of the calcaneus and was used as an index of stability of the subtalar joint. (Courtesy of Yamamoto H, Yagishita K, Ogiuchi T, et al: Subtalar instability following lateral ligament injuries of the ankle. *Injury* 29:265-268, 1998. Reprinted with permission from Elsevier Science.)

unstable ankles (Fig 2). The findings of subtalar joint stress radiography were analyzed in 23 acute and 23 chronic lateral ligament injuries of the ankle, as well as in 80 normal ankles.

Results.—Intraobserver error in measurement of the subtalar tilt angle ranged from 1.4 to 1.9 degrees at a 95% confidence level. Interobserver error was 2 degrees. Mean subtalar tilt angle was 9.7 degrees in acutely injured ankles and 10.3 degrees in chronically injured ankles, compared with 5.2 degrees in normal ankles. Talar tilt angles were 12.4 and 12.7 degrees versus 4.6 degrees, respectively.

Conclusions.—Subtalar stress radiography using the Telos equipment shows significant differences in subtalar and talar tilt angles between injured and uninjured ankles. Acute and chronic lateral ligament injuries are apparently associated with subtalar joint instability. This technique of measuring subtalar tilt angle may be useful in evaluating ankle joint stability before and after treatment of lateral ligament injuries. The subtalar and talar tilt angles are significantly correlated in normal ankles, but not in injured ankles.

▶ In many respects, the components of ankle instability remain an enigma. Clearly, the overwhelming majority of lateral ankle sprains respond well to conservative management. However, there are those few that require surgical reconstruction. I have always suspected that a major component in those requiring stabilization was associated subtalar instability.

J.S. Torg, M.D.

A Randomized, Prospective Study of Operative and Non-Operative Treatment of Injuries of the Fibular Collateral Ligaments of the Ankle
Povacz P, Unger F, Miller K, et al (Gen Hosp, Salzburg, Austria; Gen Hosp, Wels, Austria; Technical Univ, Innsbruck, Austria)
J Bone Joint Surg Am 80-A:345-351, 1998   3–49

Introduction.—The debate regarding operative versus nonoperative treatment of injuries of the fibular collateral ligaments of the ankle continues. This issue has not been addressed by a prospective clinical trial. The functional and radiographic findings of operative and nonoperative treatment of injuries of the fibular collateral ligaments of the ankle were analyzed in 146 adult patients.

Methods.—Patients were prospectively and blindly randomized to operative or nonoperative management. Patients had closed epiphyseal growth plates, were younger than 40 years, and had injuries within 24 hours before their initial examination. Stress radiographs were obtained for all patients. All 73 patients in the operative group had repair within 72 hours after the injury. Patients were instructed in proprioceptive muscle training and isometric exercises for the peroneal muscles after cast removal 6 weeks postoperatively. The 73 patients in the nonoperative group were managed via use of elastic wrap with ice and foot elevation for 3 to 7 days. A commercially available ankle brace was used after swelling subsided. Patients were instructed in the same exercises given to the operative group.

Results.—At a minimum follow-up of 2 years, no significant between-group differences were detected in the functional result or degree of joint laxity seen on stress radiographs. The mean time lost from work was 1.6 weeks and 7.0 weeks, respectively, for patients in the nonoperative and operative groups.

Conclusion.—Nonoperative treatment of a sprain of the fibular collateral ligaments of the ankle in young adults had results similar to those of operative treatment. Patients with nonoperative treatment had shorter recovery times and less lost time from work.

▶ The findings of this study are in keeping with the current opinion that fibular collateral ligament injuries of the ankle should be treated nonoperatively. Apparently, the injuries included partial and complete rupture of the fibular collateral ligament complex. Thus, in the operative group, only 2 patients had complete rupture of all 3 components of the ligament complex. Put another way, apparently all injuries were not equal. The data also indicated that there was a discrepancy between the patients' subjective feelings of instability and findings on physical and x-ray exams. That is, some patients with a stable joint had subjective sensations of instability, while those with objective instability reported no symptoms. I would suspect that the latter phenomenon is a function of physical therapy.

J.S. Torg, M.D.

Peroneus Brevis Tendon Tears: Pathophysiology, Surgical Reconstruction, and Clinical Results
Krause JO, Brodsky JW (Baylor Univ Med Ctr, Dallas; Univ of Texas, Dallas)
Foot Ankle Int 19:271-279, 1998   3–50

Background.—Chronic peroneus brevis tendon tears are more common than generally believed and are often overlooked or misdiagnosed. One series of patients with this injury was studied.

Patients and Findings.—Twenty patients with peroneus brevis tendon tears were seen during an 8-year period. Ten were men and 10 women, aged 27 to 63 years. Nine patients could not recall a specific precipitating traumatic event. Of the 11 patients who could, 4 had been injured during sports, 4 had twisted their ankles, 2 reported missteps with ankle dorsiflexion, and 1 had fallen. Persistent swelling along the peroneal tendon sheath was the most reliable diagnostic sign. Thirteen patients had been treated conservatively by at least 1 other physician before being seen first by the current authors. Patients were classified as having grade 1 tears, defined as 50% or less cross-sectional area involvement, or grade 2 tears, defined as more than 50% cross-sectional area involvement. The former were treated by tendon repair and the latter by tenodesis. Though return to maximal function was prolonged, most patients ultimately had good-to-excellent outcomes.

Conclusions.—Peroneus brevis tendon tears result from subclinical or overt subluxation of the tendon over the posterolateral edge of the fibula, which produces multiple longitudinal splits. Treatment is primarily operative and needs to address the split tendon as well as the subluxation that caused it. Débridement and repair are recommended for grade 1 injuries and excision of the damaged segment and tenodesis to the peroneus longus are recommended for grade 2 injuries. Stabilization of the etiologic subluxation must augment both procedures.

Peroneus Brevis Tendon in Normal Subjects: MR Morphology and Its Relationship to Longitudinal Tears
Rosenberg ZS, Rademaker J, Beltran J, et al (Hosp for Joint Diseases/Orthopaedic Inst, New York; Med School of Hannover, Germany; Univ of Puerto Rico, San Juan)
J Comput Assist Tomogr 22:262-264, 1998   3–51

Background.—Longitudinal splits of the peroneus brevis tendon are commonly thought to result from the compression of the peroneus brevis tendon by the peroneus longus tendon in dorsiflexion. However, this theory has not been proven. The shape of the peroneus brevis tendon and its relationship to the adjacent structures in the fibular groove during plantarflexion and dorsiflexion were studied to gain insight into this pathomechanism.

Methods.—MR images of the ankles of asymptomatic adult volunteers were obtained. Thirteen ankles were imaged in full dorsiflexion and plantarflexion.

Findings.—In 12 ankles, the peroneus brevis tendon was anterior or anteromedial to the peroneus longus tendon in the fibular groove. The peroneus brevis tendon was more flattened and compressed against the fibular groove by the overlying peroneus longus tendon in dorsiflexion than in plantarflexion. Fat planes were observed in plantarflexion between the peroneal tendons and between the peroneus brevis tendon and the fibular groove. In dorsiflexion, these planes were obliterated.

Conclusions.—The peroneus brevis tendon undergoes changes in configuration and in location as it moves from plantarflexion to dorsiflexion. These findings are consistent with the proposed mechanism of longitudinal tears of the peroneus brevis tendon.

▶ Chronic peroneal brevis tendon tears are not commonly diagnosed. These 2 articles (Abstracts 3–50 and 3–51) are complimentary. Rosenberg et al present the value of MR imaging in both diagnosing and explaining the pathomechanics of the lesion. Krause et al contribute information about the pathophysiologic mechanism to subluxation of the tendon over the posterior lateral edge of the fibula. Their point that débridement and repair should be augmented by stabilization of the subluxation is well made.

J.S. Torg, M.D.

Managing Injuries of the Great Toe
Churchill RS, Donley BG (Cleveland Clinic Found, Ohio)
Physician Sportsmed 26:29-39, 1998   3–52

Objective.—Injuries to the great toe are common, particularly in dancers, runners, and soccer players. The causes, symptoms, diagnosis, and treatment of hallux valgus, turf toe, hallux rigidus, sesamoid dysfunction, nail abnormalities, dislocations, fractures, calluses, and blisters were discussed.

Hallux Valgus.—This lateral deviation of the proximal phalanx and medial deviation of the first metatarsal is characterized by pain over the joint that is often worsened with weight bearing. Anteroposterior radiographs are diagnostic. Symptomatic relief can be provided by shoe modifications, bunion pads, night splits, and toe spacers. Continued pain and discomfort require surgery.

Turf Toe.—This hyperextension injury results in capsular injury of varying severity. Big toe pain; an antalgic gait; and painful passive motion of the first metatarsophalangeal (MTP) joint are characteristic. Radiographs may not be diagnostic. Turf toe is treated with rest, ice, compression dressings, elevation, and nonsteroidal anti-inflammatory drugs (NSAIDs).

Hallux Rigidus.—This painful, progressive loss of motion of the first MTP joint results from single or multiple incidents of trauma that causes osteophyte formation, leading to decreased range of motion of the great toe, swelling, and pain on walking and with passive and active hyperex-

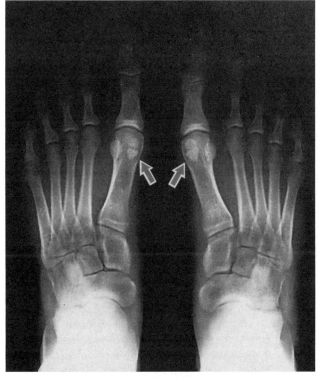

FIGURE 7.—An anteroposterior radiograph of the feet of a 25-year-old female gymnast who had no foot pain reveals bilateral bipartite sesamoids (*arrows*). The smooth, sclerotic edges are inconsistent with an acute or stress fracture, which has sharp, irregular edges. (Courtesy of Churchill RS, Donley BG: Managing injuries of the great toe. *Physician Sports Med* 26:29-39, copyright 1998. Reproduced with permission of McGraw-Hill, Inc.)

tension and maximal plantar flexion. Lateral radiographs revealing osteo-phytes are diagnostic. Treatments include rest, ice, nonsteroidal anti-in-flammatory drugs, shoe modifications, corticosteroid injections for persistent pain, and surgery to remove loose bodies.

Sesamoid Dysfunction.—Decreased range of motion of the first MTP joint and pain on dorsiflexion that is relieved by elevation are character-istic. Inflammation may or may not be present. Radiographs are usually diagnostic (Fig 7). A bone scan can distinguish between an acute fracture and a bipartite sesamoid. Treatment involves comfortable shoes and non-steroidal anti-inflammatory drugs for as long as 4 to 6 weeks. Fractures require immobilization and the use of crutches. Degenerative arthritis and osteonecrosis may require surgical excision.

Toenail Abnormalities.—For ingrown toenails, cotton is inserted be-neath the nail plate edge and changed every 5 to 7 days until the condition resolves, The patient should soak the nail twice daily in warm salt water and be instructed in nail trimming. Shoe fit should be checked. Subungual hematoma should be decompressed by penetrating the nail vertically to relieve pain.

Dislocations and Fractures.—Radiographs are diagnostic. The fracture should be immobilized and treated with rest, ice, and stiff-soled shoes. Surgery may be required for more difficult cases.

Plantar Calluses.—These result from imbalanced weight distribution. Plantar warts are painful on compression; calluses are not. Calluses are thinned by shaving and filed daily with pumice. Nonresponsive calluses may indicate an underlying structural abnormality.

Blisters.—Usually caused by new shoes, blisters should be drained with a sterile needle, if large, and covered for the first 24 hours.

Excellent Prognosis.—These conditions, with the exception of fractures and dislocations, can be managed easily and usually result in full recovery.

▶ The authors describe a taping method for turf toe injuries. They recom-mend that the tape should prevent dorsiflexion of the MTP joint beyond 30 degrees. They also state that a bipartite sesamoid may be present in 19% of the population, and 89% of these are found in the medial sesamoid. They go on to describe how a bipartite sesamoid may be differentiated from a fracture (see Fig 7).

F.J. George, A.T.C., P.T.

4 Medical Problems

Changes in Physical Fitness and Changes in Mortality
Erikssen G, Liestøl K, Bjørnholt J, et al (Central Hosp of Akershus, Norway; Univ of Oslo, Blindern, Norway; Natl Hosp, Oslo, Norway; et al)
Lancet 352:759-762, 1998   4–1

Objective.—Whereas point estimates of physical fitness are a good long-term predictor of cardiovascular mortality and all-cause mortality, they usually assume a homogeneous decline in fitness with age. Fitness patterns vary with subgroup, level of physical activity, and lifestyle. The relationships among physical fitness, changes in physical fitness, and mortality were tested in a group of apparently healthy middle-aged men.

Methods.—A cycle ergometer exercise test, physical examination, and questionnaire were given to 2,014 healthy men, aged 40 to 60 years in a 1972 to 1975 survey (survey 1). A second survey was administered to

TABLE 5.—Relative Risk of All-Cause Mortality During 13 Years' Follow-up Associated With Variables Measured at Survey 2

Characteristic	Relative Risk (95% CI) of Death (n = Events)
Age (increase of 10 years)	2·50 (1·88-3·33)†
Age-adjusted PF1 (relative to Q1 of PF1)	
Q4 (PF1)	0·60 (0·39-0·91)‡
Q3 (PF1)	0·91 (0·64-1·30)
Q2 (PF1)	0·96 (0·68-1·35)
Q1 (PF2)	1·00
Log (PF1/PF1) (increase of 0·128)*	0·70 (0·62-0·79)†
Smoking status (smokers vs non-smokers)	1·60 (1·22-2·11)†
Physical activity (active vs non-active)	0·83 (0·57-1·22)
Resting heart rate (increase of 10·1 bpm)*	1·17 (1·03-1·32)‡
Systolic blood pressure (increase of 17·7 mm Hg)*	1·15 (1·01-1·31)‡
Vital capacity (increase of 839 mL)*	0·90 (0·77-1·05)
Total cholesterol (increase of 1·2 mmol/L)*	1·05 (0·92-1·20)
Triglycerides (increase of 0·90 mmol/L)*	0·97 (0·85-1·12)
Body-mass index (increase of 2·7 kg/m2)	1·12 (1·00-1·26)
Exercise test (positive vs negative)	1·11 (0·81-1·53)

Note: Both age-adjusted physical fitness (*PF*) 1 and log (PF2/PF1) are in the model.
*Relative risk for an increase of 1 standard deviation; value of 1 standard deviation given in parentheses.
†*P* less than 0.001.
‡*P* less than 0.05.
Abbreviation: Q, quartile.
(Courtesy of Erikssen G, Liestøl K, Bjørnholt J, et al: Changes in physical fitness and changes in mortality. *Lancet* 352:759-762, copyright 1998, The Lancet Ltd.)

1,756 members of this group in 1982 (survey 2). A third survey was administered to 1,456 of the group during 1989-90 (survey 3).

Results.—The final analysis included 1,428 men followed from the date of survey 2 through December 31, 1994. At the end of the study, 234 of these men had died, 120 of cardiovascular causes and 75 of cancer. There was an inverse relationship between all-cause mortality and physical fitness (Table 5). Physical fitness was stratified by quartiles (Qs) with Q1 representing the least physically fit and Q4, the most physically fit. Using age and fitness level as predictors of death, the relative risk of death was 0.63 for Q2, 0.37 for Q3, and 0.31 for Q4, compared with Q1. Age-adjusted risk of death from all causes relative to Q1 were 0.45 for Q4, 0.48 for Q3, and 0.72 for Q2. Age-adjusted risk of death from cardiovascular causes relative to Q1 were 0.47 for Q4, 0.50 for Q3, and 0.66 for Q2.

Conclusion.—An increased level of physical fitness in men was associated with decreased all-cause and cardiovascular mortality. Improvements in fitness levels in men corresponded with improvements in risk levels. These findings may have public health policy implications.

▶ There has been only 1 previous prospective study of the relationship between an increase in fitness and changes in mortality.[1] That study reached very similar conclusions to this report, which covers a much longer period (22 years). Plainly, a long-term improvement in age-related fitness, initiated around the age of 35, carries major benefits for both overall and cardiovascular mortality. The present study controlled for a number of potentially confounding risk factors (see Table 5). Nevertheless, when such statistical adjustments are made, 1 question always remaining is whether the authors were completely successful in eliminating the impact of confounding factors. In particular, in this study, some men may have enhanced their fitness by stopping smoking, and the change in smoking behavior could conceivably have enhanced survival prospects to a greater extent than the statistical adjustment that was made for this factor.

R.J. Shephard, M.D., Ph.D., D.P.E.

Reference

1. Blair SN, Kohl HW, Barlow CE, et al: Changes in physical fitness and all-cause mortality. *JAMA* 273:1093-1098, 1995.

Intensive Lifestyle Changes for Reversal of Coronary Heart Disease
Ornish D, Scherwitz LW, Billings JH, et al (California Pacific Med Ctr, San Francisco; Univ of California, San Francisco; Univ of Texas, Houston; et al)
JAMA 280:2001-2007, 1998   4–2

Objective.—The Lifestyle Heart Trial tested whether patients with atherosclerosis could make and sustain comprehensive lifestyle changes that would reverse coronary heart disease.

Methods.—In a randomized, controlled trial conducted between 1986 and 1992, 48 patients with moderate-to-severe coronary heart disease were randomly allocated to an intensive lifestyle change group or a usual care group, and 35 completed the 5-year follow-up coronary arteriography. The intensive lifestyle change program included a 10%-fat vegetarian diet, moderate aerobic exercise, stress management training, smoking cessation, and group psychosocial support. Stenosis diameter was the outcome variable.

Results.—Over the study period, fat intake in the experimental group declined from 30% to 8.5%, cholesterol from 211 to 18.6 mg/dL, energy from 8,159 to 7724 KJ, and protein from 17% to 15%. Carbohydrates increased from 53% to 76.5%. In the control group, fat intake decreased from 30% to 25%, cholesterol from 212.5 to 138.7 mg/dL, energy from 7159 to 6581 KJ, and protein from 19% to 18%. Carbohydrates increased from 51% to 52%. Whereas patients in the experimental group lost 10.9 kg in the first year and sustained a weight loss of 5.8 kg in year 5, the body mass of the control group did not change. At 5 years, the low-density lipoprotein cholesterol levels in both groups were about 20% below baseline. Frequency of angina at 5 years was reduced by 91% in the experimental group and 72% in the control group. At 5 years, the average percentage stenosis declined by 3.1% in the experimental group and increased by 11.8% in the control group. During the trial, there were 25 cardiac events in the experimental group and 45 events in the control group (relative risk, 2.47).

Conclusion.—There was significantly more atherosclerotic regression in the experimental group than in the control group and half as many cardiac events.

▶ The original study of Dean Ornish and his colleagues,[1] showing reversal of coronary arterial occlusion over 1 year of adherence to a rigorously controlled lifestyle, attracted considerable attention. The program required more than moderate exercise; there was also a very low (10%) fat vegetarian diet, smoking cessation, and stress reduction. In many cases, it is difficult to make such lifestyle changes "stick" in the long term, and after an initial period of enthusiasm, behavior lapses. Ornish and his associates here demonstrate that given their considerable enthusiasm, patients can be persuaded to persist with a demanding regimen for 5 years, and this reaps further dividends in terms of both coronary arterial dimensions and the incidence of coronary events. The trial is relatively small in scale, and it will be interesting to see whether people can be persuaded to adhere to a similar regimen on a population-wide basis.

R.J. Shephard, M.D., Ph.D., D.P.E.

Reference

1. Ornish DM, Brown SE, Scherwitz LW, et al: Can lifestyle changes reverse coronary artherosclerosis? The Lifestyle Heart Trial. *Lancet* 336: 129-133, 1990.

Profile of Preparticipation Cardiovascular Screening for High School Athletes

Glover DW, Maron BJ (St Luke's Hosp, Kansas City, Mo; Minneapolis Heart Inst Found)
JAMA 279:1817-1819, 1998   4–3

Objective.—Interest in preparticipation screening for competitive high school athletes is increasing because of reports of sudden death in young athletes as a result of unsuspected cardiovascular disease. Preparticipation screening procedures available to high school athletes were assessed for adequacy.

Methods.—Guidelines, requirements, and screening measures of high school athletic associations from 50 states and the District of Columbia were reviewed and compared with the 1996 American Heart Association consensus panel guidelines on screening.

Results.—Whereas all jurisdictions except Rhode Island require an examination prior to athletic participation, 8 states do not have recommended history and physical questionnaire guidelines. Important cardiovascular items were included in 0% to 56% of state forms, and only 26 states required parental verification and approval of histories. Specific heart problems were addressed on only 5% to 37% of physical examination forms. Of 39 states with history and physical examination questionnaires, 16 had not revised their forms in more than 5 years and 6 had not revised their forms in more than 10 years. Seventeen of 43 state forms contained at least 9 of 13-AHA recommended items. Five of 50 states requiring preparticipation screening had no specific recommendations or requirements regarding examiners. Eleven states allow for practitioners with little or no cardiovascular training, and 25 allow examination by nonphysicians. Only 33 states recommend annual preparticipation screening.

Conclusion.—Preparticipation as it is currently practiced in U.S. high schools is unlikely to screen out potentially lethal cardiovascular problems effectively. Critically important guidelines are often missing. It is recommended that national standards be developed for preparticipation screening of high school athletes.

▶ The sudden death of a young athlete in competition has a profound societal impact. The senior researcher here has long been interested in how best to screen for the most common causes of such deaths, congenital heart conditions, especially hypertrophic cardiomyopathy. This report questions the national adequacy of preparticipation screening. Most states have approved history and physical examination questionnaires. But on perusing these questionnaires, and considering that 8 states have no questionnaires, these researchers conclude that fully 40% of state high school associations do not offer questionnaires or have screening forms that could be considered deficient by the 1996 American Heart Association scientific statement on screening. A related article concludes that a sports medicine clinic can efficiently administer preparticipation exams to a large number of athletes by using an adaptable station approach, and that the musculoskeletal component of the exam often reveals key abnormalities.[1] The senior author here has written on the good news that the courts in *Knapp v. Northwestern University* reaffirmed the primacy of the team physician in disqualifying an athlete with a medical impairment.[2]

E.R. Eichner, M.D.

References

1. Smith J, Laskowski ER: The preparticipation physical examination: Mayo Clinic experience with 2,739 examinations. *Mayo Clin Proc* 73:419-429, 1998.
2. Maron BJ, Mitten MJ, Quandt ER, et al: Competitive athletes with cardiovascular disease—The case of Nicholas Knapp. *N Engl J Med* 339:1632-1635, 1998.

Lone Atrial Fibrillation in Vigorously Exercising Middle Aged Men: Case-Control Study

Karjalainen J, Kujala UM, Kaprio J, et al (Central Military Hosp, Helsinki)
BMJ 316:1784-1785, 1998   4–4

Introduction.—Atrial fibrillation appears to be common in otherwise healthy middle-aged men who exercise vigorously. The prevalence of atrial fibrillation in middle-aged men performing intense endurance training was compared with the prevalence in men from the general population.

Methods.—Participants were 300 top level veteran orienteering runners and 495 controls. Controls had enrolled in an earlier study, were fully fit for military study at 20 years of age, and had responded in 1985 to a questionnaire on physical activity and overall health. The orienteers had been at the top of their age group in 1984. In 1995, both groups were sent questionnaires that included a question on cardiac arrhythmias. Those reporting a history of atrial fibrillation or atrial flutter were sent a more detailed questionnaire.

Results.—Orienteers had a response rate of 90%; 83% of controls responded. Compared with the general population, orienteers had much lower mortality (1.7%) than controls (8.5%), lower reported coronary heart disease since 1985 (2.7% vs. 7.5%), and fewer risk factors for atrial fibrillation. Lone atrial fibrillation was diagnosed in 5.3% of orienteers without known risk factors vs. 0.9% of controls without known risk factors. Among those with known risk factors, atrial fibrillation was also more common in orienteers than in controls (12% vs. 9%).

Conclusions.—Despite its preventive effects on coronary heart disease and premature death, vigorous long-term exercise is associated with atrial fibrillation in healthy middle-aged men. This finding may be attributed to enhanced vagal tone, atrial enlargement, and left ventricular hypertrophy.

Most of the affected orienteers responded to antiarrhythmic drugs and continued to compete.

▶ One hazard of looking at the ECG of older patients is that often there is, or appears to be, some small abnormality. As a result, many older patients face an unnecessary restriction of their physical activity. This study looked at older orienteers and found that there was a high prevalence of persistent or paroxysmal atrial fibrillation—perhaps because of vagal dominance—several times greater than in the general population. However, restriction of physical activity would have been highly inappropriate, because the mortality rate in these athletes was only about 20% of that for the general population of similar age.

R.J. Shephard, M.D., Ph.D., D.P.E.

New Walking Dependence Associated With Hospitalization for Acute Medical Illness: Incidence and Significance
Mahoney JE, Sager MA, Jalaluddin M (William S. Middleton Mem Veterans Hosp, Madison, Wis; Univ of Wisconsin, Madison)
J Gerontol 53A:M307-M312, 1998   4–5

Background.—Many elderly patients hospitalized for acute illness lose their ability to walk independently. Specific risk factors for new-onset dependence in walking have not been identified, nor do we know how long this new dependence lasts after hospital discharge. This article reviewed the incidence of new-onset walking dependence after hospitalization of elderly adults for acute medical illness, the associated risk factors, and outcomes up to 3 months after hospitalization.

Methods.—The subjects were 1,181 community-dwelling adults (59% men and 61% women) who were greater than or equal to 70 years old (mean age, 79 years) and able to walk independently before their hospitalization for acute medical illness. Within 48 hours of admission, at discharge, and 3 months after discharge, data were gathered on independent walking, the use of devices to assist walking, the reliance on other people when performing activities of daily living, and living arrangements. Subjects who could not walk across a small room without the assistance of another person were said to have walking dependence.

Findings.—At discharge, 198 subjects (16.8%) had developed new walking dependence during their hospitalization. Odds ratios (ORs) for new walking dependence were higher for subjects who had used a cane (OR, 1.5; 95% confidence interval [CI], 0.96 to 2.5), a walker (OR, 1.8; 95% CI, 1.04 to 3.2), or a wheelchair (OR, 3.2, 95% CI, 1.3 to 7.6) before hospitalization; for subjects greater than or equal to 85 years old (OR, 2.7; 95% CI, 1.5 to 4.9); for those with a primary diagnosis of cancer (OR, 2.3; 95% CI, 1.2 to 4.6); for those with more than 4 comorbid conditions (OR, 1.9; 95% CI, 1.2 to 3.0); for white subjects (OR, 1.9; 95% CI, 1.1 to 3.3); and for subjects with prehospital impairment in activities of daily living

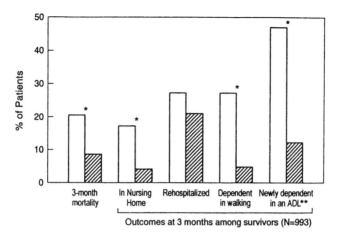

FIGURE 1.—Three-month outcomes associated with new walking dependence at hospital discharge. *Open bars*, dependent in walking at discharge; *shaded bars*, independent in walking at discharge; *P less than .001; **newly dependent in 1 or more activities of daily living (out of 5) compared to prehospitalization. (Courtesy of Mahoney JE, Sager MA, Jalaluddin M. New walking dependence associated with hospitalization for acute medical illness: incidence and significance. *J Gerontol* 53A: M307-M312, 1998. Republished with permission of the Gerontological Society of America, 1030 15th Street, NW, Suite 250, Washington, DC 20005. Reproduced by permission of the publisher via copyright Clearance Center, Inc.)

(OR, 1.4; 95% CI, 1.1 to 1.7 for each impairment). Subjects who acquired walking dependence were significantly more likely to be discharged to a nursing home and to die by 3 months after discharge than subjects who were walking independently at discharge (Fig 1). Survivors at 3 months who had new walking dependence were significantly more likely to have further limitations in activities of daily living than subjects who were walking independently at discharge. Among subjects with new walking dependence at discharge, those who used an assistive device before hospitalization were almost 5 times as likely to remain walking dependent compared to those who did not (OR, 4.87; 95% CI, 1.7 to 14.1).

Conclusions.—After hospital admission for acute medical illness, about 1 in 6 elderly who could walk independently before their hospitalization had developed walking dependence by discharge. About 1 in 4 continued to have walking dependence at 3 months, and those who used an assistive device for walking before their hospitalization were at particularly great risk for continued walking dependence. Given the poorer outcomes in subjects with walking dependence, intervention strategies are needed to prevent the loss of independent walking in the elderly.

▶ Hospital admission leads to a loss in the ability to walk independently for many elderly patients. Causes include prolonged bed rest, illness-related weakness, and a negative nitrogen balance because of poor nutrition or neoplasm. One study found that 15% of seniors who entered hospital for an acute illness subsequently required help to walk across a room,[1] and another report put the proportion who were so affected as high as 59%.[2] Much presumably depends on the age of the sample. The article by Mahoney and associates found an average figure of 16.8% in a survey of patients older than 70 years, but they also noted that an age in excess of 85 years was a risk factor for such an outcome. It is tempting for medico-legal reasons to confine elderly patients to bed; this article suggests the need to reconsider such a practice. It also indicates a number of risk factors for loss of independent walking, and it makes some good practical suggestions for increasing the potential for ambulation within a hospital, ranging from provision of appropriate clothing to ready access to assistive devices.

R.J. Shephard, M.D., Ph.D., D.P.E.

References

1. McVey LJ, Becker PM, Saltz CC, et al: Effect of a geriatric consultation team on functional status of elderly hospitalized patients: A randomized controlled clinical study. *Ann Intern Med* 110:79-84, 1998.
2. Hirsch CH, Sommers L, Olsen A, et al: The natural history of functional morbidity in hospitalized older patients. *J Am Geriatr Soc* 38: 1296-1303, 1990.

Managing Abrasions and Lacerations
Rubin A (Kaiser Permanente Sports Medicine Fellowship, Fontana, Calif)
Physician Sportsmed 26:45-55, 1998   4–6

Background.—Physicians who treat athletes must be able to quickly assess and treat skin wounds and make appropriate decisions about return to play while minimizing exposure to blood. The management of abrasions and lacerations in athletes was discussed.

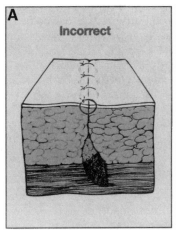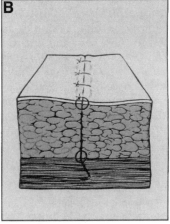

FIGURE 3.—**A,** improper wound closure—leaves dead space—a cavity where hematoma or infection can develop. **B,** with proper wound closure dead space is eliminated by placing deep, absorbable suture, such as those made from polyglycolic acid. (Courtesy of Rubin A: Managing abrasions and lacerations. *Physician Sportsmed* 26:45-55, 1998. Copyright 1998. Reproduced with permission of McGraw-Hill Inc.)

BOX.—Return to Play After an Abrasion and Laceration

When an athlete involved in a game or practice has a laceration or abrasion, the team physician must decide whether the wound is significant enough for the athlete to be excluded from play. Such decisions are not always clearcut, especially if they must be made during a game or competition.

The general guiding principle, of course, is the well-being of the athlete—including the final appearance of the wound—and others involved in the activity. Specific return-to-play considerations include:

• **Wound severity:** If the wound is a simple, superficial laceration or abrasion, the physician may close it with skin tapes and/or dress it and allow the athlete to resume play. If the laceration is more serious, the team physician must also decide whether to defer definitive treatment and treat the wound temporarily, allowing a rapid return to play, or to pull an athlete from the activity until definitive care can be provided. Return to play may be considered if an adequate temporary closure is possible and there is no associated trauma or other contraindication (as described below).

• **Type of sport:** If an athlete's wound can worsen because of forces on the skin during continued activity, he or she should be excluded from play. This is more likely in collision or contact sports.

• **Wound contamination:** If the activity increases the probability that a closed or unclosed wound will be contaminated, as might occur in swimming or rugby, a player should be sidelined.

• **Contamination of others:** If a wound cannot be protected and/or other athletes are at risk of contact with body fluids, the player should not return to play

(Courtesy of Rubin A: Managing abrasions and lacerations. *Physician Sportsmed* 26:45-55, 1998.)

Discussion.—Initial management of abrasions and lacerations includes controlling bleeding, assessing the wound site, and determining the athlete's tetanus status. Treatment of abrasions involves thorough irrigation, the use of a topical antibacterial agent, and an appropriate dressing. The treatment of lacerations include anesthetizing the area and cleaning the wound, suturing the laceration in sterile conditions (Fig 3), applying an appropriate dressing, and following up the patient in a timely manner. For some wounds, cyanoacrylate skin adhesives may be an alternative to suturing. The decision of whether the athlete may return to play is based on his or her well-being, including the final appearance of the wound, the wound severity, the type of sport, possibility of wound contamination, and contamination of other players (Box).

▶ The author recommends irrigating wounds with at least 500 mL of sterile saline under pressure through a large syringe. He recommends increasing the pressure by using an 18-gauge needle. Included is a guide for returning to activity after an abrasion or laceration.

F.J. George, A.T.C., P.T.

Comparison of the Effects of Selected Dressings on the Healing of Standardized Abrasions
Claus EE, Fusco CF, Ingram T, et al (Indiana State Univ, Terre Haute)
J Athletic Train 33:145-149, 1998   4–7

Objective.—Rapid healing of abrasions is important for athletes. Occlusive dressings have been shown to lead to more rapid healing than conventional dressings do. The healing times of abrasions and the rates of wound area reduction resulting from the use of semipermeable film, hydrocolloid, conventional method, or no dressing were compared.

Methods.—Abrasions created using sandpaper on 8 men and 6 women, aged 23 to 34, were covered with a template with circular holes. Three different dressings—a semipermeable film, a hydrocolloid, and coverlet adhesive bandage with bacitracin zinc—were randomly placed on the abraded areas in the holes. The control sites were cleansed with hydrogen peroxide and given no dressing. Wounds were cleaned, and dressings were changed and examined daily. Volunteers rated each dressing at the end of the study.

Results.—Fourteen volunteers completed the study. Whereas all dressings decreased healing time when compared with the time needed by the undressed abraded areas, there was no difference among dressings. Volunteers liked the coverlet adhesive bandage best (45%), considering it the most comfortable (36%). They thought the semipermeable film and the hydrocolloid provided the best protection. The semipermeable film and the coverlet adhesive bandage were believed to allow the wearer to conduct daily activities most easily.

Conclusion.—The semipermeable film is recommended for abrasions because it is less expensive than the hydrocolloid film and more effective than the coverlet adhesive bandage in reducing wound area.

▶ Occlusive dressings are more effective than conventional dressings in reducing the healing time of abrasions. These authors compared different occlusive dressings with each other and with a conventional dressing and concluded that there were no significant differences among the occlusive dressings. Therefore, the least expensive occlusive dressing should be used.

F.J. George, A.T.C., P.T.

An Outbreak of Methicillin Resistant *Staphylococcus aureus* Infection in a Rugby Football Team
Stacey AR, Endersby KE, Chan PC, et al (Royal Berkshire Hosp, Berks, United Kingdom; St John's Surgery, Berks, United Kingdom; Berkshire Health Authority, Reading, United Kingdom; et al)
Br J Sports Med 32:153-154, 1998   4–8

Background.—Although outbreaks of methicillin-resistant *Staphylococcus aureus* infection are common in hospitals and nursing homes, none in a community setting have been reported. An outbreak among a rugby football team is described.

Methods and Findings.—Five members of 1 team consulted the team physician about cutaneous infections unresponsive to β-lactam antibiotics prescribed by their general practitioners. All 5 were forwards who had played together in a match against a touring South Pacific team. In the 10 days after that match, the players noted large abscesses developing at various sites on their bodies, including the upper arms, back, neck, and face. The club physician obtained bacteriologic swabs from the lesions and affected sites of the players. Other team members were also screened for staphylococcal infection. Samples for analysis were also taken from 6 partly used containers of petroleum jelly from the changing room. Cultures from the affected players' lesions grew *S aureus*, resistant to penicillin and methicillin but sensitive to erythromycin, gentamicin, mupirocin, ciprofloxacin, tetracycline, and fusidic acid. The outbreak strain had an easily recognized pattern of typing. None of the other 15 squad members proved to be carrying the outbreak strain, although 7 were carrying methicillin-sensitive strains. None of the petroleum jelly containers showed methicillin-resistant *S. aureus*. The 5 affected players responded well to erthromycin or clarithromycin treatment but were removed from play until their conditions had improved. Other measures taken to control the outbreak were disinfection of training equipment and forbidding the use of communal containers of emollients.

Conclusions.—This is the first reported community outbreak of methicillin-resistant *S. aureus* outside the healthcare setting. This outbreak behaved similarly to methicillin-sensitive strains, spreading among and infecting healthy young adults in favorable conditions.

▶ This warning may also apply to wrestling teams. The antibiotic of choice seems to be clarithromycin or the like. In 1992, we covered a large outbreak of herpes gladiatorum at a high school wrestling camp in Minnesota.[1] In 1993, we reviewed other skin-to-skin infections in wrestlers, including furunculosis and tinea corporis.[2] In 1997, we reviewed other cutaneous manifestations of sports participation.[3] This report of transmission of methicillin-resistant staphylococcus infection in a rugby team expands our horizon and our concern.

E.R. Eichner, M.D.

References

1. Belongia EA, Goodman JL, Holland EJ, et al: An outbreak of herpes gladiatorum at a high-school wrestling camp. *N Engl J Med* 325:906-910, 1991. (1992 YEAR BOOK OF SPORTS MEDICINE, pp 248-249.)
2. Nelson MA: Stopping the spread of herpes simplex. A focus on wrestlers. *Physician Sports Med* 20:117-127, 1992. (1993 YEAR BOOK OF SPORTS MEDICINE, pp 447-448.)
3. Pharis DB, Tellen C, Wolf JE Jr: Cutaneous manifestations of sports participation. *J Am Acad Dermatol* 36:448-459, 1997. (1997 YEAR BOOK OF SPORTS MEDICINE, pp 429-431.)

Idiopathic Thrombocytopenic Purpura Presenting in a High School Football Player: A Case Report

Leonard JC, Rieger M (Carle Sports Medicine, Urbana, Ill)
J Athletic Train 33:269-270, 1998   4–9

Background.—Idiopathic thrombocytopenic purpura (ITP), a hemorrhagic disorder that is usually immunologic in origin, has also been associated with viral infection in children and with heroin and quinine drug use. A decreased platelet count may result in mucosal and/or deep tissue bleeding and, most important, intracranial bleeding. Thus, football players presenting with ITP-type symptoms must be removed immediately from play and referred to a physician. A case of ITP in a high school football player was presented.

>*Case Report.*—Boy, 16 years, sustained multiple contusions in a Friday evening varsity football game. Most prominent was a contusion on his chest, near the xiphoid process, which seemed to show the imprint of cleat marks. The boy also had bruises on the forearms and biceps. The team physician and athletic trainer were not overly concerned about the boy's condition. The following morning the boy participated in weight training and a 1.5-km run. On Monday he returned to school and engaged in all normal activities. However, a teammate's slap on the back resulted in ecchymosis and hemorrhage into the skin and surrounding soft tissue. At the trainer's visit, new areas of ecchymosis, not present during the postgame evaluation, were noted. The team physician was consulted, and at that time the boy reported having had an upper respiratory infection in the past 3 weeks. The neurologic examination was normal. New purpura and an increased amount of ecchymosis were observed, and the parents were contacted immediately. On further evaluation, ITP was diagnosed. Prednisone, 60 mg/day, was initiated. The boy was withheld from school for 6 days and from all sports for 30 days. He was monitored monthly for recurrence. The next season, he was able to return to football with no signs of recurrence.

Conclusions.—Athletic trainers must be aware of the signs and symptoms of ITP and its clinical presentation. Immediate intervention is needed. Traditionally, first-line treatment consists of corticosteroid medication and removal from all physical activities until the blood platelet count is normal and controlled. Because incorrect diagnosis could seriously jeopardize an athlete, the possibility of ITP must be differentiated from other disorders.

▶ This report reminds us that young athletes can develop immune thrombocytopenic purpura (ITP) that puts them at risk of bleeding. In a collision sport like football, intracranial bleeding is a feared hazard. As the authors imply, trainers and coaches should be alert to the implications of petechiae, purpura, or unusual bruising of any kind. This young man presumably had the "juvenile form" of ITP, perhaps triggered by a viral infection, that remits during corticosteroid therapy and does not recur, even when corticosteroids are tapered and stopped. On the other hand, every year or 2, I get a call from a team doctor asking about a college-age athlete with ITP. In general, it's probably safe for them to compete—even in football—if the platelet count is more than 100,000/mm^3. In adults however, ITP often recurs when corticosteroids are stopped, so splenectomy is often advised for long-term control.

In an earlier report, severe, acute ITP developed in a professional football player given quinine for muscle cramps.[1]

E.R. Eichner, M.D.

Reference

1. Powell SE, O'Brien SJ, Barnes R, et al: Quinine-induced thrombopenia. *J Bone Joint Surg* 70:1097-1099, 1988.

Sickle Cell Trait in Ivory Coast Athletic Throw and Jump Champions, 1956-1995
Bilé A, Le Gallais D, Mercier J, et al (Centre National de Médecine du Sport, Abidjan, Côte d'Ivoirie; Laboratoire Sport Santé Développement, Montpellier, France; CHU Arnaud de Villeneuve, Montpellier, France; et al)
Int J Sports Med 19:215-219, 1998   4–10

Background.—Sickle cell trait (SCT), which is widely distributed among black people, is characterized by hemoglobin S (HbS), which has a decreased affinity for oxygen. The performance of persons with SCT during brief and explosive exercise primarily involving alactic anaerobic metabolism was assessed.

Methods and Findings.—The percentage of male and female Ivory Coast track and field champions with SCT between 1956 and 1995 was investigated. Among the 122 national champions that could be contacted, 27.8% were SCT carriers. These 34 carriers had won 24.5% of national titles, and had established 43.5% of the national records. These percentages were significantly greater than the 12% prevalence of SCT in the general Ivory Coast population. The greatest percentages of record-holding SCT carriers were among athletes participating in the women's high jump (90.9%) and men's shotput events (87.5%). The top 2 national record holders and title winners—a man and a woman—were SCT carriers, whose hemoglobin S percentage and mean corpuscular volume excluded an associated alpha-thalassemia.

Conclusions.—The percentage of SCT carriers among Ivory Coast track and field champions was significantly higher than in the general population. This suggests that SCT may be a determining factor for success in brief and explosive track and field events involving mainly alactic anaerobic metabolism.

▶ As we have stated in previous reviews, rare athletes with sickle cell trait (SCT) are prone to sickling and can collapse during heroic exercise when new to altitude.[1] We have also reviewed studies suggesting that athletes with SCT may be at a disadvantage in distance races. That is, in the Ivory Coast, runners with SCT seem to be underrepresented among winners of longer races on the track and in semi-marathons. Also, in the high-altitude part of a distance race in Cameroon, SCT runners slow down more than do runners without SCT.[2] This report hints at a tradeoff: SCT athletes may have an advantage in brief and explosive track and field events. Why this should be, however, is unclear.

E.R. Eichner, M.D.

References

1. Eichner ER: Sickle cell trait heroic exercise, and fatal collapse. *Physician Sports Med* 21:51-64, 1993. (1994 YEAR BOOK OF SPORTS MEDICINE, pp 413-415.)
2. Thorsen E, Segadal K, Kambestad BK: Mechanisms of reduced pulmonary function after a saturation dive. *Eur Respir J* 7:4-10, 1994. (1995 YEAR BOOK OF SPORTS MEDICINE, pp 276-277.)

Gender Differences in Use of Stress Testing and Coronary Heart Disease Mortality: A Population-based Study in Olmsted County, Minnesota
Roger VL, Jacobsen SJ, Pellikka PA, et al (Mayo Med Ctr, Rochester, Minn; Georgetown Univ, Washington, DC)
J Am Coll Cardiol 32:345-352, 1998   4–11

Background.—The use of noninvasive procedures has been associated with the subsequent use of invasive procedures. However, no population-based data on the use of stress testing have been published. The use of exercise stress testing in relation to age and gender was investigated in a population-based setting.

Methods and Findings.—The medical records of Olmsted County, Minnesota residents undergoing exercise tests in 1987 and 1988 were reviewed. A total of 2,624 tests were performed. The crude use rate was 1,888 for 100,000 men and 703 for 100,000 women. This rate remained significantly higher in men in all age groups. The crude incidence rate of initial stress tests was 1,112 for 100,000 men and 517 for 100,000 women. The incidence increased with age among men and women. However, the incidence remained lower in women in all age groups. At the time of the initial test, women were more symptomatic and had poorer exercise performance than men did. The rate ratio of men to women for coronary heart disease mortality was 1.1. Age-adjusted rate ratios were 2.8 for stress-test use and 1.9 for coronary heart disease mortality (Table 1).

Conclusions.—The rate of stress-test use in Olmsted County was lower in women than in men. Compared with the men, women in the incidence cohort were older and more symptomatic and had poorer exercise performance.

▶ There has been much discussion in recent years about whether men and women have equal access to cardiovascular diagnostic tests and treatment. Roger and associates take the issue back 1 stage further, to exercise stress testing. Despite most of the population having medical insurance coverage, use of the procedure was 3 times more common in men, and this difference did not disappear when comparisons were restricted to the older age groups, where the risk of cardiac disease is similar in men and women.

Should women feel aggrieved at a lower frequency of stress testing? In men, a high incidence of false positive tests leads to a need for much further

TABLE 1.—Use* of Stress Tests in Olmsted County, Minnesota, 1987 to 1988

Age (yr)	Women			Men			Men/Women Rate Ratio (95% CI)	p Value
	No. of Stress Tests	Population	Rate (95% CI)	No. of Stress Tests	Population	Rate (95% CI)		
0-19	0	31,454	0 (0-0)	8	32,447	25 (8-42)		0.0080
20-29	42	18,548	226 (158-295)	71	16,645	427 (328-526)	1.9 (1.3-2.8)	0.0009
30-39	99	18,734	528 (425-638)	312	18,352	1,700 (1,513-1,889)	3.2 (2.6-4.0)	<0.0001
40-49	133	12,787	1,040 (867-1,216)	430	12,426	3,460 (3,139-3,782)	3.3 (2.8-4.1)	<0.0001
50-59	156	8,689	1,795 (1,516-2,075)	480	8,718	5,506 (5,027-5,985)	3.1 (2.6-3.7)	<0.0001
60-69	177	6,763	2,617 (2,237-2,998)	386	5,871	6,575 (5,941-7,209)	2.5 (2.1-3.0)	<0.0001
70-79	113	5,322	2,123 (1,736-2,511)	161	3,403	4,731 (4,018-5,444)	2.2 (1.8-2.8)	<0.0001
80+	28	4,041	693 (437-969)	28	1,508	1,857 (1,175-2,538)	2.7 (1.6-4.5)	<0.0001
Total	748	106,338	703 (653-754)	1,876	99,370	1,888 (1,803-1,973)	2.7 (2.5-.29)	<0.0001

*Includes all stress tests performed among local residents; each person was considered to be at risk.

Abbreviation: CI, confidence interval.

(Courtesy of Roger VL, Jacobsen SJ, Pellikka PA, et al: Gender differences in use of stress testing and coronary heart disease mortality: A population-based study in Olmsted County, Minnesota. *J Am Coll Cardiol* 32:345-352, 1998. Reprinted with permission from the American College of Cardiology.)

diagnostic investigation, with appreciable morbidity, mortality, and iatrogenic disease. Because of lower fitness levels in women, the likelihood of an adequate stress test is lower than in men, and in the age group where cardiac disease is likely, the exercise electrocardiogram is quite unreliable.[1]

R.J. Shephard, M.D., Ph.D., D.P.E.

Reference

1. Sidney KH, Shephard RJ: Training and ECG abnormalities in the elderly. *Br Heart J* 39: 1114-1120, 1977.

Evaluation of Technician Supervised Treadmill Exercise Testing in a Cardiac Chest Pain Clinic
Davis G, Ortloff S, Reed A, et al (Victoria Hosp, Blackpool, England)
Heart 79:613-615, 1998   4–12

Introduction.—Newly diagnosed patients with angina are often referred for exercise stress testing. In the United Kingdom, these tests are mainly supervised by junior doctors with various levels of cardiology experience. The efficacy and safety of having treadmill exercise tests performed independently by trained cardiac technicians were determined retrospectively.

Methods.—The study population comprised 250 patients referred with a new diagnosis of possible angina pectoris. None had a history of ischemic heart disease or contraindications to the treadmill test. Technicians who performed the tests were of senior grade and had been performing medically supervised exercise stress testing for an average of 15 years. All had been supervised for approximately 50 tests before going solo. Test results were compared retrospectively with 225 tests performed by clinical assistants and consultant cardiologists during the same period.

Results.—Patients who had testing performed by technicians or by experienced cardiology assistants and cardiologists were similar in gender distribution and mean age. A diagnostic result (positive or negative) was obtained in 76% of tests performed by technicians. Physician-supervised tests yielded similar diagnostic results (69%). Supraventricular tachycardia developed in 1 patient in the technician group during the recovery phase. The average peak work rate was lower in technician-supervised versus physician-exercised patients (7.2 vs. 8.4 mets). More tests were terminated early because of chest pain and ST segment depression in the technician group.

Conclusions.—Exercise stress testing can be performed as safely and effectively by trained technicians as by physicians. The diagnostic rate was high in the technician-supervised tests reviewed, and the complication rate low.

▶ Many hospitals and universities require physicians to provide close personal supervision of treadmill stress tests, particularly when dealing with patients who have known cardiovascular disease. However, it is logical that a technician who has been trained specifically to supervise an exercise stress test may be as effective a monitor as a physician who may have had little formal instruction in exercise testing. This report shows that a well-trained technician is as effective as an experienced cardiologist, and it urges that more effective use be made of the expertise of suitably qualified nonmedical professionals.

R.J. Shephard, M.D., Ph.D., D.P.E.

Improved Detection of Coronary Artery Disease by Exercise Electrocardiography With the Use of Right Precordial Leads
Michaelides AP, Psomadaki ZD, Dilaveris PE, et al (Univ of Athens, Greece)
N Engl J Med 340:340-345, 1999   4–13

Background.—Although it is a commonly used test, exercise ECG has low sensitivity in the detection of single-vessel coronary artery disease, even lower for the detection of right coronary artery disease. There is evidence to suggest that recordings from the right precordial leads may be useful in the detection of right coronary artery disease. The combination of right and left precordial leads was examined for sensitivity in the detection of coronary artery disease during exercise ECG.

Methods.—The study sample comprised 245 patients referred for evaluation of anginal symptoms. There were 218 men and 27 women with a

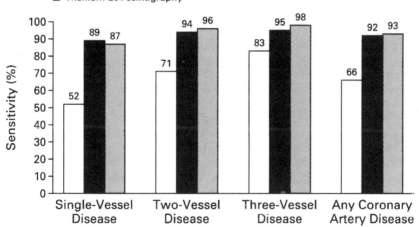

FIGURE 1.—Sensitivity of standard exercise testing with the 12-lead electrocardiogram, exercise testing with the addition of 3 right precordial leads, and ^{201}Tl scintigraphy for the detection of single-, 2-, and 3-vessel coronary artery disease and of any coronary artery disease. (Reprinted by permission of *The New England Journal of Medicine*, courtesy of Michaelides AP, Psomadaki ZD, Dilaveris PE, et al: Improved detection of coronary artery disease by exercise electrocardiography with the use of right precordial leads. *N Engl J Med* 340:340-345, copyright 1999, Massachusetts Medical Society. All rights reserved.)

mean age of 52 years. In addition to treadmill exercise ECG, each patient underwent ^{201}Tl scintigraphy and coronary arteriography. Exercise ECG was performed using the standard 12 leads and 3 right precordial leads, that is, V_3R, V_4R, and V_5R. Separate recordings and analyses were made for each set of leads. The analyses focused on the finding of exercise-induced ST-segment changes in the standard and right precordial leads.

Results.—As diagnosed by coronary arteriography, the coronary arteries were normal in 34 patients, whereas 85 had single-vessel disease, 84 had 2-vessel disease, and 42 had 3-vessel disease. Sensitivity in the detection of any coronary artery disease was 66% with standard 12-lead exercise ECG, compared with 92% for ECG with 3 additional right precordial leads and 93% with ^{201}Tl scintigraphy (Fig 1). Specificity values were 88%, 88%, and 82%, respectively. Electrocardiography with right precordial leads was also similar to ^{201}Tl scintigraphy in diagnosing disease of the left anterior descending coronary artery and the right and left circumflex coronary arteries.

Conclusion.—The combination of left and right precordial leads may enhance the value of exercise ECG for diagnosis of coronary artery disease. This technique improves sensitivity in the diagnosis of 1-, 2-, and 3-vessel disease without any loss of specificity. The use of right precordial leads is readily available and inexpensive.

▶ One major problem in diagnostic use of the exercise ECG has been the large percentage of false positive results. In a healthy population with a relatively low prevalence of disease, the false positives tend to exceed the true positive results, and diagnosis can be performed more accurately simply by tossing a coin! A low test sensitivity also leads to a substantial number of cases of coronary occlusion being overlooked. The value of any diagnostic test procedure depends, in essence, on a combination of its sensitivity and specificity. The use of right precordial leads in this study improves sensitivity from 52% to 89% for single-vessel disease, so that many fewer cases of coronary disease will be missed, but the specificity (which determines the proportion of false positive results) remains unchanged.

In my view, a false positive diagnosis in a person who is initially symptom free is a more serious error than a false negative diagnosis. The false positive test creates much unnecessary anxiety; boosts costs for the patient or health plan unnecessarily; and because of additional testing such as angiography, it causes an appreciable iatrogenic morbidity and mortality. There, thus, remains a need for a low cost, noninvasive approach with a high specificity.

R.J. Shephard, M.D., Ph.D., D.P.E.

Attenuated Physical Exercise Capacity in Smokers Compared With Non-smokers After Coronary Angioplasty Despite Similar Luminal Diameters

Jørgensen B, Endresen K, Forfang K, et al (Univ of Oslo, Norway)
Eur Heart J 19:737-741, 1998   4–14

Objective.—Exercise capacity is a measure of clinical improvement after coronary angioplasty. Because cigarette smoking is associated with a decrease in exercise capacity, and low exercise capacity is associated with increased cardiovascular mortality, the effect of smoking on exercise capacity after percutaneous transluminal coronary angioplasty was examined.

Methods.—Between April 1992 and June 1996, 334 men (77 current smokers), younger than 70 years, underwent percutaneous transluminal coronary angioplasty. Patients performed exercise tests on an electrically braked cycle ergometer 2 weeks before the procedure, and 2 weeks and approximately 19 weeks afterwards. Patients continued to receive beta blockers throughout the study.

Results.—Smokers were significantly younger than nonsmokers. There were no differences in exercise capacity between groups at baseline, but at first and second follow-up, nonsmokers had significantly increased exercise capacity and duration compared with smokers (Table 2).

Conclusion.—Whereas both smokers and nonsmokers benefited from percutaneous transluminal coronary angioplasty, exercise capacity and duration was increased substantially more in nonsmokers at all postprocedural time.

▶ It is amazing how many patients continue to smoke following cardiac surgery. I remember 1 early photo of the first 5 cardiac transplant patients in France—both the surgeon and 4 of the 5 patients were smoking. In the

TABLE 2.—Exercise Duration and Exercise Capacity in Non-smokers and Smokers at Baseline, First, and Second Follow-up

	Non-smokers (n = 257)	Smokers (n = 77)	Mean Difference	95% CI of Difference
Exercise duration (min)				
Baseline exercise test	14·9 ± 4·9	14·5 ± 5·1	0·4	−0·8 to 1·7
Follow-up exercise test 1	19·3 ± 4·4	17·2 ± 4·3**	2·1	1·0 to 3·2
Follow-up exercise test 2	18·5 ± 5·7	16·6 ± 4·9	1·9	0·5 to 3·3
Exercise capacity (W × min × kg^{-1})				
Baseline exercise test	17·6 ± 9·9	16·6 ± 8·5	1·0	−1·4 to 3·5
Follow-up exercise test 1	26·2 ± 10·5	21·0 ± 7·8**	5·2	2·6 to 7·8
Follow-up exercise test 2	25·1 ± 12·3	20·1 ± 8·7*	5·0	2·0 to 7·9

Values are means ± SD.
*P less than .01
**P less than .001 nonsmokers compared with smokers.
(Reprinted from Jørgensen B, Endresen K, Forfang K, et al: Attenuated physical exercise capacity in smokers compared with non-smokers after coronary angioplasty despite similar lumina diameters. *Eur Heart J* 19:737-741, 1998, by permission of the publisher WB Saunders Company Ltd, London.)

Toronto Rehabilitation Centre Cardiac Programme, we have found that, despite our best persuasive efforts, as many as 35% of patients—a very disappointing figure—continue to smoke, although this is less than the 80% seen before infarction. In this Norwegian series, 23% were still smoking after angioplasty. The findings offer yet 1 more reason to stop smoking. Even immediately after surgery, exercise tolerance is poorer than in non-smokers. The authors suggest that coronary vascular lesions may extend more widely in the smokers than in nonsmokers, so the benefit is less than what appears an equivalent angioplasty.

R.J. Shephard, M.D., Ph.D., D.P.E.

Improved Myocardial Ischemia Detection by Combined Physical and Mental Stress Testing
Hunziker PR, Gradel C, Müller-Brand J, et al (Univ Hosp, Basel, Switzerland)
Am J Cardiol 82:109-113, 1998   4–15

Background.—By itself, an exercise ECG or measurement of left ventricular ejection fraction (LVEF) is of limited use in the diagnosis of coronary artery disease (CAD). However, it was hypothesized that adding a measure of mental stress to the physical stress measured by the LVEF would improve the predictive value. This hypothesis was tested in people with and without CAD.

Methods.—The subjects were 10 patients with CAD (8 men and 2 women; mean age, 57) and 11 healthy controls (7 men and 4 women; mean age, 54). At baseline, the only difference between the 2 groups (other than CAD) was that the patients had a slightly but significantly lower left ventricular ejection fraction (LVEF) than the controls. Physical exercise consisted of symptom-limited cycle ergometry in three 3-minute stages. Mental exercises consisted of 9 minutes of serial subtractions by 7, starting at 2,500. Subjects performed the physical and mental exercises alone and in combination over 2 hours, with rests between tests until blood pressure and heart rate had returned to baseline. During each test, subjects rated their subjective intensity of effort, perceived psychological distress, chest pain, and dyspnea on a visual analogue scale (0-20). Radionuclide angi-

TABLE 2.—Diagnostic Value of Testing Modality for Diagnosing
Coronary Artery Disease by Radionuclide Angiography

	Mental Stress	Physical Exercise	Combined Test
Sensitivity	0.50	0.70	0.80
Specificity	0.82	0.73	0.91
Diagnostic accuracy	0.67	0.71	0.86

(Reprinted by permission of the publisher from Hunziker PR, Gradel C, Müller-Brand J, et al: Improved myocardial ischemia detection by combined physical and mental stress testing. *AMERICAN JOURNAL OF CARDIOLOGY* 82:109-113, copyright 1998 by Exerpta Medica, Inc.)

ography was used to measure LVEF, stroke volume, cardiac output, and systemic vascular resistance.

Findings.—The 21 subjects performed 63 mental stress tests and 252 physical stress tests. Maximal workrate (124 ± 37 W) was the same whether exercise was performed alone or in combination with mental stress, and both patients and controls had similar maximal workrates. Compared with mental stress alone, physical stress both alone and in combination, significantly increased mean blood pressure, heart rate, and the rate-pressure product in all subjects. Patients with CAD had a decrease in LVEF during all 3 stress modalities (lowest during the combination), whereas controls without CAD had increases in LVEF (greatest during the combination). Coronary artery disease could best be discriminated by the decrease in LVEF at peak exercise plus the decrease in LVEF during mental stress (combined sensitivity, 0.80; combined specificity, 0.91; diagnostic accuracy, 0.86) (Table 2). Subjective exercise intensity and chest pain were similar during physical exercise alone and during physical plus mental stress. However, perceived psychological distress and dyspnea were highest during the combination of physical and mental stress.

Conclusion.—The subjects responded to mental stress with a different perception of psychological distress and dyspnea. Also, the addition of mental stress to physical exercise altered circulatory responses, and led to better discrimination of CAD between patients and controls. Thus, a combination of physical and mental stress seems more useful than exercise testing alone in the noninvasive assessment of CAD.

▶ Examination of the case histories of patients who sustained their first myocardial infarction during exercise suggests that a cardiac catastrophe is particularly likely if vigorous activity is combined with psychological stress— either the excitement of intense competition or some other worrying concomitant of the activity[1] The probable mechanism is an increased secretion of catecholamines.[2] This article by Hunziker et al. confirms this finding and suggests that it can be exploited to increase the diagnostic value of an exercise stress test.

R.J. Shephard, M.D., Ph.D., D.P.E.

References

1. Shephard R.J: Sudden death: A significant hazard of exercise? *Br J Sports Med* 8:101-110, 1974.
2. Blimkie CJ, Cunningham DA, Leung FY: Urinary catecholamine excretion and lactate concentrations in competitive hockey players aged 11 to 23 years, in Lavallée H, Shephard RJ (eds): *Frontiers of Activity and Child Health*. Québec, Editions du Pélican, pp 313-321, 1977.

Response of Serum Indicators of Myocardial Infarction Following Exercise-induced Muscle Injury

Hayward R, Balog JM, Schneider CM (Univ of Arkansas, Fayetteville; Univ of Northern Colorado, Greeley)
Am J Emerg Med 16:107-113, 1998   4–16

Background.—One of the cornerstones in the diagnosis of acute myocardial infarction (AMI) is an increase in serum creatine kinase MB isoenzyme (CK-MB) activity. However, exercise-induced muscle injury can also increase CK-MB activity, which complicates the diagnosis of AMI in a patient who develops chest pain after physical activity. Other markers used to identify AMI include the total CK level and the leukocyte differential count. The changes in CK levels, CK-MB activity, and leukocyte differentials were examined in normal subjects undergoing exercises expected to cause skeletal muscle injury, and findings were compared with criteria indicating AMI.

Methods.—Twenty-one men (mean age, 35 years) refrained from exercise for 2 weeks before and 96 hours after exercise testing. Exercise testing consisted of bench-stepping a 0.5m-tall bench at a rate of 1 step/sec for 21 minutes. This task was designed to cause eccentric injury to the left knee extensor muscles and the right ankle plantar flexor muscles. Blood was sampled at baseline and up to 96 hours after exercise and tested for CK levels (normal, 23 to 170 U/L), CK-MB activity (normal, 23 to 169 U/L), total leukocyte counts (normal 4.8 to 10.8 $\times 10^9$ cells/L), and total lymphocyte counts (normal 0.96 to 3.40 $\times$ 10^9 cells/L).

Findings.—Immediately and up to 24 hours after exercise, serum CK levels were significantly increased compared with baseline. Serum CK levels peaked at 12 hours (80% greater than baseline), then declined steadily but always stayed higher than baseline. Of the 168 total CK assays performed, 49 (29%) showed abnormally elevated levels. CK-MB activity was similar to that of total CK, also peaking at 12 hours. Of the 168 CK-MB assays performed, 47 (28%) showed abnormally elevated levels. The leukocyte count increased significantly both immediately and up to 12 hours after exercise, with the peak increase occurring immediately after exercise (21% greater than baseline). The lymphocyte count increased significantly both immediately and at 12 hours after exercise, with the peak increase occurring immediately after exercise (25% increase, 38% of the level of leukocytes). The data were examined in light of various criteria used to determine AMI (Table 1). One of these criteria states a cutoff value for the lymphocyte percentage relative to leukocytes of 20.3% and a cutoff value for CK-MB activity of 13 U/L. Individually, 1.8% of the lymphocyte collection points fell below the lymphocyte cutoff, and 11% of the CK-MB collection points fell below the CK-MB activity cutoff. When these 2 cutoffs were considered together, however, at no collection point did the lymphocyte percentage and CK-MB activity fall below these cutoff values.

Conclusions.—CK-MB activity greater than or equal to 13 U/L in conjunction with a lymphocyte percentage relative to leukocytes of less than

TABLE 1.—Criteria Used in Determination of Acute Myocardial Infarction

	Total CK	CK-MB	Comment
Criterion A		>10 U/L	CK-MB > 5% of total CK
Criterion B		≥13 U/L	CK-MB increase > 50% last 4-12 hours
Criterion C	>191 U/L	CK-MB > 24 U/L	CK-MB 5.5-20% of total CK
Criterion D			Relative lymphocyte percentage <20.3% of total leukocytes
Criterion E		≥13 U/L	Relative lymphocyte percentage <20.3% of total leukocytes

(Courtesy of Hayward R, Balog JM, Schneider CM. Response of serum indicators of myocardial infarction following exercise-induced muscle injury. *Am J Emerg Med* 16:107-113, 1998.)

20.3% can reduce the misdiagnosis of AMI in patients who have recently exercised.

▶ Although a classical myocardial infarction can often be diagnosed on symptoms and signs alone, the diagnosis is difficult in a substantial proportion of cases. In such cases, considerable reliance has been placed on changes in the cardiac isoenzyme of creatine kinase (CK-MB). Unfortunately, concentrations of this isoenzyme are increased by eccentric exercise,[1,2] leading to diagnostic difficulties when investigating chest pain in a person who has engaged in a bout of vigorous physical activity.[3,4] Recently, the differential leukocyte count has been suggested as a second, independent marker of myocardial injury.[5] This also can be markedly affected by a bout of vigorous exercise in the absence of myocardial infarction.[6] Nevertheless, this study suggests that a combination of CK-MB determination and differential leukocyte count allows the detection of an infarction, with zero risk of a false-positive result.

R.J. Shephard, M.D., Ph.D., D.P.E.

References

1. Staron RS, Hikida RS, Murray TF, et al: Assessment of skeletal muscle damage in successive biopsies from strength-trained and untrained men and women. *Eur J Appl Physiol* 65: 258-264, 1992.
2. Miles M, Schneider CM: Creatine kinase isoenzyme MB may be elevated in healthy young women after submaximal eccentric exercise. *J Lab Clin Med* 122: 197-201, 1993.
3. Ordonez-Llanos J, Serra-Grima R, Gonzalez-Sastre F: Diagnostic specificity of creatine kinase-MB isoenzyme in physically active subjects. *Circulation* 89: 1447-1448, 1994.
4. Schneider CM, Dennehy CA, Rodearmel SJ, et al. The effects of physical activity on creatine kinase and the isoenzyme CK MB. *Ann Emerg Med* 25: 520-524, 1995.
5. Thomson SP, Gibbons RJ, Smars PA, et al. Incremental value of the leukocyte differential and the rapid creatine kinase-MB isoenzyme for the early diagnosis of myocardial infarction. *Ann Intern Med* 122: 335-341, 1995.

6. Shephard RJ: *Physical Activity, Training and the Immune Response*. Carmel, Ind: Cooper Publications, 1997.

Congestive Heart Failure: Training for a Better Life
Clark JR, Sherman C (Medical Fitness, Charlottesville, Va)
Physician Sportsmed 26:49-56, 1998   4–17

Objective.—Although patients with congestive heart failure (CHF) were once counseled to avoid exercise, it is now known that patients with CHF who exercise regularly improve their exercise tolerance, functional status, and quality of life.

Causes of Exercise Intolerance.—Impaired heart pumping provides less blood to muscles, accompanying pulmonary congestion interferes with alveolar oxygen transport, and weakened respiratory muscles impair ventilation. Elevated catecholamines increase vascular resistance, and increased renin output leads to pulmonary edema. Muscle atrophy and decreases in mitochondrial volume also decrease exercise capacity.

Demonstrated Exercise Benefits.—In patients with CHF who exercise, exercise tolerance improves by 26% to 37%. Quality-of-life improvements include improved ability to return to work, to remain asymptomatic during activity, and to experience minimal impairment in daily life. Functional benefits include significant improvements in walking speed, peak oxygen uptake, resting heart rate, peak power output, single-leg blood flow, a reversal of mitochondrial decline, and improvement in peripheral oxidative capacity. Exercise also benefits patients with concomitant coronary heart disease and hypertension, improves lipid profiles, and reduces the risk of diabetes. Less intensive programs have also established the benefit of exercise.

The Exercise Prescription.—The maximum benefit is obtained when patients gradually work up to exercising at 60% to 80% of maximum heart rate for 20 to 40 minutes 3 to 5 times a week after a long warm up. Strength training using light weights and many repetitions is also beneficial. Patients should discontinue exercise and seek medical attention if they experience angina, increased breathlessness, weight gain, or leg swelling. Angiotensin-converting enzyme inhibitors, vasodilators, and diuretics improve exercise capacity. Because vasodilators can cause a drop in blood pressure, dizziness, and loss of consciousness, they should not be taken before or after exercise. Water intake and sodium consumption should be carefully regulated.

When Is Exercise Contraindicated?.—Exercise can be contraindicated in the presence of obstructive valvular disease, severe aortic stenosis, viral or autoimmune myocarditis, exercise-induced arrhythmias, unstable angina, or uncompensated heart failure.

Conclusion.—A systematic, individualized exercise training program should be part of almost every CHF patient's treatment.

▶ This useful article covers a new concept, one developing over the past decade. In the old days, patients with CHF were told to avoid exercise to delay disease progression and promote diuresis induced by bed rest. Today, however, many patients are counseled to exercise prudently. Indeed, as covered here, research finds that exercise offers much gain at little risk. An exercise program in the face of CHF can improve functional status and quality of life and, possibly, reduce the risk of death. This article also covers contraindications to exercise in CHF, such as obstructive valvular disease or active myocarditis. It is accompanied by a 1-page practical guide to exercise—1 suitable for handing out to patients with CHF.

E.R. Eichner, M.D.

Early Development of EMG Localized Muscle Fatigue in Hand Muscles of Patients With Chronic Heart Failure
Buonocore M, Opasich C, Casale R (Rehabilitation Inst of Montescano, Italy)
Arch Phys Med Rehabil 79:41-45, 1998   4–18

Introduction.—Fatigue and exercise intolerance are common in patients with chronic heart failure (CHF), but these symptoms do not exhibit a direct correlation with the degree of cardiac failure. The cause of muscle fatigue is thought to be a not well-defined muscle function impairment. A group of patients with CHF underwent electromyography (EMG) to determine whether the development of localized muscle fatigue in small muscles of the hand is accelerated in CHF.

Methods.—Study participants were 11 men with a mean age of 48 years and a mean duration of CHF of 4.1 years. Etiologies were idiopathic in 4, valvular in 1, and coronary heart disease in 6. Controls were 10 sedentary age-matched men who had coronary heart disease without heart failure. All participants were right-handed and had no history of neurologic or vascular disorders. The frequency compression of EMG signal power spectrum during isometric contractions, a commonly accepted index of localized muscle fatigue, was compared in the 2 groups.

Results.—Patients with CHF tended to have higher intercepts and steeper slopes than controls at 40% of maximal voluntary contraction (MVC), but the differences were not statistically significant. Mean intercepts were 196.5 Hz for CHF patients and 177.3 Hz for controls; mean slopes were -0.90 Hz/sec and -0.81 Hz/sec, respectively. At 80% of MVC, however, patients with CHF had significantly higher intercepts and significantly lower slopes than controls. When passing from 40% to 80% MVC, there was a small increase in intercept values and a dramatic decrease in slope values among patients with CHF. In contrast, intercepts in controls were stable and slopes decreased considerably less.

Conclusions.—During the high level of contraction (80% of MVC), patients with CHF exhibited early development of localized muscle fatigue, suggesting an increased glycolytic metabolism. Muscle impairment appears not to be limited to large muscles, but occurs as well in the small muscles of the hand that are generally not included in rehabilitative programs.

▶ The metabolic demand of the interosseous muscles is extremely small, and it might be thought that even in a patient with severe congestive heart failure, there would be little difficulty in providing an adequate blood supply to prevent fatigue of these muscles. However, when the muscle is contracting at 80% of its maximal force, the local blood flow is occluded by the muscle contraction unless there is a large increase in systemic blood pressure, and the patient with congestive heart failure does not tolerate the necessary increase in after-loading of the left ventricle. Blood flow is inadequate, anaerobic work requires glycolysis, and the accumulation of lactate rapidly causes fatigued muscles.

R.J. Shephard, M.D., Ph.D., D.P.E.

The Effect of Exercises on Walking Distance of Patients With Intermittent Claudication: A Study of Randomized Clinical Trials
Brandsma JW, Robeer BG, van den Heuvel S, et al (Dutch Natl Inst of Allied Health Professions, Amersfoort, The Netherlands)
Phys Ther 78:278-288, 1998   4–19

Background.—Does an exercise program improve walking distance in patients with intermittent claudication of the lower extremity because of peripheral arterial occlusive disease? Numerous studies have addressed this question, with greatly varying test groups and methodologies. These authors performed a meta-analysis of randomized clinical trials to distil the effect that walking exercises have on the distance walked by patients with intermittent claudication.

Methods.—Searches of the MEDLINE and Dutch National Institute of Allied Health Professionals databases, and of the reference lists in the articles thus identified revealed 82 articles that assessed the effect of walking exercises on walking distance via treadmill testing. Outcomes were compared with a control group (either placebo, a different intervention, or no intervention). Of the 82 articles reviewed, 10 randomized clinical trials were selected for meta-analysis, based on an exhaustive checklist of information relative to this patient group. The authors rated the methodological quality of these 10 studies on a 100-point scale that weighed the study population, intervention, effect measurement, and data presentation/analysis.

Findings.—In the 10 studies examined, all of the groups were small (25 subjects or fewer) and most of the subjects were men (75% or more). Furthermore, half the studies involved an untreated control group. Comparison groups in the other 5 studies included those receiving medications or percutaneous transluminal angioplasty. The intensity, duration, and content of exercise programs varied greatly in these studies, as did the maximum walking distances before study entry and during treadmill test-

TABLE 3.—Exercise Variables and Effect on Walking Distance or Time

Author	Exercise Program	Frequency Duration (at Institution)	Home Program	Group*	Outcome Variable†	Preexercise	Postexercise	Percentage of Change	Remarks
Larsen and Lassen[37]	Walking only	6 mo	1 h, daily	A C	MWT	102 s 114 s	210 102	+106 −10	
Dahllöf et al[38]	"Physical training" or dynamic leg exercises	3 times/wk, 30 min 3 mo	No	A C	MWD PWD	300 m 100 m	600 225	±100 ±125	Distances estimated from figures in article No changes in control group
Ernst and Matrai[39]	Treadmill	Twice daily, 5 times weekly 2 mo	Twice daily walks	A B	MWD PWD MWD PWD	125 ± 50 m 59 ± 37 m 129 ± 50 m 64 ± 41 m	281 ± 91 120 ± 52 149 ± 93 76 ± 44	+122 +104 +16 +18	Significant improvement as compared with baseline and control values
Kiesewetter et al[29]	"Extensive physical exercises"	5 times/weekly 60 min 6 wk	No	A E	PWD	Not available	Not available	+28 +40	Short-duration program
Lundgren et al[40]	"Dynamic leg exercises," walking included	3 times/weekly 30 min Minimum 6 mo	"Encouraged" to exercise at home	A F G	MWD	183 ± 22 m 209 ± 20 m 180 ± 20 m	276 ± 66 361 ± 73 474 ± 81	+51 +73 +163	Low-intensity program

TABLE 3 (cont.)

Author	Exercise Program	Frequency Duration (at Institution)	Home Program	Group*	Outcome Variable†	Preexercise	Postexercise	Percentage of Change	Remarks
Creasy et al[41]	Walking and other dynamic leg exercises	Twice weekly/ 30 min 6 mo	Yes	A F	MWD	120 ± 28 m 127 ± 37 m	± 375 ± 225	±210 ±70	Further improvement at 9 mo C: deterioration at 9 mo
Hiatt et al[42]	Treadmill	3 times/ weekly/ 60 min 3 mo	No	A B	MWT	6.4 ± 1.7 min 6.0 ± 2.0 min	13.9 ± 3.5 7.1 ± 2.9	+165 +20	Compare time with Larsen and Lassen[37] and Mannarino et al[43]
Mannarino et al[43]	Daily walking or other exercises	Twice weekly 6 mo	1 h daily	A D E	PWT	91 ± 41 s 101 ± 35 s 90 ± 44 s	171 ± 56 137 ± 41 197 ± 52	+90 +35 +120	Compare time with Hiatt et al[44]; time difference because of differences in treadmill test: slope/speed
Hiatt et al[44]	Treadmill or strengthening exercises only, or combination	3 times/ weekly/ 60 min 3 mo	No	A B H	MWT	9.6 ± 5.7 min 6.5 ± 2.9 min 7.4 ± 3.3 min	14.7 ± 7.3 8.5 ± 5.2 7.3 ± 2.7	+74 +36 0	Crossover after 3 mo for further improvement in A; in B and H, improvement after crossover comparable to first 3 mo in A

*Group A, walking exercises; Group B, untreated; Group C, placebo drug; Group D, drugs; Group E, drugs and walking exercises; Group F, surgery; Group G, surgery and walking exercises; Group H, strength training lower extremities only.

†MWT, maximum walking time; MWD, maximum walking distance; PWD, pain-free walking distance; PWT, pain-free walking time.

(Reprinted from Brandsma JW, Robeer BG, van den Heuvel S, et al: The effect of exercises on walking distance of patients with intermittent claudication: A study of randomized clinical trials. *Phys Ther* 78:278-288, 1998, with permission of the American Physical Therapy Association.)

ing. Improvement in walking was reported variously as improvement in pain-free or maximum walking distance or time. Despite the large variance in how the studies assessed the effect of walking exercises, all 10 studies showed a positive effect, with a mean percentage improvement of 105% (range, 28% to 210%) (Table 3). The mean methodologic quality score for these 10 studies was 62.5 (range, 47 to 75).

Conclusions.—For patients with intermittent claudication, walking exercises can greatly improve pain-free or maximum walking distance and time. The randomized clinical trials examined had many methodologic flaws, however, including a lack of heterogeneity between study groups and the inclusion of patients with comorbidities. Further research is needed to determine the best duration, frequency, intensity, and type of walking program for these patients, and to determine the effects of improved walking distance and time on patients' overall quality of life.

▶ Much controversy continues regarding the effectiveness of exercise programs in the treatment of peripheral vascular disease. Costly surgical treatments often are adopted without any consideration of the possible improvements from a progressive exercise program. It is thus useful to have a carefully conducted meta-analysis that examines randomized clinical trials of exercise in patients with intermittent claudication. The authors of the meta-analysis scored all articles carefully for quality, and it is interesting that only 10 of 82 articles identified by their literature search merited inclusion in the final analysis. Even among the 10 papers selected, the quality of studies varied between 47 and 75 on a score of 0 to 100, and the reported benefit in terms of walking distance or endurance time showed gains ranging from 28% to 210%. Nevertheless, all studies showed at least some benefit. Patients with peripheral vascular disease should certainly be encouraged to exercise regularly, and this message should also be passed on to some of the surgeons involved in treating this population.

R.J. Shephard, M.D., Ph.D., D.P.E.

Circadian Variation in Acute Ischemic Stroke: A Hospital-based Study
Lago A, Geffner D, Tembl J, et al (Hospital Universitari La Fe, Valencia, Spain; Hospital General, Castellón, Spain)
Stroke 29:1873-1875, 1998   4–20

Objective.—The reason why ischemic stroke occurs more frequently in the early morning is not known. Data from a hospital-based stroke registry were examined to determine whether strokes occur more often at certain times of the day and whether different types of stroke may have different circadian variations.

Methods.—Time of symptom onset was determined for a consecutive series of 1,223 patients (527 women), aged 15 to 97 years, with ischemic stroke who were admitted at 2 reference hospitals in Spain from March

1994 and May 1996. Demographic differences and risk factors for stroke and their relationship to stroke onset time were analyzed statistically.

Results.—Of 1,049 patients with known symptom onset data, 25.6% had onset on awakening, 28.4% had lacunar stroke, 28.9% had presumed thrombotic stroke, 18.8% had presumed embolic stroke, and 17.9% had undetermined stroke. The differences in diurnal variation between presumed thrombotic and presumed embolic stroke and between lacunar and presumed embolic stroke were significant. For all strokes, there was a peak between 6 AM and noon. When patients were redistributed to the previous time frame (12:00 AM to 6 AM) based on waking time, the difference was no longer significant. There was also no significant difference in onset between first ever and recurring stroke.

Conclusion.—Thrombotic and lacunar strokes occur more frequently during sleeping hours than do embolic strokes. These results suggest that the circadian rhythm of arterial blood pressure may be disturbed in these patients.

▶ This study extends the evidence for a "morning increase" in stroke. It shows that all types of ischemic stroke (lacunar, thrombotic, embolic)—whether first-ever or recurrent—are most common between 6 AM and noon. This jibes with much evidence that most other ischemic events—angina, myocardial infarction, sudden cardiac death—are also more common in the morning. Most endogenous functions have circadian rhythms; on balance, the "stage seems set" for thrombosis or ischemia in the morning.[1] Yet the debate rages: Is it morning *exercise* that's risky, or just *morning*? Some researchers argue that it's the exercise[2]; others argue the opposite.[1] Research here will continue.

Meanwhile, experts agree that the benefits of exercise—at *any* time—vastly outweigh the risks. And mounting evidence suggests that regular physical activity reduces the risk of stroke. In the most recent study—a 14-year follow-up of some 11,000 Harvard men—walking 20 km or more a week was tied to a 30% lower risk of stroke.[3]

E.R. Eichner, M.D.

References

1. Eichner ER: Circadian rhythms: The latest word on health and performance. *Phys Sports Med* 22:82-93, 1994.
2. 1995 Year Book of Sports Medicine, pp 470-472.
3. Lee IM, Paffenbarger RS Jr: Physical activity and stroke incidence: The Harvard Alumni Health Study. *Stroke* 29:2049-2054, 1998.

The Effect of Exercise Training on the Severity and Duration of a Viral Upper Respiratory Illness

Weidner TG, Cranston T, Schurr T, et al (Ball State Univ, Muncie, Ind)
Med Sci Sports Exerc 30:1578-1583, 1998   4–21

Objective.—Although many athletes continue to compete and exercise with viral upper respiratory illnesses (URI), research has failed to establish conclusively whether exercise training during a URI prolongs or intensifies the illness. The effect of exercise training on the severity and duration of a viral URI was assessed in students in a school of physical education.

Methods.—Fifty subjects, aged 18 to 29 years, who were HRV 16 antibody–free were randomly assigned to an exercise (N = 34, 17 males) or a nonexercise (N = 16, 7 males) group. Those in the exercise group exercised to 70% of heart rate reserve. Individuals were inoculated on 2 consecutive days with HRV 16. The exercise group exercised at 70% heart rate for 40 minutes every other day for 10 days, completing a 13-item symptom severity test every 12 hours. Symptom severity scores were compared for the 2 groups.

Results.—There was no difference between groups with respect to symptom severity, preexercise and postexercise cold symptom severity scores, mucous weight measurements, or physical activity profiles.

Conclusion.—Moderate exercise does not appear to increase the symptoms and duration of viral URI.

▶ This study indicates that moderate exercise does not increase the symptoms or duration of the common cold. The key word here for most athletes and coaches is *moderate*. About 1% to 2% of the subjects had a fever over 100F.

F.J. George, A.T.C., P.T.

Exercise Effects on IFN-β Expression and Viral Replication in Lung Macrophages After HSV-1 Infection

Kohut ML, Davis JM, Jackson DA, et al (Univ of South Carolina, Columbia)
Am J Physiol 275:L1089-L1094, 1998   4–22

Background.—Previous reports have suggested that overexertion may predispose to infection. In a previous study, the authors found that exercising to fatigue suppressed alveolar macrophage intrinsic antiviral resistance to herpes simplex virus type 1 (HSV-1); mortality is higher in mice that exercise before HSV-1 exposure than in control mice. This study assessed viral replication and IFN-β production as indicators of lung macrophage resistance to HSV-1 after exercise.

Methods.—One group of mice ran on a treadmill until fatigue, after which alveolar macrophages were removed for incubation with HSV-1. Another group of mice were studied as nonexercising controls. Interferon-β mRNA content in alveolar macrophages was measured by reverse

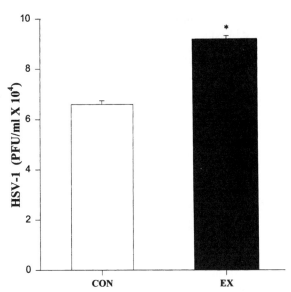

FIGURE 3.—Number of plaque-forming units (*pfu*)/mL obtained from supernatant of HSV-1-infected alveolar macrophages from exercising and control mice. Supernatants were collected at 48 hours postinfection. *Significantly higher vs. controls, *P* less than 0.05. *Abbreviations: Ex*, exercising; *Con*, control. (Courtesy of Kohut ML, Davis JM, Jackson DA, et al: Exercise effects on IFN-β expression and viral replication in lung macrophages after HSV-1 infection. *Am J Physiol* 275:L1089-L1094, 1998. Copyright The American Physiological Society.)

transcriptase-rapid polymerase chain reaction. A bioassay was used to measure IFN release, and plaque titration to assess viral replication within the macrophage.

Results.—Alveolar macrophages from exercising mice showed greater IFN-β mRNA levels than those from nonexercising mice. In infected macrophages, the level of IFN release and the number of infectious viral particles in supernatant was higher for the exercise group (Fig 3). The increased IFN-β mRNA level appeared to reflect greater viral replication.

Conclusions.—This experiment demonstrates reduced resistance to infection with HSV-1 in mice that are exercised to fatigue, a difference that probably reflects a greater degree of viral replication. Circulating catecholamines increase in response to exercise, possibly contributing to immunosuppression of macrophage antiviral function.

▶ The potential adverse effects of over-strenuous exercise on the resistance to infection have long been suspected, but the evidence, particularly self-reports of symptoms indicative of viral illness, has mostly been indirect.[1,2] Such reports are inherently unreliable, and it is good to have some direct in vitro evidence that viruses are replicating more rapidly in infected alveolar macrophages. It is hard to quantify the level of stress in small mammals, but running uphill at increasing speeds for 2.5 to 3 hours, until the treadmill speed cannot be matched even after prodding, seems rather akin to running a marathon, which is the level of stress reported to have an adverse effect on human runners.

R.J. Shephard, M.D., Ph.D., D.P.E.

References

1. Nieman DC, Johanssen LM, Lee JW, et al: Infectious episodes in runners before and after the Los Angeles marathon. *J Sports Med Phys Fitness* 30: 316-328, 1990.
2. Shephard RJ: *Physical Activity, Training and the Immune Response.* Carmel, Ind, Cooper Publications, 1997.

Evidence for Mast Cell Activation During Exercise-induced Bronchoconstriction

O'Sullivan S, Roquet A, Dahlén B, et al (Karolinska Institutet, Stockholm; McMaster Univ, Hamilton, Canada)
Eur Respir J 12:345-350, 1998   4–23

Purpose.—Up to 80% of patients with asthma experience exercise-induced bronchoconstriction (EIB). The pathophysiology of EIB is uncertain, but bronchoconstricting mediators may be released in response to hyperosmolar triggering of mast cells and other inflammatory mediators. The involvement of mast cell activation in EIB was examined.

Methods.—The study included 12 nonsmoking patients with mild asthma and a history of EIB. All performed 5 minutes of cycle ergometer exercise at 80% of maximum workrate. The occurrence of EIB was as-

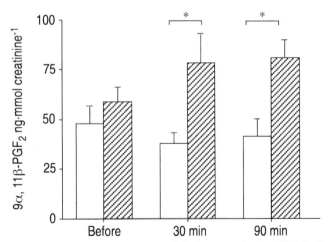

FIGURE 2.—Mean (+SEM) urinary excretion of $9\alpha,11\beta$-prostaglandin $(PG)F_2$ in the responder (*shaded bars*) and nonresponder (*white bars*) groups after 5 minutes of exercise. Asterisk indicates P less than 0.05, significant increase in levels of $9\alpha,11\beta$-PGF_2 in the responder group at 30 and 90 minutes compared with the nonresponders at the same time points. The concentration of $9\alpha,11\beta$-PGF_2 in the responder group at 90 minutes was also significantly increased (P less than 0.05) above baseline levels. (Courtesy of O'Sullivan S, Roquet A, Dahlén B, et al: Evidence of mast cell activation during exercise-induced bronchoconstriction. *Eur Respir J* 12:345-350, 1998.)

sessed by pulmonary function markers; a positive response was defined as a greater than 15% reduction in forced expiratory volume in 1 second. Before and 30 and 90 minutes after exercise, urine samples were taken for immunoassay to measure the mast cell markers $9\alpha,11\beta$-prostaglandin (PG)F_2 and Nτ-methylhistamine. Also measured was urinary leukotriene (LT)E_4, which indicates changes in whole-body cys-LT production.

Results.—Exercise-induced bronchoconstriction occurred in 7 of the 12 patients; the others showed stable pulmonary function. Patients with EIB showed a significant increase in urinary $9\alpha,11\beta$-PGF$_2$, compared with nonresponders; the difference was significant at both 30 and 90 minutes (Fig 2). The 2 groups were no different in Nτ-methylhistamine or LTE$_4$ excretion.

Conclusion.—Adult asthmatics with EIB have increased urinary excretion of the mast cell marker $9\alpha,11\beta$-PGF$_2$ in response to exercise. The findings demonstrate the association between mast cell activation and EIB in asthmatic patients. $9\alpha,11\beta$-PGF$_2$ appears to be a useful and sensitive mast cell marker.

▶ One problem in detecting mediators of EIB has been that the production of many of the substances of interest is augmented by exercise alone. Further, in the usual mild case of EIB, any response is much smaller than with the usual allergens. The substantial increase of urinary 9α, 11β-PGF$_2$ (a metabolite of prostaglandin D$_2$) in individuals in whom bronchospasm develops provides a strong pointer to involvement of mast cell–released prostaglandins in EIB. The absence of significant change in urinary excretion of N-methyl histamine agrees with earlier work[1,2] and suggests that $9\alpha,11\beta$-PGF$_2$ may be a more sensitive marker of mast cell activation than histamine metabolites.

Nevertheless, the present study found no increase in urinary leukotrienes, although another recent report has found a 2-fold increase in a group of asthmatics after an exercise challenge.[3] This points to the dangers of basing studies on small samples; given the effectiveness of cys-LT receptor antagonists, the conclusion of Reyes et al.[3] seems more credible, and leukotriene antagonists seem the most promising current development in the treatment of EIB.

R.J. Shephard, M.D., Ph.D., D.P.E.

References

1. Zimmermann A, Urbanek R, Kühr J, et al: Harnausscheidung des N-Methylhistamins (Urinary Excretion of N-Methyl Histamine). *Monatsschr Kinderheilkd* 140: 51-56, 1992.
2. Granerus G, Simonsson BG, Skoogh B-E, et al: Exercise-induced bronchoconstriction and histamine release. *Scand J Resp Dis* 52: 131-136, 1971.
3. Reiss TF, Hill JB, Harman E, et al: Increased urinary excretion of LTE4 after exercise and attenuation of exercise-induced bronchospasm by montelukast, a cysteinyl leukotriene receptor antagonist. *Thorax* 52: 1030-1035, 1997.

Effects of a 5-Lipoxygenase Inhibitor, ABT-761, on Exercise-induced Bronchoconstriction and Urinary LTE₄ in Asthmatic Patients

Lehnigk B, Rabe KF, Dent G, et al (Krankenhaus Groβhansdorf, Germany; Abbott Labs, Abbott Park, Ill)

Eur Respir J 11:617-623, 1998   4–24

Objective.—Increased urinary levels of leukotriene E_4 (LTE_4) have been found in asthmatic children after exercise. Because 5-lipoxygenase (5-LO) inhibitors have been shown to reduce bronchoconstriction in exercise-induced asthma (EIA), the effect of a single dose of the novel 5-LO inhibitor, ABT-761, on EIA and on urinary LTE_4 excretion was investigated in a placebo-controlled, double-blind, randomized, 2-period cross-over study.

Methods.—Either oral ABT-761 or placebo was administered to 10 patients with EIA 5 hours before exercise. Tests were conducted on 2 occasions at least a week apart. Lung function parameters, whole blood and urinary leukotriene B_4 (LTB_4) release, and plasma ABT-761 levels were measured at baseline, before exercise, and several times until 4 hours after exercise.

Results.—ABT-761 decreased post-exercise forced expiratory volume at 1 second (FEV_1) significantly more than placebo (27.1% vs. 19.9%). ABT-761 significantly inhibited the fall in FEV_1 after exercise by 6.47% at 5 minutes, 10.2% at 10 minutes, 15.5% at 15 minutes, and 8.07% at 30 minutes. After ABT-761 administration, the mean area under the curve,

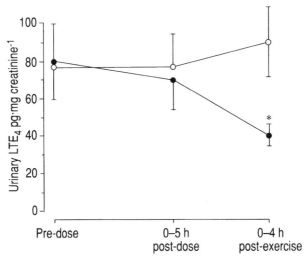

FIGURE 3.—Mean ± standard error of the mean leukotriene E_4 (*LTE₄*) concentrations in the urine of patients treated with placebo (*open circle*) or ABT-761 (*black circle*). There were no significant differences between LTE_4 levels for the 3 time periods within either group. Asterisk indicates *P* less than 0.05 compared with placebo. (Courtesy of Lehnigk B, Rabe KF, Dent G, et al: Effects of a 5-lipoxygenase inhibitor, ABT-761, on exercise-induced bronchoconstriction and urinary LTE₄ in asthmatic patients. *Eur Respir J* 11:617-623, 1998.)

representing the overall effect of exercise between 1 and 45 minutes, was significantly reduced. Return to baseline FEV_1 was significantly shorter after ABT-761 treatment than after placebo treatment (15.5 vs. 28.1 minutes). ABT-761 treatment significantly inhibited the release of LTB_4 in all patients. Urinary LTE_4 was significantly lower after ABT-761 treatment than after placebo treatment (40.1 vs. 89.8 pg/mg creatinine) (Fig 3). Inhibition of LTB_4 was significantly associated with a reduced post-exercise FEV_1 decline. ABT-761 was generally well-tolerated.

Conclusion.—ABT-761 attenuates exercise-induced asthma by inhibiting 5-LO production.

▶ Exercise-induced bronchospasm is a major problem in winter sports. Some skating programs report that as many as 20% to 25% of children are affected. The etiology is far from clear, and in addition to exercise and cold exposure, there have been suspicions that pollution of arenas may contribute to the phenomenon. In recent years, attention has also focused on the leukotrienes LTC_4, LTD_4, and LTE_4. These metabolites of arachidonic acid are produced in mast cells by the action of the enzyme 5-LO. Together, they form what was once described as the "slow reacting substance" of anaphylaxis, and they contribute particularly to the late component of exercise-induced bronchoconstriction.

Concentrations rise in the urine when asthmatic children undertake exercise.[1] It is, thus, logical to attempt to counter EIB with drugs that block 5-LO. This paper not only demonstrates empirically the effectiveness of 1 such blocking agent, it also relates the improvement in condition to the decrease in enzyme activity. Despite almost complete blockage of the enzyme, there is still some EIB, suggesting that the leukotrienes are but 1 piece of the EIB puzzle.

R.J. Shephard, M.D., Ph.D., D.P.E.

References

1. Kikawa Y, Miyanomae T, Inoue Y, et al: Urinary leukotriene E4 after exercise challenge in children with asthma. *J Allergy Clin Immunol* 89:1111-1119, 1992.

Montelukast, a Leukotriene-Receptor Antagonist, for the Treatment of Mild Asthma and Exercise-induced Bronchoconstriction
Leff JA, Busse WW, Pearlman D, et al (Merck Research Labs, Rahway, NJ; Univ of Wisconsin, Madison; Colorado Allergy and Asthma Clinic, Aurora; et al)
N Engl J Med 339:147-152, 1998   4–25

Objective.—The release of inflammatory mediators such as leukotrienes is stimulated in exercise-induced bronchoconstriction. The effect of once-daily montelukast, a leukotriene receptor antagonist, on airway hyperresponsiveness to exercise and methacholine challenges and on the overall

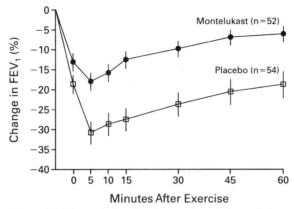

Minutes After Exercise

FIGURE 2.—Mean ± SEM changes in forced expiratory volume is 1 second after exercise challenge after 12 weeks of treatment with montelukast or placebo. Treatment with montelukast was associated with a significant ($P = .002$) reduction in exercise-induced bronchoconstriction. (Reprinted by permission of *The New England Journal of Medicine* courtesy of Leff JA, Busse WW, Pearlman D, et al: Montelukast, a leukotriene-receptor antagonist, for the treatment of mild asthma and exercise-induced bronchoconstriction. *N Engl J Med* 339:147-152, copyright 1998, Massachusetts Medical Society.)

clinical condition of patients with mild asthma was investigated in a 12-week, placebo-controlled, parallel-group study.

Methods.—After a 2-week washout/placebo period, either 10 mg montelukast (N = 54) or placebo (N = 56) was administered once daily at bedtime for 12 weeks to 110 asthma patients, aged 15 to 45 years, with exercise-induced bronchoconstriction. Exercise challenges were performed 20 to 24 hours after dosing at baseline; at weeks 4, 8, and 12; and after a 2-week washout period. Methacholine challenges were performed at baseline, at weeks 4 and 12 on nonexercise days, and after a 2-week washout period. The area under the curve (AUC) for forced expiratory volume is 1 second (FEV_1) in the first 60 minutes after exercise was the primary end point.

Results.—Six patients in the montelukast group and 7 in the placebo group did not complete the study. Montelukast provided significantly more protection against bronchoconstriction during exercise than did placebo (Fig 2). Compared with placebo, montelukast significantly improved AUC (47.4%), and, after 12 weeks of therapy, it significantly improved the maximal postexercise decrease in FEV_1 and significantly shortened the time for lung function to return to within 5% of preexercise FEV_1 at all time points. After 12 weeks of montelukast therapy, patients' global assessment of asthma control improved significantly. Montelukast patients were significantly less likely to require β-agonist rescue. Montelukast patients exhibited no rebound effect during the washout period. Methacholine challenge results were not significantly different between groups. The frequency of adverse effects was similar between groups.

Conclusion.—Montelukast provided significantly more protection than placebo against exercise-induced bronchoconstriction in asthma patients. There was no rebound effect during the washout period.

▶ In contrast to Lehnigk et al (Abstract 4–24), Leff and associates counter the action of leukotrienes by blocking their receptor sites. The immediate benefit seems similar to that obtained by blocking 5-lipoxygenase, with the severity of exercise-induced bronchospasm being approximately halved. The authors claim that tolerance to the medication did not develop over a 12-week period, although this claim must be viewed with some scepticism, as they offer no good explanation as to why this should be the case, and others have demonstrated that the body can compensate for use of this class of medication by upregulating leukotriene receptors.[1]

R.J. Shephard, M.D., Ph.D., D.P.E.

Reference

1. Adelroth E, Inman MD, Summers E, et al: Prolonged protection against exercise-induced bronchoconstriction by the leukotriene D4 receptor antagonist cinalukast. *J Allergy Clin Immunol* 99: 210-215, 1997.

Exertional Dyspnoea in Patients With Airway Obstruction, With and Without CO_2 Retention

Cloosterman SGM, Hofland ID, van Schayck CP, et al (Univ of Nijmegen, The Netherlands)
Thorax 53:768-774, 1998   4–26

Background.—Cardiopulmonary disease is commonly associated with dyspnea, which can be disabling. The mechanisms underlying this symptom are not well understood. The association between dyspnea and the load on the ventilatory muscles, chemical drive, and ventilatory indices was studied in patients with obstructive pulmonary disease during an incremental exercise test.

Methods.—Fifty patients with a broad range of obstructive pulmonary disease were included. Twenty-two patients had CO_2 retention, and 28 did not. The incremental exercise test was performed on a cycle ergometer.

Findings.—Dyspnea was significantly correlated with the increase in inspiratory time tension index (TTIi) overall and in patients without CO_2 retention. In patients with CO_2 retention, dyspnea was significantly correlated with $\Delta PaCO_2$. This factor, along with $\Delta VE\%MVV$ and $\Delta(VT/Ti)$ were associated with a *P* value of ≤ 0.10 overall and in patients without CO_2 retention. Analysis of covariance suggested that the relationship between dyspnea score and $\Delta PaCO_2$ differed significantly between the 2 groups, being more marked in the patients with CO_2 retention (Table 4).

Conclusions.—The main determinant of exertional dyspnea in normocapnic or hypocapnic patients with pulmonary disease appears to be the mechanical load and length-tension inappropriateness on ventilatory

TABLE 4.—Correlations Between Changes in Dyspnea Score and Changes in Other Indices for the Total Group and for the 2 Subgroups Independently

| | Pearson correlation coefficient | | |
	Total ($n = 50$)	Without CO_2 ($n = 28$)	With CO_2 ($n = 22$)
ΔPa_{O_2}	−0.1416	−0.2577**	−0.0487
ΔPa_{CO_2}	0.1135	−0.0378	0.4951*
$\Delta TTli$	−0.2272*	−0.3143*	−0.1467
$\Delta TTle$	0.0614	0.0619	0.0652
ΔBE	−0.0214	0.0864	−0.1976
$\Delta VE\%MVV$	0.2068**	0.1690	0.2490
ΔVE	0.0248	0.1043	−0.1066
$\Delta Work$	0.0663	0.0109	0.2267
$\Delta Ptot$	0.1502	0.1124	0.1922
ΔV_T	−0.0351	−0.0787	−0.0303
$\Delta(V_T Ti)$	0.2019**	0.2044	0.2057
$\Delta(Pi/Ti)$	0.1735	0.0685	0.2658
$\Delta Ptot\%$	0.0132	−0.1396	0.1741

Pa_{O_2}, Pa_{CO_2} = arterial oxygen and carbon dioxide tension; TTli, TTle = inspiratory and expiratory time tension index; BE = base excess; VE = minute ventilation; MVV = maximal voluntary ventilation; Ptot = total amplitude–pressure; V_T = tidal volume; Ti = inspiratory time; Pi = inspiratory pressure. *$P \leq 0.05$; **$P \leq 0.10$.

(Courtesy of Cloosterman SGM, Hofland ID, van Schayck CP, et al: Exertional dyspnoea in patients with airway obstruction, with and without CO_2 retention.*Thorax* 53:768-774, 1998.)

muscles. The occurrence of hypercapnia seems to override all other inputs for dyspnea.

▶ Dyspnea is an important symptom, and indeed, is often the factor limiting effort in older individuals as well as those with cardiac or respiratory disease. However, arguments over its physiological basis continue.[1] Contributing factors include the mechanical load on the chest muscles, the drive from the respiratory centers, hypercapnia, hypoxia, and metabolic acidosis.[2] Some suggest that the sensation of dyspnea differs between athletes and patients, being more unpleasant in the latter.[3] Although athletes may be able to suppress unpleasant sensations to achieve their competitive goals, the present observations provide some support for this hypothesis, suggesting there may be a differing physiological basis for dyspnea as carbon dioxide begins to accumulate.

R.J. Shephard, M.D., Ph.D., D.P.E.

References

1. Anonymous: The enigma of breathlessness. *Lancet* 891-892, 1986.
2. Gandevia SC, Killian K, McKenzie DK et al: Respiratory sensations, cardiovascular control, kinaesthesia and transcranial stimulation during paralysis in humans. *J Physiol* 470: 85-107, 1993.
3. Shephard RJ: *Aerobic Fitness and Health*. Champaign, Ill, *Human Kinetics Publishers*.

Physical Activity and Breast Cancer Risk in a Cohort of Young Women

Rockhill B, Willett WC, Hunter DJ, et al (Harvard Med School, Boston)
J Natl Cancer Inst 90:1155-1160, 1998   4–27

Introduction.—Increased physical activity has been suggested as a means of primary prevention of breast cancer. There is no agreement regarding the critical time of exposure or level of intensity of activity needed to influence breast cancer risk. The association between physical activity at each of 2 different times in life and breast cancer risk was assessed using data from the Nurses' Health Study II, a prospective investigation of women who were aged 25 to 42 years of age in 1989.

Methods.—On the baseline survey, respondents were asked, "While in high school, and between the ages 18 and 22 years, how often did you participate in strenuous physical activity at least twice a week?" The answers to this question were averaged to determine a measure of late adolescent activity (Table 3). Women were also questioned at baseline about the number of hours per week they currently spent in various nonoccupational activities (Table 4).

Results.—During 6 years of follow-up, invasive breast cancer was detected in 372 women. Women who were physically active in late adolescence did not have a decreased risk of receiving a diagnosis of invasive breast cancer. High levels of recent nonoccupational physical activity also were not associated with decreased risk of breast cancer.

Conclusion.—These data do not support a link between physical activity in late adolescence or in the recent past and breast cancer risk among young women. Future investigation should focus on improving the evaluation of lifetime physical activity and determining whether there is a dose-dependent relationship or an optimal time period, frequency, or intensity of physical activity with respect to diminished breast cancer risk.

▶ The association between regular physical activity and protection against all-cause cancer or colonic cancer is now well established, but the influence of exercise on the risk of breast cancer remains more controversial. Postu-

TABLE 3.—Average Level of Vigorous Physical Activity During High School and Between Ages 18 and 22 Years and Relative Risks (RRs) of Breast Cancer (95% Confidence Intervals [CIs]

	Person-years of Observation (N = 518 297)	No. of Subjects with Breast Cancer (N = 372)	Age-adjusted RR (CI)	Multivariate-adjusted* RR (CI)
Never	90 489	77	1.0	1.0
1-3 mo/y	109 639	70	0.9 (0.6-1.2)	0.9 (0.6-1.2)
4-6 mo/y	126 440	93	1.1 (0.8-1.4)	1.1 (0.8-1.4)
7-9 mo/y	112 962	78	1.1 (0.8-1.5)	1.1 (0.8-1.5)
10-12 mo/y	78 768	54	1.1 (0.8-1.6)	1.1 (0.8-1.6)

*Estimates adjusted for age at baseline, age at menarche, history of benign breast disease, history of breast cancer in mother and/or sister, recent alcohol consumption, height, oral contraceptive history, and parity and age at first birth (combination variable).

(Courtesy of Rockhill B, Willett WC, Hunter DJ, et al: Physical activity and breast cancer risk in a cohort of young women. *J Natl Cancer Inst* 90:1155-1160, 1998, by permission of Oxford University Press.)

TABLE 4.—Average Hours Per Week of Percent (1989) Moderate Plus Vigorous Physical Activity and Relative Risk (RR) of Breast Cancer (95% Confidence Interval [CIs])

	Person-years of Observation (N = 518 297)	No. of Subjects with Breast Cancer (N = 372)	Age-adjusted RR (CI)	Multivariate-adjusted* RR (CI)
<1 h/wk	174 787	124	1.0	1.0
1.0-1.9 h/wk	89 896	65	1.1 (0.8-1.4)	1.1 (0.8-1.4)
2.0-3.9 h/wk	111 716	82	1.1 (0.8-1.4)	1.1 (0.8-1.4)
4.0-6.9 h/wk	68 399	48	1.0 (0.8-1.5)	1.0 (0.7-1.4)
≥7.0 h/wk	73 499	53	1.1 (0.8-1.6)	1.1 (0.8-1.5)

*Estimates adjusted for age at baseline, age menarche, history of benign breast disease, history of breast cancer in mother/sister, recent alcohol consumption, height, oral contraceptive history, and parity and age at first birth (combination variable).

(Courtesy of Rockhill B, Willett WC, Hunter DJ, et al: Physical activity and breast cancer risk in a cohort of young women. *J Natl Cancer Inst* 90:1155-1160, 1998, by permission of Oxford University Press.)

lated mechanisms for protection of the exerciser against breast tumors include a decreased exposure to circulating ovarian hormones, and (after the menopause) a decreased synthesis of carcinogenic estrogens. Nevertheless, the difference of opinion concerning benefit is shown by a recent meta-analysis,[1] which found the variance weighted geometric mean risk of a sedentary lifestyle to be 1.22 (95% confidence interval 1.00-1.50) for premenopausal women, and 1.25 (0.98-1.61) for women after menopause. Perhaps because of the hormonal mechanism, protection is more apparent for moderate activity (risk ratio 1.41 [1.17-1.69]) than for low-intensity activity (1.26 [1.03-1.55]). The article by Rockhill and associates, which appeared after the meta-analysis, found no benefit from physical activity either as a late adolescent or as an adult. In agreement with the findings of the meta-analysis, the authors conclude that the absence of benefit may reflect the relatively low level of physical activity in the general population. To obtain benefit with a suppression of estrogen production, it is probably necessary to pursue exercise at a vigorous competitive level.

R.J. Shephard, M.D., Ph.D., D.P.E.

Reference

1. Shephard RJ, Futcher R: Physical activity and cancer: How may protection be maximized? *Crit Rev Oncogen* 8: 219-272, 1997.

Exercise-induced Anxiolysis: A Test of the "Time Out" Hypothesis in High Anxious Females
Breus MJ, O'Connor PJ (Univ of Georgia, Athens)
Med Sci Sports Exerc 30:1107-1112, 1998   4–28

Background.—Research shows that a single bout of exercise results in a small decrease in state anxiety scores in individuals without anxiety disorders. The effects of acute exercise in individuals with anxiety problems have not been widely studied.

Methods and Findings.—Fourteen female undergraduates with high trait anxiety participated in the current study. They completed 4 conditions in random order: exercise-only, consisting of 20 minutes of cycling followed by 20 minutes of recovery; study-only, consisting of 40 minutes of studying while sitting on a cycle ergometer; exercise/study, consisting of 20 minutes of cycling while studying, followed by 20 minutes of studying while sitting on the cycle ergometer; and control, in which participants sat quietly on an ergometer for 40 minutes. State anxiety was determined before and after each condition. State anxiety was decreased after the exercise-only condition. However, it was not decreased after exercising while studying.

Conclusions.—Female undergraduates with high state anxiety experience significant decreases in state anxiety after low-intensity cycling for 20 minutes. However, these reductions appear to occur because such exercise provides time away from daily worries.

▶ It has long been recognized that a bout of exercise has a short-term anxiolytic effect, with the greatest benefit in those who begin an exercise bout with a significant level of anxiety. However, the mechanisms behind the anxiolytic response have remained unclear. One of the most reasonable explanations, supported by the present study, is that exercise provides "time out" from daily worries. This has several practical corollaries. If the main reason for exercising is to reduce anxiety, then the intensity of effort is probably less important than the environment in which the activity is performed: many people will find a walk in pleasant countryside more beneficial than exercise in a noisy gymnasium. Further, the benefit from exercise will not be unique: for some people, other leisure pursuits may provide an equally effective time-out, although those pursuits are unlikely to carry other health dividends associated with regular exercise. Finally, time-out is likely to be less effective if a person is fussing about adhering to a complicated exercise prescription than if simply enjoying a modest bout of physical activity.

R.J. Shephard, M.D., Ph.D., D.P.E.

Effects of Exercise on Cognitive and Motor Function in Chronic Fatigue Syndrome and Depression
Blackwood SK, MacHale SM, Power MJ, et al (Edinburgh Univ, Scotland; Oxford Univ, England)
J Neurol Neurosurg Psychiatry 65:541-546, 1998   4–29

Background.—Patients with chronic fatigue syndrome (CFS) report physical and mental fatigue that worsens on exertion. Whether cognitive and motor responses to vigorous exercise in patients with CFS differ from those in individuals with depression and healthy individuals was determined.

TABLE 5.—Median (Range) Changes in Cognitive Test Performance, Cardiovascular Indices, and Subjective Scores From Assessments Before to After Exercise

	Controls	CFS	MDD	Kruskal-Wallis	Final Test
Digit span (forwards)	0.0 (−2 to 1)	−0.5 (−2 to 2)	0.0 (−2 to 0)	$\chi^2 = 1.2$, p = 0.6	
Digit span (backwards)	0.0 (−2 to 2)	0.0 (−2 to 2)	0.0 (−1 to 2)	$\chi^2 = 0.4$, p = 0.8	
Digit symbol substitution	2.5 (−6 to 8)	0.0 (−2 to 3)	1.0 (0 to 2)	$\chi^2 = 3.2$, p = 0.2	
Word fluency	−3.5 (−15 to 3)	−2.0 (−9 to 2)	−3.5 (−10 to 2)	$\chi^2 = 0.01$, p = 0.9	
Telephone search	−1.0 (−6 to 1)	−4.0 (−7 to −1)	−1.0 (−6 to 1)	$\chi^2 = 7.2$, p = 0.03	CFS>MDD, p = 0.03 CFS>CON, p = 0.02
Lottery	0.0 (−1 to 7)	−4.5 (−9 to 0)	−1 (−8 to 4)	$\chi^2 = 11.0$, p = 0.004	CFS>CON, p = 0.001
Change in heart rate	6.0 (−6 to 18)	1.5 (−6 to 10)	4 (0 to 12)	$\chi^2 = 0.9$, p = 0.6	
Change in systolic BP	−1.0 (−14 to 10)	1.0 (−20 to 8)	3 (−6 to 10)	$\chi^2 = 1.8$, p = 0.4	
Change in diastolic BP	−3.5 (−12 to 10)	−1.0 (−8 to 10)	1.0 (−6 to 10)	$\chi^2 = 2.1$, p = 0.4	
Change in perceived effort	0.0 (−3 to 1)	1.5 (−3 to 3)	−0.5 (−3 to 2)	$\chi^2 = 4.2$, p = 0.1	
Change in physical fatigue	0.0 (−2 to 3)	1.0 (−3 to 5)	2.0 (−6 to 6)	$\chi^2 = 4.2$, p = 0.1	
Change in mental fatigue	0.5 (−3 to 2)	1 (−5 to 4)	0.5 (−4 to 4)	$\chi^2 = 1.1$, p = 0.6	
Change in mood	0.0 (−4 to 0)	0.0 (−2 to 5)	0.5 (−4 to 3)	$\chi^2 = 4.4$, p = 0.1	

Note: Negative values in cognitive and cardiovascular scores indicate a decline in test performance from trial 1 to trial 2. Negative values in subjective ratings indicate a drop in perceived rating of effort, fatigue, or negative mood—that is, improved subjective experience.

Abbreviations: CFS, chronic fatigue syndrome; MDD, major depression disorder; CON, controls.

(Courtesy of Blackwood SK, MacHale SM, Power MJ, et al: Effects of exercise on cognitive and motor function in chronic fatigue syndrome and depression. *J Neurol Neurosurg Psychiatry* 65:541-546, 1998.)

Methods.—Ten individuals in each group underwent cognitive and muscle strength testing before and after treadmill exercise. At each stage of testing, cardiovascular functioning and perceived effort, fatigue, and mood were measured.

Findings.—At baseline, depressed individuals performed worst on the cognitive tests. During treadmill exercise, patients with CFS had greater ratings of perceived effort and fatigue than either control group, whereas depressed patients had lower mood scores. After exercise, patients with CFS had a greater reduction on everyday tests of focused and sustained attention than healthy individuals, and greater deterioration on the focused attention task than the depressed patients. The groups did not differ in cardiovascular or symptom measures obtained during cognitive testing (Table 5).

Conclusions.—Patients with CFS are particularly sensitive to the effects of exertion on effortful cognitive functioning, despite subjective and objective evidence of effort allocation in CFS. This suggests that patients with CFS have a decreased memory capacity, a higher demand to monitor cognitive processes, or both.

▶ Moderate exercise is the 1 type of therapy that seems to have some benefit in CFS.[1] On the other hand, it has also long been recognised that excessive exercise can worsen this condition, and the present demonstration of impaired cognition after a brief stress test to 85% of maximal heart rate strengthens such warnings. The authors of this report advance the interesting hypothesis that such problems may arise because the patient with CFS has a greater need to monitor both physical tasks that would otherwise be automatic and simple mental tasks. The corollary of this view is that the condition could be helped by encouraging patients to adopt a more automatic (cerebellar) approach to simple types of physical activity.

R.J. Shephard, M.D., Ph.D., D.P.E.

Reference

1. Fulcher KY, White PD. Randomised controlled trial of graded exercise in patients with the chronic fatigue syndrome. *BMJ* 314:1647-1652, 1997.

5 Physical Activity and Exercise

Comparison of Lifestyle and Structured Interventions to Increase Physical Activity and Cardiorespiratory Fitness: A Randomized Trial
Dunn AL, Marcus BH, Kampert JB, et al (Cooper Inst for Aerobics Research, Dallas; Brown Univ, Providence, RI; Baylor College of Medicine, Houston; et al)
JAMA 281:327-334, 1999   5–1

Introduction.—Despite the well-known health benefits of exercise, it is estimated that 60% of the population is inactive or has an inadequate level of physical activity. One recommended approach to increasing physical activity is lifestyle programs that concentrate on integrating moderate-intensity physical activity into everyday life. This lifestyle approach was compared with a traditional structured exercise program.

Methods.—The 2-year study included 235 men and women with a mean age of 46 years. The subjects were sedentary—with reported physical activity levels of less than 36 kcal/kg/day for men and 34 kcal/kg/day for women—and moderately overweight. They were randomized to either a lifestyle physical activity program—which used small-group cognitive and behavioral strategies to help in accumulating at least 30 minutes of moderate physical activity per day, or a traditional, structured, fitness center–based exercise program. Each group received 6 months of intensive intervention followed by 18 months of maintenance intervention. Physical activity effects were assessed using the 7-Day Physical Activity Recall and peak oxygen consumption during maximal treadmill exercise. Changes in plasma lipid profile, blood pressure, and body composition were assessed as well.

Results.—At the 24-month assessment, both groups showed significant and similar improvements in physical activity and cardiorespiratory fitness. The adjusted mean increase in activity level was 3.52 kJ/kg/day (0.84 kcal/kg/day) in the lifestyle group and 2.89 kJ/kg/day (0.69 kcal/kg/day) in the structured activity group. The increases in peak oxygen consumption were 0.77 and 1.34 mL/kg/min, respectively. Blood pressure decreased by a mean of 3.63/5.38 mm Hg in the lifestyle group and 3.26/5.14 mm Hg in the structured activity group. Although body mass did not decline

175

significantly in either group, percentage of body fat decreased by 2.39% in the lifestyle group and 1.85% in the structured activity group. There were no significant changes in lipid levels.

Conclusion.—A behaviorally based lifestyle intervention like the 1 evaluated in this study can significantly improve physical activity level and physical fitness in sedentary adults. The benefits in terms of cardiorespiratory fitness, blood pressure, and body composition are comparable to those of a traditional structured exercise program. Such lifestyle programs may help to overcome the traditional barriers to increased physical activity.

▶ There has recently been a great deal of interest in the potential for incorporating physical activity into everyday living—what Health Canada has called the "Active Living" approach.[1] Critical review of work site and community fitness programs has suggested that their impact on the average person is small, whether assessed in terms of the physical activity generated or resultant changes in markers of physical fitness.[2,3] Problems include a high dropout rate and (in the case of community programs) the time needed to travel to and from the fitness center. The incorporation of physical activity into everyday life certainly reduces the time commitment needed for exercising, and it also eliminates a need for special clothing, equipment, and membership fees.

The big question is whether the main activity of everyday life (walking) is pursued with sufficient vigor to enhance health. This depends, in part, on the age of the individual and, in part, on the speed of walking; particularly in younger individuals, walking is unlikely to be of much benefit unless a rapid pace is adopted. The study by Dunn and colleagues is the first experimental comparison of the 2 apporaches, and it certainly suggests that active living is as effective as structured interventions in enhancing the health of initially very sedentary older adults.

R.J. Shephard, M.D., Ph.D., D.P.E.

References

1. Shephard RJ: Physiological responses to structured vs. lifestyle activities, in Leon AS (ed): *Physical Activity and Cardiovascular Health: A National Consensus.* Champaign, Ill, Human Kinetics, 1997.
2. Dishman RK, Oldenburg B, O'Neal H, et al: Worksite physical activity interventions. *Am J Prev Med* 15:344-361, 1998.
3. Shephard RJ: Do work-site exercise and health programs work? *Physician and Sportsmedicine* 27:48-72, 1999.

A Systematic Review of Physical Activity Promotion in Primary Care Office Settings

Eaton CB, Menard LM (Brown Univ, Pawtucket, RI)
Br J Sports Med 32:11-16, 1998   5–2

Objective.—The positive health effects of physical activity are well known. Yet 70% of Britons and 60% of Americans are sedentary. Whether office-based counseling from primary care physicians would increase physical activity is unknown. Results are presented of a systematic review that investigated evidence that physical activity counseling in primary care office practice is efficacious and evaluated the generalizability of these results to normal primary care office practice.

Methods.—A computerized search of MEDLINE, Dialog(R) of Dissertation Abstracts and Sci Li Reference from 1961 to 1997 turned up 20 relevant articles. Eight trials (13,981 individuals from 203 practices) met the criteria for the presence of control groups, for doctor's office interventions, and for exercise behavior assessment ≥4 weeks after intervention, from which odds ratios could be calculated.

Results.—Although 5 trials showed positive effects on physical activity efforts after physician intervention, one had only a 28% response, another had a potential selection bias due to use of nonparticipants as the control group, a third abandoned randomization, and the remainder did not comply with the exercise duration and frequency recommendations. Four of 4 short-term trials showed positive results, 3 of 3 single–risk-factor trials had positive results, and 2 of 3 randomized trials gave positive results. One of 4 large, long-term trials yielded positive results.

Conclusion.—The limited evidence available suggests that promotion of physical activity by office-based physicians works. Office-based physicians should do more to promote physical activity.

▶ Dr. Terence Kvanagh and I have recently been questioning the offspring of patients enrolled in our cardiac program, and we have been surprised to find that, even in this high-risk group, family physicians make little effort to enhance lifestyle by suggesting an increase in physical activity and adoption of a prudent diet. This is particularly unfortunate, since the majority of patients still respect the advice of their doctors, and as this article from Eaton and Menard demonstrates, physical activity promotion can be remarkably effective in a primary care office setting. There seems to be 2 reasons why more physicians do not engage in health promotional activities: (1) the time required for counseling is not adequately compensated in current fee schedules, and (2) a lack of background in sports medicine, preventive medicine, and exercise prescription inhibits physician involvement. Both factors could be corrected—the latter by a change in medical school curricula and the organization of refresher courses on exercise prescription for established practitioners.

R.J. Shephard, M.D., Ph.D., D.P.E.

Barriers to Physical Activity Promotion by General Practitioners and Practice Nurses

McKenna J, Naylor P-J, McDowell N (Univ of Bristol, UK; Ministry of Health, Victoria, BC, Canada)
Br J Sports Med 32:242-247, 1998   5–3

Background.—Physical activity is beneficial in preventing and treating many health problems. General practitioners (GPs) and practice nurses (PNs) have a role in promoting physical activity. The barriers to activity promotion by GPs and PNs were reported.

Methods.—A confidential questionnaire was mailed to 574 GPs and 272 PNs in 118 general practices in southwest England. Response rates exceeded 70%.

Findings.—Sixty-nine percent of GPs and PNs said that they regularly promote physical activity in their practices. GPs reporting lack of time or lack of incentives as barriers were less likely to discuss physical activity regularly with their patients. GPs who exercised themselves were more likely to promote exercise among patients. The strongest predictor of exercise promotion for PNs was personal physical activity stage (Table 3).

TABLE 3.—All Staff: Logistic Regression Results to Predict Active Promoting Staff From Preactive Staff Using Five Barrier Variables and Dichotomized Own Activity Stage of Change

Variable	β	Wald (z)	Significance	Odds Ratio	95% Confidence Interval
Barriers					
Lack of time (1-5)	−0.39	13.17	0.0003	0.67	0.55 to 0.84
Lack of success (1-5)	0.01	0.02	0.86	1.01	1.01 to 1.24
Lack of resources (1-5)	0.02	0.06	0.79	1.02	1.02 to 1.26
Lack of protocols (1-5)	−0.00	0.00	0.99	0.99	1.00 to 1.24
Lack of incentives (1-5)	−0.25	5.88	0.01	0.77	0.77 to 0.95
Demographic					
Own activity stage of change (1 or 2)	1.21	30.00	0.0001	3.38	2.17 to 5.19
Age (years) (1-4)*	−0.08	0.21	0.64	0.91	1.33 to 1.57
Years in current role (1-4)†	−0.05	0.07	0.78	0.94	1.38 to 1.52
List size (1-4)‡	−0.20	2.24	0.13	0.81	1.26 to 1.31
Hours of PA promotion training (1-2)§	0.01	0.2	0.79	1.02	1.02 to 1.24
GP:patient ratio (1-4)‖	0.49	2.91	0.06	1.24	1.05 to 1.63
PN:patient ratio (1-4)¶	−0.09	0.45	0.50	0.90	1.20 to 1.43
Duration of consultations (min) (1-4)**	0.46	6.11	0.01	1.58	1.08 to 1.71
Constant	1.21	2.15	0.14		

N=470.

All variables labeled 1-4 were divided into quartiles to achieve this grouping. Quintiles 1 to 4 for each variable.

*Age: up to 37 years, 37.1 to 42 years, 42.1 to 48 years, more than 48 years.

†Years in current role: up to 8, 8.1 to 15 years, 15.1 to 22 years, more than 22 years.

‡List size: up to 5,500 patients, 5,501 to 7,500 patients, 7,501 to 10,856 patients, more than 10,856 patients.

§Hours of exercise promotion training: up to 3.75 hours, more than 3.75 hours.

‖GP to patient ratio: up to 1,612.5, 1,612.6 to 1,850, 1,851 to 2,033.3, more than 2,033.3.

¶PN to patient ratio: up to 2,200 patients, 2,201 to 3,000 patients, 3,001 to 3,833.3 patients, more than 3,833.3 patients.

**Duration of patient consultations: up to 8.5 minutes, 8.6 to 10 minutes, 10.1 to 12.5 minutes, more than 12.5 minutes.

Variables shown in bold indicate significant ($P<0.05$) predictors.

Abbreviations: GP, general practitioner; *PN*, practice nurse.

(Courtesy of McKenna J, Naylor P-J, McDowell N: Barriers to physical activity promotion by general practitioners and practice nureses. *Br J Sports Med* 32:242-247, 1998.)

Conclusions.—GPs who exercise are 3 times more likely to regularly encourage patients to exercise than GPs who are not beginning or maintaining physical activity. This variable quadruples the likelihood of PNs promoting physical activity.

▶ A number of early reports suggested that a disappointingly low proportion of family physicians were encouraging their patients to exercise,[1-4] and it is encouraging to see that this situation is now changing. As in many areas of behavior, actions speak louder than words. The physician or nurse who is already committed to exercise is perceived more favorably,[5] and is a more effective advocate than the health practitioner who is not personally involved in a physical activity program. It is particularly interesting that the behavior of the health provider has a much greater impact than the commonly cited barriers to physical activity, such as lack of time on the part of the health care provider.

Time is certainly an important consideration when giving advice on exercise, and in the case of nurses, even a small increase in the time allowed per patient (1-2 minutes) increased the likelihood that advice would be offered.

R.J. Shephard, M.D., Ph.D., D.P.E.

References

1. Godin G, Shephard RJ: An evaluation of the potential role of the physician in influencing community exercise behavior. *Am J Health Prom* 4:255-259, 1990.
2. Iversen D, Fielding J, Crow R, et al: The promotion of physical activity in the U.S. population: The status of programs in medical, worksite, community and school settings. *Publ Health Rep* 100:212-224, 1985.
3. Wechsler H, Levine S, Idelson R, et al: The physician's role in health promotion—A survey of primary care practitioners. *N Engl J Med* 308:97-100, 1983.
4. Wyshak G, Lamb GA, Lawrence RS, et al: A profile of the health promoting behavior of physicians and lawyers. *N Engl J Med* 303:104-107, 1983.
5. Belcher DW, Berg AO, Inui TS: Practical approaches to providing better preventive care: Are physicians a problem or a solution? *Am J Prev Med* 4:27-48, 1988.

Advice on Exercise From a Family Physician Can Help Sedentary Patients to Become Active

Bull FC, Jamrozik K (Univ of Western Australia, Nedlands, Perth)
Am J Prev Med 15:85-94, 1998   5–4

Background.—Lack of physical activity is an important public health problem. The impact of family physicians' (FPs') verbal advice combined with supporting written information on physical activity level among patients seen in a primary care setting was studied.

Methods.—Of 6,351 sedentary adults in FP practices who completed a screening questionnaire, 763 were assigned to a treatment or control group. The FPs provided verbal advice on exercise to the patients, who were then mailed a pamphlet on exercise within 2 days. Physical activity level was assessed at 1, 6, and 12 months after the initial visit. Follow-up

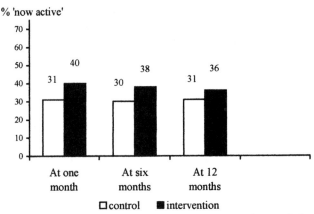

FIGURE 2.—Proportion of subjects "now active" at follow-up at 1, 6, and 12 months by experimental group with nonresponders treated as sedentary. (Courtesy of Bull FC, Jamrozik K: Advice on exercise from a family physician can help sedentary patients to become active. *Am J Prev Med* 15:85-94, copyright 1998 by Elsevier Science Inc.)

data on 70%, 60%, and 57% of the patients, respectively, were available. All patients not responding to telephone interviews were considered sedentary.

Findings.—At 1 month, 40% of the patients in the combined intervention group reported doing some physical activity, compared with 31% in the control group, a significant difference. At 6 months, 38% and 30%, respectively, reported that they were "now active." At 12 months, the corresponding percentages were 36% and 31% (Fig 2).

Conclusions.—This FP intervention effectively increases physical activity levels among patients in a primary care setting. These findings underscore the potential contribution of FPs to national goals for reducing physical inactivity.

▶ The good news from this study is that the FP can make a difference in the exercise habits of a large random sample of sedentary patients, given a brief (30-60 minutes) training period by an expert in health promotion. The test of impact of the simple regimen (discussion of a health questionnaire, advice on exercise, and a follow-up pamphlet mailing) is a conservative one, because control subjects are presumed to have been uninfluenced by completion of the health questionnaire and those who do not respond to follow-up questionnaires are assumed to have reverted to a sedentary lifestyle. Nevertheless, 1 month after receiving advice, the number of sedentary individuals who became active was 40%, compared with 31% of the control subjects who merely completed a health questionnaire.

The bad news is that it is very easy for good habits to disappear with time; the difference in the percentage of active individuals relative to the control group drops to 8% at 6 months, and 5% at 12 months. However, most patients will be back to see their FP within a year, and this offers the opportunity to reinforce the exercise message.

R.J. Shephard, M.D., Ph.D., D.P.E.

Cost-effectiveness of a Primary Care Based Physical Activity Intervention in 45-74 Year Old Men and Women: A Randomised Controlled Trial
Stevens W, Hillsdon M, Thorogood M, et al (London School of Hygiene and Tropical Medicine; West London Health Promotion Agency, Middlesex, England)
Br J Sports Med 32:236-241, 1998   5–5

Background.—The positive effects of physical activity on health and disease have recently been substantiated. Because a high proportion of the general population is seen in primary care settings each year, the cost-effectiveness of a primary care–based intervention to increase activity levels among inactive adults was explored.

Methods.—Seven hundred fourteen inactive persons seeking care at 2 West London general practices were randomly assigned to an intervention or control group. Intervention consisted of consultation with an exercise development officer and a personalized 10-week program to increase regular physical activity level, combining health club and home-based exercise.

Findings.—The intervention reduced the proportion of patients classified as sedentary by 10.6% compared with the control group at 8 months. In addition, the mean number of episodes of physical activity per week increased compared with the control group. The cost of moving a patient from the sedentary to the active group was £650. The cost of moving a patient to the activity level now commonly recommended for health was about £2500 (Table 6).

Conclusions.—A primary care–based intervention can effectively promote moderate physical activity among previously sedentary persons aged 45 to 74 years. The most important cost variable was the process of recruitment. A high uptake rate would maximize the cost-effectiveness of

TABLE 6.—Cost-effectiveness of the Intervention

	Reduction in No. of Sedentary People	Increase in No. of People Who Are Active	Movement Into Higher Level of Physical Activity
Total cost	£24 043	£24 043	£24 043
Gross shift (%)	11.2	5.8	21
Net shift (%)	10.6	2.7	20
People equivalent*	38	10	73
Cost per person	£623	£2498	£327

*N = 363.
(Courtesy of Stevens W, Hillsdon M, Thorogood M, et al: Cost-effectiveness of a primary care based physical activity intervention in 45-74 year old men and women: A randomized controlled trial. *Br J Sports Med* 32:236-241, 1998.)

the intervention. With more effective recruiting methods, unit costs could be reduced by half.

▶ This program's impact on exercise behavior seems similar to that achieved by family physician counseling, except an exercise development officer at one of Britain's publicly funded leisure centers carried out this intervention. The costs of shifting people from sedentary to more active behavior appear relatively high, although the estimates may be somewhat inflated, because there is an assessment for design and production of a questionnaire (which presumably would be available in a subsequent trial). Also if the development officer were not conducting a research study, he or she might have time to deal with a larger number of sedentary people. Further, it is admitted that costs would have been lower if more people could have been recruited to the present study. Given the apparent similarity of exercise response rate between the development officer, the family physician, and the registered nurse, it would be interesting to compare costs for these 3 types of individuals, and possibly also for other well-qualified staff. It is also important to note that the data are for 1 development officer— others might be more or less effective. Several alternative cost assessments are cited in the present analysis; if we assume that the objective is to get a sedentary person doing something, the cost is £623 per person (about $1,250), but if we look at the cost of moving someone who is already taking some activity to the level recommended in recent reports,[1] the alarming figure of £2,498 (about US $5,000) is obtained. Plainly, such figures could hardly be sustained on a population-wide basis.

One important issue that must be decided is whether it is sufficient to get people doing something, in the short term,[2] or whether the CDC/ACSM recommendation must be met rapidly, which seems to have a fourfold impact on the costs of exercise promotion.

R.J. Shephard, M.D., Ph.D., D.P.E.

References

1. Pate RR, Pratt M, Blair SN, et al: Physical activity and public health: A recommendation from the Centers for Disease Control and Prevention and the American College of Sports Medicine. *JAMA* 273:402-407, 1995.
2. Haskell WL: Health consequences of physical activity: Understanding and challenges regarding dose response. *Med Sci Sports Exerc* 26:649-660, 1994.

Six-Month Physical Activity and Fitness Changes in Project *Active*, a Randomized Trial
Dunn AL, Garcia ME, Marcus BH, et al (Cooper Inst for Aerobics Research, Dallas; Vanderbilt Univ, Nashville, Tenn; Brown Univ, Providence, RI; et al)
Med Sci Sports Exerc 30:1076-1083, 1998   5–6

Introduction.—A sedentary lifestyle is associated with low cardiorespiratory fitness and increased morbidity and mortality. In the elderly, physical inactivity leads to loss of function and other nonfatal health problems. A need for alternatives to structured exercise programs, which are not widely adopted, led to the development of a lifestyle physical activity approach. The 6-month outcome was reported for this program, known as Project Active.

Methods.—Project Active is a randomized clinical trial designed to evaluate 2 different physical activity interventions: a new, lifestyle treatment and a standard, structured treatment. The lifestyle treatment consists of a behavioral, group process intervention designed to help participants integrate more physical activity into their daily routines. The 235 participants were healthy but sedentary and aged 35 to 60 years. Clinical measurements were obtained at baseline and after 6 months of intervention.

Results.—Those in Project Active were given membership in a state-of-the-art health club and asked to exercise at least 3 days a week for 30 minutes. They also met regularly with a health psychologist. Both lifestyle and structured groups significantly increased their energy expenditure over baseline, and both spent significantly less time sitting and significantly more time walking and stair climbing. The goal of increasing physical activity 12.5 kJ·kg^{-1} (3 kcal·kg^{-1}) was achieved by 21% of the lifestyle group and 14% of structured participants. Increases in moderate activity from baseline were significantly greater in the lifestyle group. Compliance was good in both groups.

Conclusions.—In this group of sedentary men and women, both the structured exercise intervention and the intensive lifestyle intervention succeeded in increasing physical activity and fitness during a 6-month period. The lifestyle approach is an option that may benefit some individuals more than the structured approach.

▶ There has been much talk about "active living" in recent years. The suggestion is to incorporate the physical activity needed for health into our normal daily lives. Although the suggestion is logical, it has to date had little formal appraisal. Here, a well-designed, randomized, clinical trial shows that during a 6-month period, the active living intervention is as effective as a formal exercise program in increasing physical activity and enhancing fitness. There remains a need for longer-term observations, because dropouts from the formal program are likely to increase progressively with time. Because of lower opportunity costs, the lifestyle approach is more likely to be sustained in the long term.

R.J. Shephard, M.D., Ph.D., D.P.E.

Scaling of Submaximal Oxygen Uptake With Body Mass and Combined Mass During Uphill Treadmill Bicycling

Heil DP (Univ of Massachusetts, Amherst)
J Appl Physiol 85:1376-1383, 1998   5–7

Background.—During uphill bicycling at a given ground speed and inclination, heavier cyclists are believed to expend less energy than lighter cyclists relative to their body mass (M_B). This is because the bicycle and gear as part of the combined mass (M_C) are proportionally a smaller part of the M_C for heavier cyclists. Therefore, submaximal oxygen intake ($\dot{V}O_2$) should be directly proportional to M_C but less than proportional to M_B. This study tested this hypothesis during uphill treadmill bicycling.

Methods.—The subjects were 25 competitive cyclists (23 men and 2 women; mean age, 24.7). Peak $\dot{V}O_2$ was tested at the first visit by having subjects pedal to exhaustion on an incremental cycle. On the second visit, the subject's M_B (mean, 73.9 ± 8.8 kg) and M_C (mean, 85.0 ± 9.0) were measured. Then $\dot{V}O_2$ was again measured while subjects were tested on 4 treadmill grades (1, 2, 3, and 4 degrees, or 1.7%, 3.5%, 5.2%, and 7.0% inclines) for 6 minutes each at a fixed treadmill speed of 3.46 m/sec. Net oxygen intake ($\dot{V}O_{2(net)}$) during exercise was calculated by subtracting the subject's resting $\dot{V}O_2$ from the peak $\dot{V}O_2$. Then the $\dot{V}O_{2(net)}$ data were pooled during multiple log–linear regression analysis, and differences in treadmill grade and dynamic friction were controlled to arrive at the exponents for M_B and M_C.

Findings.—Mean $\dot{V}O_{2(net)}$ differed significantly between the 4 grades (1.10 ± 0.17, 1.67 ± 0.22, 2.26 ± 0.25, and 2.88 ± 0.32 L/min for the 1-, 2-, 3-, and 4-degree slopes). Statistical regression of $\dot{V}O_{2(net)}$ on M_C showed that $\dot{V}O_{2(net)}$ increased in proportion to M_C raised to the power 0.99. Statistical regression of $\dot{V}O_{2(net)}$ on M_B showed that $\dot{V}O_{2(net)}$ increased in proportion to M_B raised to the power 0.89.

Conclusion.—During uphill bicycling, $\dot{V}O_{2(net)}$ is directly proportional to the combined mass of the cyclist, the bicycle, and any other equipment (ie, M_C). This scaling relationship exists independently of grade and road speed. The $\dot{V}O_{2(net)}$ scaled less than proportionally with the cyclist's mass (ie, M_B) because the extra mass associated with gear is proportionally lighter for heavier cyclists.

▶ Methods of scaling biological data to allow for differences in M_B have long fascinated exercise scientists. Although theoretical arguments can be advanced for the use of various exponents of M_B, in many tasks the M_B must be displaced. It is thus most logical to express data per unit of M_B. In a number of sports such as cycling, the competitor must not only displace M_B against gravity but must also move a machine, and in such a situation, it is an advantage to have a large M_B; the weight of the machine then accounts for a relatively small fraction of the mass to be displaced. This report provides experimental proof of this concept, based on data collected during fixed-speed uphill treadmill cycling.

R.J. Shephard, M.D., Ph.D., D.P.E.

Sustained Submaximal Exercise Does Not Alter the Integrity of the Lung Blood-Gas Barrier in Elite Athletes
Hopkins SR, Schoene RB, Henderson WR, et al (Univ of California, San Diego; Univ of Washington, Seattle)
J Appl Physiol 84:1185-1189, 1998   5–8

Background.—When capillary pressure increases during exercise, the extreme thinness of the pulmonary blood-gas barrier results in high mechanical stresses in the capillary wall. In a previous study of elite cyclists, 6 to 8 minutes of maximal exercise increased blood-gas barrier permeability, causing increased concentrations of red blood cells, total protein, and leukotriene B_4 in bronchoalveolar lavage (BAL) fluid. The hypothesis that stress failure of the barrier occurs only at the highest level of exercise was tested.

Methods.—Six healthy athletes underwent BAL after 1 hour of exercise at 77% maximal oxygen consumption. Eight healthy nonathletes who did not exercise before BAL made up a control group.

Findings.—Compared with control participants, the athletes did not have greater concentrations of red blood cells, total protein, or leukotriene B_4. However, prolonged exercise was associated with increased concentrations of surfactant apoprotein A and with a higher surfactant apoprotein A-to-phospholipid ratio.

Conclusions.—The integrity of the blood-gas barrier is apparently affected only by maximal physiologic stresses. Such a result would be expected if the blood-gas barrier is regulated continuously to meet all but the most extreme physiologic stresses.

▶ Bleeding from the lung during racing is common in thoroughbred horses and can also occur in Shetland ponies and greyhound dogs. It has been reported—in association with pulmonary edema—in human athletes, especially ultramarathoners and swimmers as well.[1,2] These authors earlier found that in elite athletes brief, maximal exercise results in higher concentrations of red blood cells and protein in fluid from BAL. The conclusion was that intense exercise can impair the pulmonary blood-gas barrier in elite athletes.[3] Intense exercise can evoke mechanical stress failure of lung capillaries, leading to hemoptysis. This article shows that 1 hour of submaximal exercise is not sufficient stress to cause the lung capillaries to fail. In other words, heavy but submaximal exercise would not be likely to cause hemoptysis.

E.R. Eichner, M.D.

References

1. McKechnie JK, Leary WP, Noakes TD, et al: Acute pulmonary oedema in two athletes during 90-km running race. *S Afr Med J* 56:261-265, 1979.
2. Weiler RD, Shupak A, Goldenberg I, et al: Pulmonary oedema and haemoptysis induced by strenuous swimming. *BMJ* 311:361-362, 1995.
3. Hopkins SR, Schoene RB, Henderson WR, et al: Intense exercise impairs the integrity of pulmonary blood-gas barrier in elite athletes. *Am J Respir Crit Care Med* 155:1090-1094, 1997.

Cardiac Responses to Exercise in Child Distance Runners
Rowland T, Goff D, Popowski B, et al (Baystate Med Ctr, Springfield, Mass; Univ of Massachusetts, Amherst)
Int J Sports Med 19:385-390, 1998   5–9

Objective.—Trained athletes have a higher maximal stroke volume, probably because of a larger resting end-diastolic volume and a continuous rise in stroke volume during progressive exercise, whereas nonathletes have plateaus in stroke volume above low-to-moderate exercise intensities. Cardiovascular dynamics during exercise in children have not been well studied, although it is known that well-trained child endurance runners do not have "athlete's heart." Doppler echocardiography was used to characterize cardiac variables in response to progressive exercise in trained child distance runners and compared with those of nontrained children and of adults.

Methods.—Eight trained prepubertal male runners, aged 9 to 13 years, and 14 male prepubertal nontrained but active controls performed cycle testing at a constant rate of 50 rpm with initial and incremental workloads of 25 W in 3-minute stages to exhaustion. Patterns of heart rate, stroke

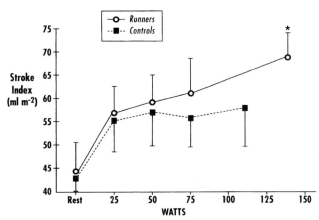

FIGURE 2.—Changes in stroke index during progressive exercise in child distance runners (N = 8) and nontrained controls (N = 14). *Asterisk* indicates *P* less than 0.05 for runners versus controls. (Courtesy of Rowland T, Goff D, Popowski B, et al: Cardiac responses to exercise in child distance runners. *Int J Sports Med* 19:385-390, copyright 1998, Georg Thieme Verlag.)

volume, cardiac output, aortic flow velocity, and systolic ejection time were determined by Doppler echocardiography.

Results.—Stroke index and cardiac index were significantly higher in runners than in controls (68 vs 58 mL/m^2 and 11.05 vs 13.09 L/min/m^2, respectively) (Fig 2). Mean stroke indices for both groups were comparable at baseline. As work intensity increased, stroke index increased in runners but remained stable in controls. As heart rate increased, ejection time decreased by 24% in runners and by 15% in controls.

Conclusion.—Trained child runners have a higher maximal stroke volume than untrained child runners but lack the larger resting stroke volume found in adult athletes.

▶ "Athlete's heart" in adults confers a greater stroke volume and cardiac output at top exercise. The higher peak stroke volume in adult athletes stems from a larger resting end-diastolic volume and a steady rise in stroke volume during progressive exercise. Conversely, stroke volume in nonathletes plateaus as exercise progresses.

This study reminds us that athlete's heart was defined in adult, male athletes. Children are different. For example, prior research shows that child runners do not have left ventricular enlargement comparable to adult athletes. This study finds no difference in resting stroke volume of child athletes vs. nonathletes. In other words, child athletes lack the larger resting stroke volume of adult athletes. Yet, as in adult athletes, child runners had a steady rise in stroke volume as workload increased, whereas child nonathletes did not.

Do differences in athlete's heart in children versus adults reflect training duration or biological influence? Probably both. For example, a study of 600 elite female athletes finds the features of athlete's heart differ between adult female and male athletes. That is, left ventricular cavity size does not increase as much in females. More striking, in female athletes, left ventricular wall thickness rarely, if ever, exceeds normal limits. So distinguishing athlete's heart from hypertrophic cardiomyopathy seems a problem only in male athletes.[1]

E.R. Eichner, M.D.

Reference

1. Pellicia A, Maron BJ, Culasso F, et al: Athlete's heart in women: Echocardiographic characterization of highly trained elite female athletes. *JAMA* 276:211-215, 1996.

Seven-Year Change in Graded Exercise Treadmill Test Performance in Young Adults in the CARDIA Study

Sidney S, Sternfeld B, Haskell WL, et al (Kaiser Permanente Med Care Program, Oakland, Calif; Stanford Univ, Calif; Univ of Minnesota, Minneapolis; et al)

Med Sci Sports Exerc 30:427-433, 1998   5–10

Background.—Previous studies of changes in physical fitness have had some methodological flaws. Seven-year changes in physical fitness in a population of young, racially diverse men and women are reported.

Methods.—Change in exercise treadmill test performance was evaluated in 1,962 participants, aged 18 to 30 years at baseline. Both blacks and whites were represented in this cohort. The participants completed symptom-limited graded exercise treadmill tests at baseline and 7 years later.

Findings.—During the 7 years, mean test duration declined by 9.5%. The decline was 13.6% among black men, 11.1% among black women, 7.4% among white men, and 7% among white women. Mean time to heart rate 130, which measures submaximal performance, declined by 11.3% overall—16.9% in black men, 12.3% in black women, 10% in white men, and 6.1% in white women. Baseline body mass index and physical activity did not significantly predict test duration change in any race or gender group. However, changes in body mass index and activity did. A 7-year weight gain of more than 20 lb, occurring in 31% of the cohort, was correlated with an 18.5% decline in mean duration and a 21.8% decline in mean time to heart rate.

Conclusions.—Fitness apparently declines during young adulthood in both black and white women and men. These changes in fitness are associated with changes in weight and in physical activity levels.

▶ This article provides epidemiologic proof of our national decline. In a 7-year follow-up of young adults, fitness declined in all race and both gender groups, with black men showing the largest decline and white women the smallest decline. The change in fitness correlated strongly with weight change and also with change in physical activity. A weight gain of 20 lb was tied to a fitness decline of about 20%. This article also suggests that, with the exception of black women, a similar decline in fitness has occurred in young adults aged 25 to 30, surely because nearly everybody these days is sitting around too much and getting fat.

E.R. Eichner, M.D.

Effects of Respiratory Muscle Work on Cardiac Output and Its Distribution During Maximal Exercise

Harms CA, Wetter TJ, McClaran SR, et al (Univ of Wisconsin, Madison)
J Appl Physiol 85:609-618, 1998   5–11

Background.—Recent research has shown that changes in the work of breathing during maximal exercise affect blood flow and vascular conductance in the leg. This study determined the effects of changes in the work of breathing on cardiac output (CO) during maximal exercise.

Methods.—Eight men performed repeated 2.5-minute bouts of cycle exercise at VO_{2max}. Inspiratory muscle work was performed either at unmodified levels, decreased by a proportional-assist ventilator or increased through resistive loads.

Findings.—Stroke volume, CO, and pulmonary O_2 consumption did not differ between standard and loaded trials at VO_{2max}. However, these values were lower than standard figures with inspiratory muscle unloading at VO_{2max}. Loading and unloading did not affect the arterial-mixed venous O_2 difference (Fig 7).

Conclusions.—Respiratory muscle work normally expended during maximal exercise has 2 significant effects on the cardiovascular system. First, up to 14% to 16% of the CO is directed to the respiratory muscles. Second, local reflex vasoconstriction significantly compromises blood flow to leg locomotor muscles.

▶ Many people do not realize the heavy demands that respiratory muscles place on circulation and oxygen transport during vigorous exercise.[1,2] The present findings are for healthy and relatively fit young cyclists, with a

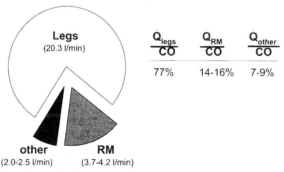

FIGURE 7.—Distribution of total CO among legs, respiratory muscles (RM), and other metabolically active tissues (skin, heart, brain, kidneys, and liver) at VO_{2max}. CO is the mean value measured in our subjects at VO_{2max} control (26.5 ± 0.8 L/min). Leg blood flow (Qlegs) was also measured under control conditions at VO_{2max} (20.3 L/min). Respiratory muscle blood flow (QRM) at VO_{2max} was assumed to be equal to measured fall in CO obtained with respiratory muscle unloading at VO_{2max} and extrapolated to zero Wb (26.5 − 22.3 = 4.2 L/min). Range of blood flows to RM (14% to 16%) and to other nonskeletal muscle tissues (Qother; 7% to 9%) represents values based on our present measurements for RM extrapolated to zero levels for Wb (16% and 7%) and those values that take into account published values for nonskeletal muscle blood flow (14% and 9%). (Courtesy of Harms CA, Wetter TJ, McClaran SR, et al: Effects of respiratory muscle work on cardiac output and its distribution during maximal exercise. *J Appl Physiol* 85:609-618, 1998.)

maximal oxygen intake of 62 mL/[kg.min]; the demands of the respiratory muscles may be somewhat less in more sedentary young adults who do not push their chests to maximal performance. On the other hand, the costs of breathing are likely to be even greater in the older individual whose respiratory system has deteriorated because of many years of exposure to air pollutants, cigarette smoke, and bronchial disease.

The measurement of CO during maximal exercise with respiratory unloading is an ingenious approach. Yet the authors themselves admit that part of the observed decrease in CO during unloading may reflect changes in intrathoracic pressure and thus venous return, rather than a reduction in the work of the chest muscles. The estimate that 14% to 16% of total CO is diverted to the chest muscles in a healthy young adult may be an overestimate. Nevertheless, it certainly emphasizes the importance of minimizing respiratory work rates. In the subjects tested by Harms and associates, the oxygen consumption available to the working muscles is likely to have been less than 48 mL/[kg.min] rather than the 62 mL/[kg.min] seen in the maximal oxygen intake test, with a corresponding limitation in the performance of useful external work.

R.J. Shephard, M.D., Ph.D. D.P.E.

References

1. Shephard RJ. Oxygen cost of breathing during vigorous exercise. *Q J Exp Physiol* 51:336-350, 1966.
2. Aaron EA, Seow KC, Johnson BD, et al: Oxygen cost of exercise hyperpnea: Implications for performance. *J Appl Physiol* 72:1818-1825, 1992.

Reversible Ischemic Colitis in a High Endurance Athlete
Lucas W, Schroy PC III (Boston Med Ctr)
Am J Gastroenterol 93:2231-2234, 1998   5–12

Objective.—Long-distance runners experience a variety of gastrointestinal problems, but hemorrhage is relatively rare. A rare case of severe ischemic colitis was reported in an elite marathon runner.

> *Case Report.*—Woman, 30 years, with moderately severe hematochezia and abdominal pain was evaluated after completing a marathon. She had lower abdominal cramps and bloody diarrhea after completing 4 miles of the race. Her condition improved and then worsened at the end of the race, and she passed blood without stool. She had practiced by running 180 miles/week at an altitude of 10,000 feet. The patient had mild left lower-quadrant tenderness, enlarged external hemorrhoids, bright red blood, a leukocyte count of 26,000/mm³, a hematocrit of 48.9%, and a serum creatinine phosphokinase value of 1,287 U/mL. A sigmoidoscopy showed patchy erythema, friability, exudate in the proximal rec-

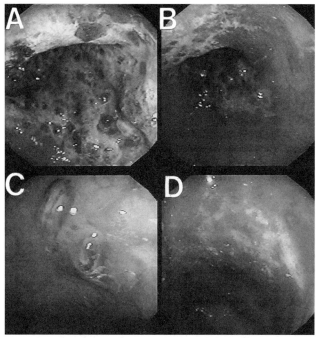

FIGURE 1.—Endoscopic findings of ischemic colitis. Sigmoid colon with segmental narrowing, marked hyperemia, submucosal hemorrhage, nodularity, and fibrinopurulent exudate (**A, B**). Focal inflammatory changes in rectum (**C**). Region of moderately severe segmental colitis in rectosigmoid junction (**D**). (Courtesy of Lucas W, Schroy PC III: Reversible ischemic colitis in a high endurance athlete. *Am J Gastroenterol* 93:2231-2234, copyright 1998 by Elsevier Science Inc.)

tum, and severe nodular hemorrhagic segmental colitis in the sigmoid colon (Fig 1). Ischemic injury was confirmed by biopsy (Fig 2).

The patient was treated with vigorous IV hydration, and her symptom resolved within 24 hours. She was given clear liquids on day 2 and then a regular diet. She remained asymptomatic. MR arteriography/venography revealed normal anatomy and flow within the abdominal aorta and mesenteric vessels. Stool samples were negative for pathogens. Results of a hypercoagulation workup were negative. A day 4 sigmoidoscopy showed improvement of ischemic changes in the rectum but not in the sigmoid. The patient was discharged on day 4. Sigmoidoscopy at 6 weeks showed complete resolution of colitis, with no recurrence at 24 months.

Discussion.—Mesenteric blood flow decreases by as much as 80% during intensive exercise, primarily because of high sympathetic tone. Symptoms generally improve in conditioned vs unconditioned athletes with exercise. A literature review turned up 6 cases, 5 of which resolved similarly and 1 which required subtotal colectomy for perforation. The ischemia that occurred in the proximal colon in 5 of the 6 patients reflects

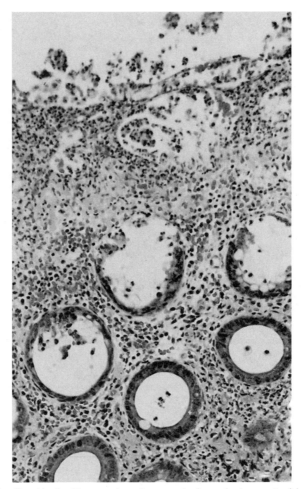

FIGURE 2.—Sigmoid colon biopsy specimen demonstrating hemorrhagic necrosis of the mucosa with stromal hemorrhage, crypt effacement, and mucopurulent exudate; hematoxylin-eosin; original magnification, ×95. (Courtesy of Lucas W, Schroy PC III: Reversible ischemic colitis in a high endurance athlete. *Am J Gastroenterol* 93:2231-2234, copyright 1998 by Elsevier Science Inc.)

ischemic colitis in other low-flow states, probably because of a vasospastic reflex and shunting. Segmental involvement has not been previously reported.

In the case presented here, the use of oral contraceptives may have exacerbated the condition because they have been linked to spontaneous ischemic colitis. The patient also had mild polycythemia resulting from high-altitude training. The ischemic process probably began during training and worsened during the race because of shunting of mesentery blood, chronic dehydration, and, possibly, small-vessel occlusive disease or anatomical anomalies.

▶ This elite female runner experienced bloody diarrhea at the 4-mile mark of a highly competitive marathon, yet hung tough for 22 miles to finish, after which she passed frank blood without stool. She had severe ischemic colitis. Fortunately, with conservative therapy, she recovered fully. It is not widely known that ischemic colitis is a hazard of distance racing. Mesenteric blood flow can fall by 80% during peak exercise. Dehydration likely augments the problem of perfusing the gut during a long race. Yet some athletes will not stop despite dire warning signals. I know of 3 endurance athletes (1 recreational runner, 2 elite triathletes) in whom—during distance races—ischemic colitis so severe developed that they ended up with subtotal colectomy!

E.R. Eichner, M.D.

Sensitivity of Reticulocyte Indices to Iron Therapy in an Intensely Training Athlete
Ashenden MJ, Dobson GP, Hahn AG (Australian Inst of Sport, Canberra; James Cook Univ of North Queensland, Townsville, Australia)
Br J Sports Med 32:259-260, 1998   5–13

Objective.—Iron-deficiency anemia is a particular problem for female athletes. Because low serum ferritin values are not a reliable indication of iron deficiency anemia, other more accurate measures are desirable. Whether automated blood cell counters that analyze reticulocytes are sensitive to iron deficiency in intensely training athletes was assessed.

Case Report.—Woman, 18, a female international-level volleyball player, had a hemoglobin concentration of 11.4 g/dL and a

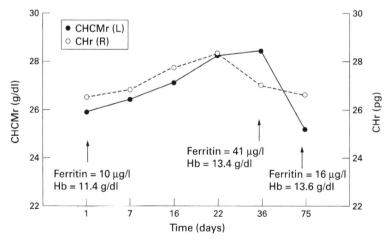

FIGURE 1.—Concentration (*CHCMr*, left axis) and amount (*CHr*, right axis) of hemoglobin in reticulocytes of an iron-deficient female volleyball player receiving oral iron supplementation. *Abbreviation: Hb*, serum hemoglobin. (Courtesy of Ashenden MJ, Dobson GP, Hahn AG: Sensitivity of reticulocyte indices to iron therapy in an intensely training athlete. *Br J Sports Med* 32:259-260, 1998.)

serum ferritin value of 10 µg/L. She did not eat red meat. She was prescribed 350 mg/day of Ferrogradumate and encouraged to eat red meat 2 or 3 times a week. Earlobe blood samples were monitored weekly. Mean corpuscular hemoglobin concentration (CHCMr) and hemoglobin content (CHr) progressively increased (Fig 1). At day 75, ferritin values plummeted almost to baseline values with no decrease in hemoglobin. The patient had decreased her iron tablet intake to once per week. CHCMr and CHr increased within 7 days of supplementation and declined when iron intake declined.

Conclusion.—Monitoring reticulocyte indices by a simple pinprick test is an accurate and sensitive method for monitoring the effects of iron therapy.

▶ This advance enables sports medicine doctors to follow the size and hemoglobin content of reticulocytes, or "newborn" red cells. If an athlete is truly iron deficient and is treated with iron, an increase in size (and hemoglobin) of reticulocytes should occur before an increase in blood hemoglobin level—the time-honored way to monitor reversal of iron-deficiency anemia. One case report with no statistical testing proves little. Yet Figure 1 suggests that charting reticulocytes can confirm a response to iron in a week or 2, whereas confirmation by hemoglobin level may take a month or more. This difference in timing is trivial for most athletes, but could be key in monitoring world-class athletes before competition.

E.R. Eichner, M.D.

Iron Supplementation in Athletes: Current Recommendations
Nielsen P, Nachtigall D (Universitäts-Krankenhaus Eppendorf, Hamburg, Germany)
Sports Med 26:207-216, 1998   5–14

Objective.—The relevance of iron deficiency in athletes is unclear. A review of studies describing iron supplementation in athletes, on the assumption that intensive physical activity is a risk factor for iron deficiency, and recommendations for diagnostic evaluation and treatment are presented.

Iron Metabolism in Humans.—Most iron in the human body is involved in oxygen transport, but some is used for electron transport. Iron loss is balanced by intestinal absorption, primarily in the duodenum.

Iron Deficiency in Athletes.—Accurate studies of iron deficiency in women athletes is complicated by the fact that all menstruating women are at risk of iron deficiency. Studies with male athletes have shown that increased physical activity results in lower serum ferritin levels, increased intestinal iron absorption, increased iron elimination rates, and depleted iron stores in liver and bone marrow. Iron storage depletion is exacerbated by gastrointestinal blood loss, increased iron loss in urine, intestinal iron malabsorption, and iron malnutrition.

Nutritional Iron Status in Athletes.—Although dietary iron intake is adequate for male athletes, it typically is not for female athletes or for females in general.

Iron Supplementation in Athletes.—Iron supplementation is beneficial in individuals with iron deficiency, but its effect on nonanemic athletes is not clear. Pharmaceutical iron preparations have a low iron availability. There are dosage restrictions on iron supplements because adverse effects are dose dependent. Iron supplementation must be continued for 3 months in iron-depleted individuals. Overtraining can increase plasma ferritin levels and mimic iron deficiency.

Recommendations for Studying Iron Supplementation in Nonanemic Athletes.—Intervention studies are easier to perform in female athletes, but physical activity effects are easier to study in male athletes. Iron supplementation studies are best done in distance runners because they have the highest iron requirement. Iron supplements must be standardized. Performance testing should be done only after allowing appropriate equilibration times. Blood-testing methods and conditions should be standardized.

Recommendations for Optimized Iron Supplementation.—Iron supplementation decisions should be made on an individual basis after standard blood cell counts and serum ferritin levels have been determined. Supplementation should begin for athletes with scrum ferritin levels of less than 35 μg/L and should continue for 2 to 3 months at 100 mg/day. Improved performance after iron supplementation has not been demonstrated. Increased risk of acute myocardial infarction or cancer with increased iron supplementation has not been shown. Iron supplementation in individuals with hemochromatosis is dangerous.

▶ This is a thoughtful article by a group that did novel research emphasizing gastrointestinal blood loss as the main cause of the slightly negative iron balance in male distance runners compared with controls.[1] In this follow-up overview, they agree with the consensus that "... studies in clearly non-anemic athletes do not show iron supplementation to produce any significant changes in physical capacity." But they argue for controlled supplementation of iron for all athletes with low ferritin levels, on 2 grounds: (1) it will prevent iron deficiency, and (2) it will reverse nonspecific upregulation of intestinal metal ion absorption and so prevent hyperabsorption of potentially toxic lead and cadmium. I can't quibble with this stance.

E.R. Eichner, M.D.

Reference

1. Keller HR, Maggiorini M, Bärtsch P, et al: Simulated descent ε dexamethasone in treatment of acute mountain sickness: A randomized trial. *BMJ* 310:1232-1235, 1995. (1996 Year Book of Sports Medicine, pp 405-407).

The Haematological Response to an Iron Injection Amongst Female Athletes

Ashenden MJ, Fricker PA, Ryan RK, et al (Australian Inst of Sport, Canberra; James Cook Univ of North Queensland, Townsville, Australia)
Int J Sports Med 19:474-478, 1998   5–15

Objective.—Although iron supplementation increases ferritin levels in female athletes with very low levels, concentrations of hemoglobin do not always improve. Small changes in hemoglobin mass can be determined precisely by measuring reticulocyte parameters. The changes in red blood cell parameters in female basketball players with very low ferritin levels were monitored after iron injection.

Methods.—Eleven female basketball players, with an average age of 18 years, were randomly allocated to iron or to a control group. After determination of total hemoglobin mass, the treatment group (n = 6) received an injection of 0.5 mL of Ferrum H and returned the next day for another injection of 2 mL of Ferrum H. Reticulocyte parameters were measured at weeks 1 and 2 after injection. Total hemoglobin mass was determined again 3 weeks after the beginning of treatment. Complete blood cell counts were determined from venous blood samples drawn at that time.

Results.—After a 2-week break in training, and before treatment, the athletes' ferritin levels had increased considerably (treatment group, 35.0 µg/mL vs control, of 36.4 µg/mL). The earlier values had been 23.8 µg/mL and 31.0 µg/mL, respectively. Serum ferritin levels had declined in both groups by 28% at week 1 and 38% overall (Fig 1). Ferritin in 1 individual increased from 9 to 10.3 µg/mL after injection.

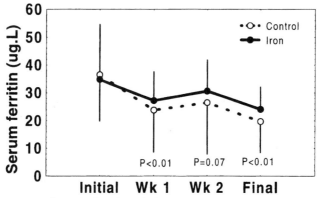

FIGURE 1.—Serum ferritin levels in female basketball players during the 3 weeks after a 2.5-mL IM iron treatment (125 mg of elemental iron). Analysis using a 2 × 2 (treatment × time) analysis of variance with repeated measures over time, Scheffe post hoc analysis ($P < 0.05$). P values reflect significance of changes relative to initial measures for iron and control groups combined. (Courtesy of Ashenden MJ, Fricker PA, Ryan RK, et al: The haematological response to an iron injection amongst female athletes. *Int J Sports Med* 19:474-478, copyright 1998, Georg Thieme Verlag.)

Conclusion.—Although iron injections failed to increase ferritin levels, athletes were able to maintain normal red blood cell production. Low ferritin levels apparently do not always indicate iron depletion. That hemoglobin concentrations did not rise after treatment also suggests that red blood cell production was properly maintained. Ferritin levels dropped with the onset of physical training, were unaffected by iron injections, and increased during training breaks for both the treatment and control groups. Iron injections do not benefit athletes with low ferritin levels but no clinical signs of iron deficiency.

▶ These authors seem surprised that female athletes with moderately low ferritin levels (5 of the 6 treated with iron had ferritin values less than 40 μg/L) did not show any increase in hemoglobin level 3 weeks after the injection of iron. Of course they didn't. They were not anemic! And their ferritin levels were not that low for female athletes—not nearly low enough to limit erythropoiesis. Another lesson is the variation in serum ferritin level by level of training. When these athletes stopped training, ferritin levels rose because plasma volumes fell (hemoconcentration). And when they resumed training, ferritin levels fell (even in those treated with iron), largely because ferritin was diluted by a rise in plasma volume.

The predictable conclusion: "...iron injections are of no haematological benefit to athletes with low ferritin in the absence of clinical signs of iron deficiency." An analysis of 10 clinical studies of ferritin and performance concludes correctly that "...iron supplementation can raise serum ferritin levels, but increases in ferritin concentration, unaccompanied by increases in hemoglobin concentration, have not been shown to increase endurance performance."[1] Amen.

E.R. Eichner, M.D.

Reference

1. Garza D, Shrier I, Kohl HW III, et al: The clinical value of serum ferritin tests in endurance athletes. *Clin J Sport Med* 7:46-53, 1997.

Coagulation and Thrombomodulin in Response to Exercise of Different Type and Duration
Weiss C, Welsch B, Albert M, et al (Univ of Heidelberg, Germany)
Med Sci Sports Exerc 30:1205-1210, 1998   5–16

Background.—In healthy people, exercise induces activation of the coagulation cascade, which results in thrombin formation, indicated by increasing plasma levels or prothrombin fragment 1 + 2 and thrombin-antithrombin II complexes. The current study determined whether exercise duration affects exercise-induced activation of coagulation and assessed the role of mechanical factors.

Methods.—Eleven male triathletes performed stepwise maximal and 1-hour maximal exercise by swimming, cycling, and running. Changes in

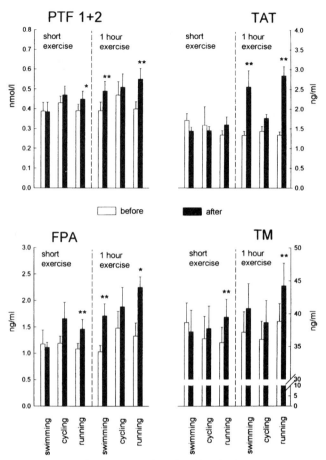

FIGURE 2.—Pre-exercise and postexercise values of prothrombin fragment 1+2 (*PTF 1+2*), throm-bin-antithrombin III complexes (*TAT*), fibrinopeptide A (*FPA*), and plasma levels of thrombomodulin (*TM*) in 11 male endurance-trained triathletes subjected to a stepwise maximal exercise test and a 1-hour maximal exercise test, each in swimming, cycling, and running. Values represent mean ± standard error, *P less than 0.05, and **P less than 0.01 for differences before vs. after exercise (Wilcoxon test). (Courtesy of Weiss C, Welsch B, Albert M, et al: Coagulation and thrombomodulin in response to exercise of different type and duration. *Med Sci Sports Exerc* 30:1205-1210, 1998.)

hemostatic variables and plasma thrombomodulin, a marker of endothe-lial cell activation, were documented.

Findings.—Regardless of exercise type, changes in markers of thrombin and fibrin formation were more marked after 1 hour of exercise than after stepwise maximal exercise. Hemostatic variables increased to the highest levels after running and resulted in substantial fibrin formation, indicated by increased fibrinopeptide A, after 1 hour of exercise. Plasma thrombo-modulin increased significantly only after running (Fig 2).

Conclusions.—Prolonged exercise is needed for exercise-induced activa-tion of coagulation resulting in thrombin and fibrin formation. Endothelial cell activation may play a role, possibly because of mechanical factors associated with running.

▶ This group of authors continues their fine research. It is known that exercise increases fibrinolysis acutely and that active men have more brisk baseline fibrinolysis than inactive men.[1,2] In theory, however, exercise can also be pro-thrombotic, by increasing platelet count and activating coagulation. In an earlier study this group found some activation of coagulation and fibrinolysis after a 2-hour marathon, but the net effect seemed anti-thrombotic.[2] In another study,[3] the authors found that moderate exercise increases only plasmin (anti-thrombotic) and that heavy exercise generates more plasmin than thrombin or fibrin (net effect anti-thrombotic). Now the authors show that exercise-induced thrombin and fibrin formation—and platelet activation—are related to duration and type of exercise. Pro-thrombotic markers are more pronounced after 1-hour exercise (than after stepwise maximal exercise), and after running (than after swimming or cycling). The authors speculate that mechanical injury to the endothelium during running may contribute to hemostatic changes.

E.R. Eichner, M.D.

References

1. Szymanski LM, Pate RR, Durstine JL: Effects of maximal exercise and venous occlusion on fibrinolytic activity in physically active and inactive men. *J Appl Physiol* 77:2305-2310, 1994. (1995 YEAR BOOK OF SPORTS MEDICINE, pp 451-453.)
2. Szymanski LM, Pate RR: Effects of exercise intensity, duration and time of day on fibrinolytic activity in physically active men. *Med Sci Sports Exerc* 26:1102-1108, 1994. (1995 YEAR BOOK OF SPORTS MEDICINE, pp 468-470).
3. Bartsch P, Welsch B, Albet M, et al: Balanced activation of coagulation and fibrinolysis after a 2-H triathlon. *Med Sci Sports Exerc* 27:1465-1470, 1995. (1996 YEAR BOOK OF SPORTS MEDICINE, pp 243-244.)
4. Weiss C, Seitel G, Bärtsch P: Coagulation and fibrinolysis after moderate and very heavy exercise in healthy male subjects. *Med Sci Sports Exerc* 30:246-251, 1998. (1998 YEAR BOOK OF SPORTS MEDICINE, pp 307-310.)

Exercise Training Enhances Basic Fibroblast Growth Factor-induced Collateral Blood Flow

Yang HT, Ogilvie RW, Terjung RJ (State Univ of New York, Syracuse; Med Univ of South Carolina, Charleston)
Am J Physiol 274:H2053-H2061, 1998   5–17

Background.—Exercise plays an important role in the management of peripheral arterial insufficiency. Increased physical activity increases capillary density within muscles and may increase collateral blood flow. The stimulus for remodeling of the collateral vessels may be increased pressure, flow, or both, resulting in increased wall tension, shear, or both. This process may also play a role in the increased collateral blood flow in rats induced by basic fibroblast growth factor (bFGF). The effects of exercise on bFGF-induced collateral vessel development were studied in rats.

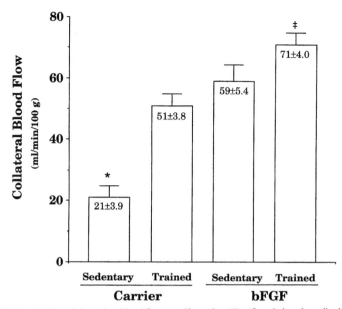

FIGURE 2.—Collateral-dependent blood flow to calf muscles. *Significantly less than all other groups
($P < 0.001$); ‡significantly greater than carrier-trained group ($P < 0.05$). (Courtesy of Yang HT, Ogilvie
RW, Terjung RJ: Exercise training enhances basic fibroblast growth factor-induced collateral blood flow.
Am J Physiol 274:H2053-H2061, 1998. Copyright The American Physiological Society.)

Methods and Results.—Bilateral ligation of the femoral arteries was
performed in Sprague-Dawley rats. This was followed by 2 weeks of
treatment with bFGF, 1 µg/day, or carrier solution given by intra-arterial
infusion through osmotic pumps. Within each treatment group, some
animals were kept sedentary while others performed daily walking exercise
for 4 weeks. The exercise groups showed significantly increased citrate
synthase activity in active muscle. Microsphere studies showed significant
increases in blood flow to the entire hindlimb in response to bFGF infusion, with still greater increases in the exercise animals treated with bFGF.
Areas of the distal hindlimb that depended on collateral flow showed the
greatest increases in blood flow. The increase in blood flow to the calf
muscle was 140% in exercising, non–bFGF-treated rats; 180% in sedentary, bFGF-treated rats; and 240% in exercising, bFGF-treated rats (Fig 2).
As collateral blood flow increased, so did calf muscle performance.

Conclusions.—This study in rats suggests that treatment with exogenous bFGF plus moderate exercise produces dramatic increases in collateral-dependent blood flow and muscle performance. The findings support
the hypothesis that the mechanism of collateral vessel enlargement involves hemodynamic factors. bFGF could be a useful treatment for peripheral arterial insufficiency, and the collateral response could be enhanced by the addition of physical activity.

▶ Sports physicians have debated for many years the extent to which an increase of collateral blood flow contributes to the exercise-induced improvement of prognosis in the patient with coronary or peripheral vascular atherosclerosis. In the case of peripheral vascular disease, part of the benefit of exercise may be linked to an increased expression of vascular endothelial growth factor[1]; this is probably expressed in response to local ischemia, and stimulates the development of the capillary bed within the skeletal muscles. However, ischemia seems unlikely in the collateral vessels; it is possible that exercise, by increasing wall tension, or shear, or both, stimulates vascular enlargement.[2] There is a similar response to bFGF; the present data show that the combination of exercise and bFGF produces a larger increase in collateral flow than either element alone.

R.J. Shephard, M.D., Ph.D., D.P.E.

References

1. Breen, EC, Johnson EC, Wagner H, et al: Angiogenic growth factor mRNA responses in muscle to a single bout of exercise. *J Appl Physiol* 81:355-361, 1996.
2. Ito WD, Arras M, Scholz D, et al: Angiogenesis but not collateral growth is associated with ischemia after femoral artery occlusion. *Am J Physiol* Vol No.:H1255-H1265, 1997.

Overtraining and Immune System: A Prospective Longitudinal Study in Endurance Athletes

Gabriel HHW, Urhausen A, Valet G, et al (Univ of the Saarland, Saarbrücken, Germany; Max-Planck-Inst for Biochemistry, Martinsried/Munich, Germany)
Med Sci Sports Exerc 30:1151-1157, 1998   5–18

Background.—Exercise-induced leukocytosis has been well documented. The current longitudinal study determined the impact of the overtraining syndrome on immune parameters.

Methods.—Immunophenotypes of peripheral leukocytes during severe training were assessed prospectively during a mean of 19 months. Leukocyte membrane antigens in endurance athletes were immunophenotyped by dual-color flow cytometry and analyzed during overtraining syndrome (in 15 athletes) and on several occasions in the absence of staleness symptoms (in 70 athletes).

Findings.—Cell counts of neutrophils, T, B, and natural killer (NK) cells did not differ between overtrained and unaffected athletes at physical rest or after a short-term highly intensive cycle ergometer exercise session at 110% of individual anaerobic threshold. Eosinophils were reduced during overtraining. In addition, activated T cells were slightly increased during overtraining, though not above the normal range. Cell-surface expression of CD45RO on T cells but not cell concentrations of CD45RO$^+$ T cells were increased during overtraining syndrome. The syndrome could be classified with a specificity of 92% and sensitivity of 93% (Fig 3).

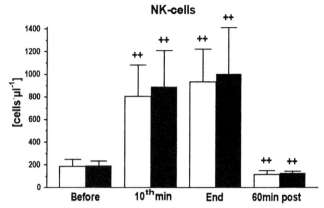

FIGURE 3.—Natural killer (NK)-cell (CD3⁻CD16/CD56⁺) counts. (Courtesy of Gabriel HHW, Urhausen A, Valet G, et al: Overtraining and immune system: A prospective longitudinal study in endurance athletes. *Med Sci Sports Exerc* 30:1151-1157, 1998.)

Conclusions.—Overtraining syndrome does not result in clinically important changes in immunophenotypes in peripheral blood. An immunosuppressive effect cannot be detected.

▶ The hunt for markers of overtraining continues. Last year this YEAR BOOK covered a prospective study of 16 hormonal, immunologic, or hematologic variables in swimmers who overtrained. Among these 16 markers, few changed much; the authors made a weak case for low urinary norepinephrine as a marker of those who "overreached."[1] This article also shows how vexing it is to find markers of overtraining. Cyclists and triathletes were studied 5 times over 19 months. These athletes were judged "overtrained" on a minority of occasions, and the diagnosis was subjective. Basically, athletes were "overtrained" when doctors said they were. When participants were "overtrained," they rated the stress test as more difficult and performed less well on it. But there were no differences (during "overtraining") in the exercise-induced rises in blood counts of NK cells, B cells, and T cells. Nor were there any signs of immunosuppression or any clinically relevant differences in immunophenotype profiles of blood lymphocytes. Why were the eosinophil counts lower during "overtraining?" Probably from higher blood cortisol levels (not measured). The authors argue unconvincingly that immunophenotyping could have a role in diagnosing overtraining.

E.R. Eichner, M.D.

Reference

1. 1998 YEAR BOOK OF SPORTS MEDICINE, pp 314-315.

Effects of Mode and Carbohydrate on the Granulocyte and Monocyte Response to Intensive, Prolonged Exercise

Nieman DC, Nehlsen-Cannarella SL, Fagoaga OR, et al (Appalachian State Univ, Boone, NC; Loma Linda Univ, Calif; Univ of South Carolina, Columbia)
J Appl Physiol 84:1252-1259, 1998   5–19

Background.—Carbohydrate supplementation may affect stress hormones and the neutrophil and monocyte response to exercise. Exercise mode may have an impact on the inflammatory response and reactive oxygen species generation. The effect of supplemental carbohydrate on the immune response to 2.5 hours of intensive running or cycling in triathletes was investigated.

Methods.—Ten triathletes participated in the study. They served as their own control group and ran or cycled for 2.5 hours at about 75% maximal O_2 uptake, ingesting carbohydrate or placebo. During the 2.5-hour exercise bouts, carbohydrate or placebo was ingested every 15 minutes. Blood samples were obtained 15 minutes before exercise, immediately after exercise, and at 1.5, 3, and 6 hours after exercise.

Findings.—The pattern of change for granulocyte and monocyte phagocytosis and oxidative burst activity differed significantly between the carbohydrate and placebo conditions. Postexercise values were lower during the carbohydrate trials. Little difference between the running and

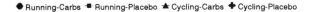

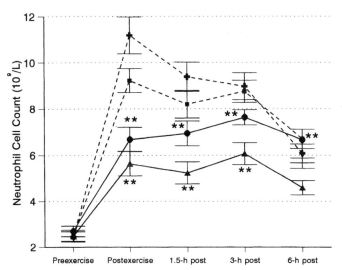

FIGURE 1.—Pattern of change in blood neutrophil counts over time was influenced by carbohydrate versus placebo ingestion $(P < 0.001)$ and slightly by exercise mode $(P = 0.02)$. *Abbreviation: Post,* postexercise. *$P < 0.013$, change from pre-exercise, carbohydrate vs. placebo, same mode. (Courtesy of Nieman DC, Nehlsen-Cannarella SL, Fagoaga OR, et al: Effects of mode and carbohydrate on the granulocyte and monocyte response to intensive, prolonged exercise. *J Appl Physiol* 84:1252-1259, 1998.)

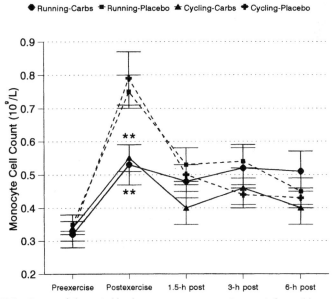

● Running-Carbs   ✚ Running-Placebo   ▲ Cycling-Carbs   ✚ Cycling-Placebo

FIGURE 2.—Pattern of change in blood monocyte counts over time was influenced by carbohydrate versus placebo ingestion ($P < 0.001$) and slightly by exercise mode ($P = 0.03$). *Abbreviation: Post,* postexercise. *$P < 0.013$, change from pre-exercise, carbohydrate vs. placebo, same mode. (Courtesy of Nieman DC, Nehlsen-Cannarella SL, Fagoaga OR, et al: Effects of mode and carbohydrate on the granulocyte and monocyte response to intensive, prolonged exercise. *J Appl Physiol* 84:1252-1259, 1998.)

cycling modes was noted. Compared with placebo, carbohydrate ingestion was associated with greater plasma levels of glucose and insulin, lower plasma levels of cortisol and growth hormone, and lower blood neutrophil and monocyte cell counts (Figs 1, 2, and 4).

Conclusions.—These findings indicate that carbohydrate ingestion reduces hormonal and immune responses associated with stress and lessens detrimental effects on various tissues through the indiscriminate action of reactive oxygen species. Additional research is needed to define the clinical significance of these findings on host protection against various pathogens.

▶ Last year we reviewed research by this group showing that during running, sports drinks like a carbohydrate beverage (Gatorade) (vs. placebo) keep glucose higher and stress hormones lower and so cause lesser swings in blood levels—but not activity—of natural killer (NK) cells.[1] This report extends the research. Mode of exercise (running vs cycling) mattered not, but a carbohydrate beverage (vs placebo) significantly raised plasma glucose levels, decreased cortisol and growth hormone levels, and attenuated increases in blood neutrophils and monocytes. Also, for 6 hours after running, an increase in blood granulocyte and monocyte phagocytosis (of *Staphylococcus aureus*) was seen, with levels somewhat lower after Gatorade (carbohydrate ingestion). A carbohydrate beverage also diminished the increase in granulocyte and monocyte oxidative burst activity after exercise. Because cortisol enhances phagocytosis, the authors think a carbohydrate beverage

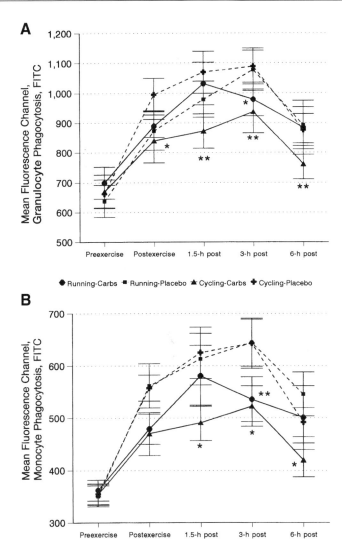

FIGURE 4.—Pattern of change in blood granulocyte (**A**) and monocyte (**B**) phagocytosis over time was influenced by carbohydrate vs. placebo ingestion ($P = .05$ and $P = .01$, respectively) and slightly by exercise mode ($P = 0.04$ and $P = 0.12$, respectively). *Abbreviation: Post*, postexercise. *$P < .05$, †$P < .013$, change from pre-exercise, carbohydrate versus placebo, same mode. (Courtesy of Nieman DC, Nehlsen-Cannarella SL, Fagoaga OR, et al: Effects of mode and carbohydrate on the granulocyte and monocyte response to intensive, prolonged exercise. *J Appl Physiol* 84:1252-1259, 1998.)

reduces phagocytosis by keeping glucose higher and therefore cortisol lower. In another article exploring this model, a carbohydrate beverage diminished pro-inflammatory and anti-inflammatory cytokine responses to exercise.[2] Whether any of these changes is clinically key is unclear.

E.R. Eichner, M.D.

References

1. Nieman DC, Menson DA, Garner EB, et al: Carbohydrate affects natural filler cell redistribution but not activity after running. *Med Sci Sports Exerc* 29:1318-1324, 1997. (1998 YEAR BOOK OF SPORTS MEDICINE, pp 320-321.)
2. Nieman DC, Nehlsen-Cannarella SL, Fagoaga OR, et al: Influence of mode and carbohydrate on the cytokine response to heavy exertion. *Med Sci Sports Exerc* 30:671-678, 1998.

Influence of Carbohydrate Status on Immune Responses Before and After Endurance Exercise
Mitchell JB, Pizza FX, Paquet A, et al (Texas Christian Univ, Fort Worth)
J Appl Physiol 84:1917-1925, 1998   5–20

Background.—Acute bouts of strenuous exercise induce changes in the immune system, depressing functional responses and altering the number of circulating leukocytes. The exact cause of such changes is not well

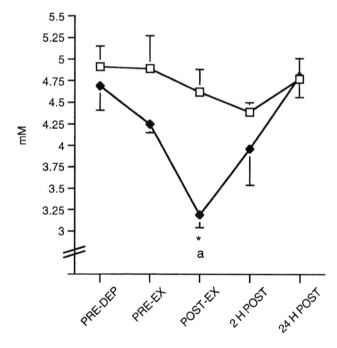

TIME POINT

FIGURE 1.—Blood glucose responses. *Square*, high-carbohydrate condition (*HiCHO*); *diamond*, low-carbohydrate condition (*LoCHO*). *Abbreviations: Pre-dep*, predepletion; *Pre-EX*, pre-exercise; *Post* and *post-EX*, postexercise. *LoCHO is significantly different from HiCHO at designated time. ^aSignificant difference from predepletion and 24-hour post-EX values within LoCHO condition. In this and other figures, all significances are P less than 0.05. (Courtesy of Mitchell JB, Pizza FX, Paquet A, et al: Influence of carbohydrate status on immune responses before and after endurance exercise. *J Appl Physiol* 84:1917-1925, 1998.)

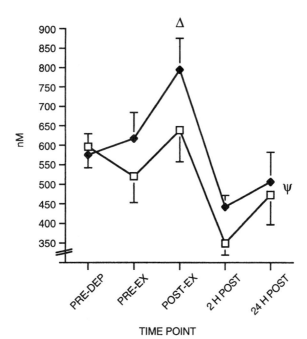

TIME POINT

FIGURE 4.—Serum cortisol responses. *Square*, high-carbohydrate condition (*HiCHO*); *diamond*, low-carbohydrate condition (*LoCHO*); ψ, main effect for condition; *triangle*, significant main effect for time, with postexercise value different from 2 and 14-hours postexercise in both conditions. (Courtesy of Mitchell JB, Pizza FX, Paquet A, et al: Influence of carbohydrate status on immune responses before and after endurance exercise. *J Appl Physiol* 84:1917-1925, 1998.)

understood. The current study determined the effect of carbohydrate (CHO) status on immune responses after long exercise.

Methods.—On 2 occasions, 10 men completed a glycogen-depleting bout of cycle ergometry followed by 48 hours of a high-CHO or low-CHO diet. After 48 hours, the men completed a 60-minute ride at 75% maximal oxygen uptake (EX). Blood samples were obtained before depletion, before and after EX, and at 2 and 24 hours after EX. Samples were assayed for leukocyte number and function, glucose, glutamine, and cortisol.

Findings.—Glucose response was significantly greater in the high-CHO than in the low-CHO condition post-EX. Glutamine was significantly greater in the high-CHO than in the low-CHO condition at all assessments. Throughout the trial, cortisol concentrations were significantly higher in the low-CHO than in the high-CHO condition. Post-EX lymphocyte proliferation was significantly depressed, though it did not differ between conditions and was unassociated with increases in cortisol. At the post-EX and 2-hour post-EX assessments, circulating numbers of leukocytes, neutrophils, lymphocytes, and lymphocyte subsets were significantly greater in the low-CHO than in the high-CHO condition (Figs 1, 4, and 6).

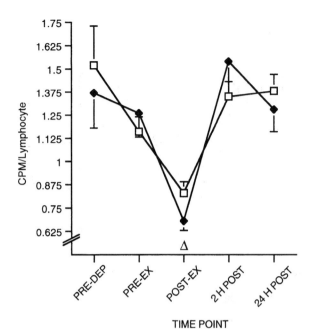

TIME POINT

FIGURE 6.—Counts per minute (*CPM*) per lymphocyte. *Square*, high-carbohydrate condition (*Hi-CHO*); *diamond*, low-carbohydrate condition (*LoCHO*); *triangle*, significant main effect for time, with postexercise value different from all other time points in both conditions. (Courtesy of Mitchell JB, Pizza FX, Paquet A, et al: Influence of carbohydrate status on immune responses before and after endurance exercise. *J Appl Physiol* 84:1917-1925, 1998.)

Conclusions.—Exercise and diet manipulation alter the number of circulating leukocytes in men. However, such manipulation does not appear to affect the reduction in lymphocyte proliferation after exercise.

▶ The high-CHO diet kept the plasma glutamine level higher during the ride, but did not affect the decrease in lymphocyte proliferation post-exercise. Other findings here are similar to those of Nieman et al (Abstract 5–19).[1] That is, compared to a low-CHO diet, a high-CHO diet (plus a carbohydrate drink during exercise) kept blood glucose higher and so cortisol lower during the ride. Surely in part because of higher cortisol levels, the low-CHO group developed higher blood counts for leukocytes, neutrophils, and lymphocytes. So 2 groups of researchers agree that consuming CHOs before or during endurance exercise can decrease the resulting immune stress. What we don't know is whether this finding is clinically important.

E.R. Eichner, M.D.

N-Acetylcysteine Does Not Affect the Lymphocyte Proliferation and Natural Killer Cell Activity Responses to Exercise

Nielson HB, Secher NH, Kappel M, et al (Univ of Copenhagen)
Am J Physiol 275:R1227-R1231, 1998   5–21

Objective.—Exercise is associated with reduced mitogen-induced lymphocyte proliferation and increased natural killer (NK) cell activity. During recovery, NK cell activity falls below resting values. Impaired lymphocyte function also occurs, perhaps in association with low cellular

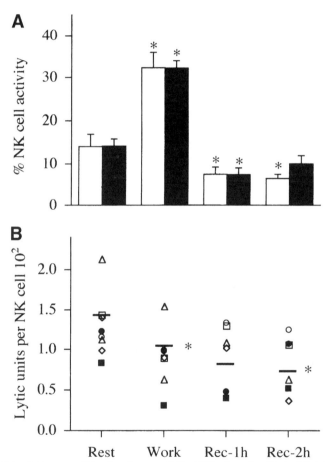

FIGURE 1.—**A**, Percentage ^{51}Cr release by natural killer (NK) cell–mediated lysis of K-562 target cells at an effector-to-target ratio of 50:1 (%NK activity). Values are means with SE at rest, during, and 1 (*Rec-h*) and 2 hours (*Rec-2h*) after maximal exercise with either placebo (*open bars*) or N-acetylcysteine (*solid bars*). **B** includes individual (*symbols*) and average values (*horizontal bars*) for lytic units on a per CD16+ cell basis (*placebo trial*). *Different from rest, *P* less than .05. (Courtesy of Nielson HB, Secher NH, Kappel M, et al: N-Acetylcysteine does not affect the lymphocyte proliferation and natural killer cell activity responses to exercise. *Am J Physiol* 275:R1227-R1231, 1998, copyright The American Physiological Society.)

glutathione concentration and an effect of reactive oxygen species. This study analyzed the effect of N-acetylcysteine (NAC) on exercise-induced reductions in lymphocyte proliferation and NK cell activity.

Methods and Findings.—Fourteen male oarsmen were randomized to receive 6 days of treatment with NAC, 6 g/day, or placebo. The response to a 6-minute exercise of intense ergometer rowing was assessed. Both groups showed increased concentrations of lymphocytes in the peripheral blood, including increased percentages of CD16+ cells. Lymphocyte proliferation was unchanged during exercise. Although phytohemagglutinin-stimulated proliferation decreased during exercise, NAC treatment had no significant effect. During exercise, NK cell activity was increased, but decreased below rest levels at 1 and 2 hours (Fig 1). However, when NK cell activity was expressed as lytic units per CD16+ cell, it was reduced both during and after exercise, and was unaffected by NAC.

Conclusions.—Treatment with NAC does not eliminate impairment of NK cell activity and mitogen-stimulated lymphocyte proliferation in response to maximal exercise. Thus, exercise does not reduce cellular cysteine and glutathione to levels critical for lymphocyte function. The reduction in NK cell activity may reflect an effect of reactive oxygen species, which either is not inhibited by NAC or does not reach a level sufficient to affect NK cell function.

▶ As we often review,[1] by laboratory markers at least, intense exercise is briefly "immunosuppressive." This study extends laboratory support for "immunosuppression" and explores whether oxidative damage to immune cells is involved. The hypothesis was that cysteine, which enhances NK cell activity in vitro and, by increasing intracellular glutathione levels, increases lymphocyte proliferation, would blunt exercise-induced immunosuppression. But results were negative. Brief, intense rowing did evoke brief immunosuppression. That is, the rowing reduced NK cell activity (per cell) and also reduced phytohemagglutinin-stimulated lymphocyte proliferation. But taking oral NAC for 3 days before rowing had no effect. So either oxidative damage plays no role in such immunosuppression, or oral cysteine is unable to offset it. As I've said before, any clinical import of these mild and brief perturbations in immune markers remains unclear.

E.R. Eichner, M.D.

Reference

1. Nieman DC, Henson DA, Garner EB, et al: Carbohydrate affects natural killer cell redistribution but not activity after running. *Med Sci Sports Exerc* 29:1318-1324, 1997. (1998 YEAR BOOK OF SPORTS MEDICINE, pp 320-326.)

Reservation Card for the Year Book

Yes! I would like my own copy of *Year Book of Sports Medicine*® at the price of **$77.95** (**$86.00** outside the U.S.) plus sales tax, postage, and handling. Please begin my subscription with the current edition according to the terms described below.* I understand that I will have 30 days to examine each annual edition.

Name _____

Address _____

City _____ State _____ ZIP_____

Method of Payment

Check (in U.S. dollars, drawn on a U.S. bank, payable to *Year Book of Sports Medicine*®)

❑ VISA   ❑ MasterCard   ❑ Discover   ❑ AmEx   ❑ Bill me

Card number _____ Exp. date: _____

Signature _____

Prices are subject to change without notice.   PMC-365

Subscribe to the related journal in your field!

Yes! Begin my one-year subscription to *Journal of Shoulder and Elbow Surgery* (6 issues).

Name _____

Institution _____

Address _____

City _____ State _____

ZIP/PC _____ Country _____

Specialty _____
(Students/residents, please list Institution)

Method of payment

Enclose payment (check or credit card number) and we'll send an extra issue FREE!

❑ Check (in U.S. dollars, drawn on a U.S. bank, and payable to *Journal of Shoulder and Elbow Surgery*)

❑ VISA   ❑ MasterCard   ❑ Discover
❑ AmEx   ❑ Bill me   Exp. date_____

Card #_____

Signature _____

*Includes Canadian GST

Individual/student subscriptions must be in the name of, billed to, and paid for by the individual.

Canada/Int'l prices include airmail postage.
Prices subject to change without notice.

Subscription prices (through 9/30/99)

		USA	Canada*	Int'l
Individuals	❑	$116.00	$154.08	$144.00
Institutions	❑	143.00	182.97	171.00
Students, residents	❑	60.00	94.16	88.00

J032991YC

Your Year Book service guarantee:

When you subscribe to the *Year Book*, you will receive advance notice of future annual volumes about two months before publication. To receive the new edition, you need do nothing—we'll send you the new volume as soon as it is available. If you want to discontinue, the advance notice allows you time to notify us of your decision. If you are not completely satisfied, you have 30 days to return any *Year Book*.

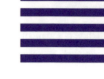
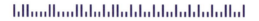

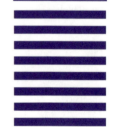
Want to speed up the process?

To order a *Year Book* or *Advances*,
you also may call 1-800-426-4545

To subscribe to a journal today,
call toll-free in the U.S.:
1-800-453-4351
or fax 314-432-1158
Outside the U.S., call: 314-453-4351

Visit us at: *www.mosby.com/periodicals*

Mosby, Inc.
Subscription Services
11830 Westline Industrial Drive
St. Louis, MO   63146 U.S.A.

 Mosby

Cognitive Orientations in Marathon Running and "Hitting the Wall"

Stevinson CD, Biddle SJH (Univ of Exeter, England)
Br J Sports Med 32:229-235, 1998   5–22

Background.—The concepts of cognitive association and dissociation in marathon runners have been investigated. An associative strategy involves concentration on the task of running and on bodily sensations, whereas a dissociative strategy involves distraction from the task of running and bodily sensations. In interviews of marathon runners by various investigators, some runners have reported that they tend to associate during a marathon immediately before noticing an injury. Some elite marathon runners have described "the wall" as a myth and say that symptoms of "the wall" can be avoided by associating with their body and adjusting their pace. Some non-elite marathon runners have reported that "hitting the wall" was inevitable but could be endured by dissociating from the pain. Other marathon runners have reported that cognitive strategy was not related to "hitting the wall."

Such studies are problematic because it is difficult to find out what people are thinking while they are running and because associative and dissociative thoughts are often defined in different ways. The relationship between the cognitive strategies of runners during a marathon and "hitting the wall" was examined. Methodological issues were investigated, and a classification system for the cognitions of marathon runners was developed.

Methods.—Questionnaires were sent to 100 non-elite marathon runners. Of these, 66 were returned and could be analyzed. Fifty-six men and 10 women participated. A classification system was developed for identifying thoughts as associative or dissociative. The classification system had 2 dimensions: task relevance and direction of attention. Thoughts directly relevant to task performance—such as monitoring physical sensations or calculating split times—were considered associative. These were further classified as internal or external. For example, monitoring physical sensations was considered internal, but calculating split times was considered external. Thoughts that were not directly relevant to task performance, such as daydreaming or observing scenery, were considered dissociative, and these were also divided into internal or external. For example, daydreaming was considered internal, but observing scenery was considered external.

Results.—Of the 66 respondents, 35 reported that they "hit the wall." This was associated with men significantly more than with women. Most respondents reported that their thoughts were internally associative during the race. Internally dissociative thoughts were the least common. Runners who "hit the wall" reported more internal dissociation than other runners, suggesting a hazardous situation when sensory feedback is blocked. Internal association was related to "hitting the wall" earlier, suggesting that physical symptoms may be magnified by concentrating on them. External dissociation was related to "hitting the wall" later, perhaps because of a degree of distraction while the runner was still focusing on the race.

Discussion.—The most common thought category of marathon runners was inward monitoring. These findings do not support the assertion that non-elite marathon runners tend to dissociate during a race. The results indicate that runners should avoid inward distraction during a race to increase the likelihood of completing a marathon. Total distraction is not recommended because it blocks awareness of the pace and warning signals from the body. Inward attention is important if it is not excessive, for example, making brief, regular checks on bodily sensations, rather than constant monitoring. Runners should focus most of their attention externally.

▶ Seminal research has suggested that non-elite marathoners "dissociate" (block out sensory input and pain) but that elite marathoners "associate" (heed and adjust to what their bodies tell them). Subsequent research tends to agree that elite marathoners associate. One elite runner explained it this way: "I don't worry if I start feeling bad during a race, because I know everyone else is feeling worse." But research on what non-elite marathoners think has brought mixed results. This study of non-elite marathoners suggests men are more apt to "hit the wall" than women and gives insight on thinking during the run. It ends with practical advice: (1) avoid inward distraction; if you don't read your body at all, you are more apt to run too fast early and hit the wall; (2) but don't pay too much attention to your body; if you do, you will magnify symptoms and seem to hit the wall earlier and for longer; and (3) focus most attention externally, both on task-related things (eg, mile splits, aid stations) and on task-unrelated things (outward distractors such as scenery, crowd, other runners). This combination of occasional inward monitoring and steady outward monitoring seems the best for maximizing performance and enjoying the race.

E.R. Eichner, M.D.

Impact of Rapid Weight Loss on Cognitive Function in Collegiate Wrestlers

Choma CW, Sforzo GA, Keller BA (Ithaca College, NY)
Med Sci Sports Exerc 30:746-749, 1998   5–23

Objective.—Rapid weight loss (RWL) involving dehydration and starvation can lead to hypoglycemia. Neuroglycopenia, secondary to hypoglycemia, can cause impaired cognitive function. Whether RWL in athletes can result in neuroglycopenia has not been studied. Whether RWL affects cognitive function and mood state in collegiate wrestlers during the competitive season was investigated.

Methods.—Five cognitive testing procedures and mood and hypoglycemic profiles were completed by 14 male college-aged wrestlers 1 week before RWL, during RWL, and after rehydration. Findings were compared

TABLE 2.—Selected Cognitive and Physiologic Data at 3 Points for Wrestlers and Controls

Variable	Group	Baseline	RWL	Rehydration
Story recall	Wrestlers	12.1 ± 3.3	10.1 ± 2.4*	13.0 ± 2.1
(# recalled)	Controls	11.8 ± 1.9	12.4 ± 1.8	12.4 ± 2.1
Digit span	Wrestlers	13.6 ± 1.1	12.5 ± 2.1*	14.5 ± 1.2
(# recalled)	Controls	13.5 ± 1.2	13.7 ± 1.5	13.5 ± 1.5
Glucose	Wrestlers	84.8 ± 5.4	71.1 ± 19*	88.2 ± 15.7
(mg·dL⁻)	Controls	88.1 ± 9.3	85.0 ± 8.1	83.0 ± 9.9
Plasma vol. (mL)	Wrestlers	53.2 ± 1.9	47.3 ± 4.1*	53.3 ± 2.3
	Controls	53.3 ± 3.3	53.8 ± 3.3	53.1 ± 3.4

Wrestlers (n = 14) and Controls (n = 15).
*$P < 0.05$, between-group difference.
Abbreviation: RWL, rapid weight loss.
(Courtesy of Choma CW, Sforzo GA, Keller BA: Impact of rapid weight loss on cognitive function in collegiate wrestlers. *Med Sci Sports Exerc* 30:746-749, 1998.)

with those from 15 control off-season college athletes. Glucose, hemoglobin, hematocrit, plasma volume, and body weight were measured at each point.

Results.—Wrestlers lost an average of 6.2% of body mass during RWL. After RWL, wrestlers scored significantly lower than controls on digit span and story recall tests, scored significantly more negatively on 5 of 6 mood tests, had a lower blood glucose with more hypoglycemic symptoms, and had an 11.0% decrease in plasma volume (Table 2). Plasma volume and mood state returned to baseline levels after rehydration.

Conclusion.—RWL affects cognitive function and mood state in collegiate wrestlers. The effects are reversible after rehydration.

▶ The practice of RWL in wrestling is plainly undesirable, and various arguments have been marshalled in an attempt to persuade competitors to avoid such behavior. Commonly, the focus has been on a persistent loss of muscle strength after rehydration. However, some wrestlers may be persuaded by this demonstration of a deterioration in mood state and cognitive ability. The basis for the impaired intellectual function seems a 15% decrease in blood glucose; glucose is an essential metabolite for the brain. We have previously commented that a glycopenia induced by repeated isometric contractions may also impair the tactical performance of dinghy sailors.[1] Given such changes develop with only a 15% drop in blood glucose, there is probably a need to monitor blood glucose levels in any sport that requires clear thinking.

R.J. Shephard, M.D., Ph.D., D.P.E.

Reference

1. Niinimaa V, Wright G, Shephard RJ, et al: Characteristics of the successful dinghy sailor. *J Sports Med Phys Fitness* 17:83-96, 1977.

6 Metabolism, Nutrition, Fluids, Environment

Effects of Exercise on Appetite Control: Implications for Energy Balance
King NA, Tremblay A, Blundell JE (Univ of Leeds, England; Univ of Laval, Quebec)
Med Sci Sports Exerc 29:1076-1089, 1997   6–1

Introduction.—Increased physical activity is recommended as a means of preventing obesity, although there is concern that exercise might lead to an increase in food intake. It has been difficult, however, to determine with accuracy the effects of physical activity on energy intake and energy balance. There may be a rise in energy intake, a suppression of energy intake, or an exercise-induced change in food choice or nutrient selection. A number of studies pertaining to these issues were reviewed.

Acute Effects of Exercise on Energy Intake.—One study of lean men found a brief suppression of subjective hunger after high-intensity exercise, whereas another reported that obese individuals increased their energy intake. Although hunger may be suppressed immediately after intense exercise, the period of reduced appetite appears to be too brief to affect energy intake significantly (Table 1).

Cross-sectional Studies.—In an early and frequently cited study (Mayer et al., 1956), mill workers were classified as being sedentary, moderately active, or highly active. The sedentary workers ate more than the moderately active workers and as much as those who were highly active. A study of lean, highly active individuals found that they had increased energy intake and had relatively higher carbohydrate intakes.

Longitudinal Studies.—Most studies indicate that there is not a compensatory increase in energy intake in response to interventions in physical activity. A few studies report hypophagia in response to exercise. There are a number of reports in which, during a period of increased activity, energy intake was highest on days of lowest activity and least on days of greatest physical activity.

TABLE 1.—Short-term Effects of Exercise on Energy Intake

Author	Sex	Lean/Obese	Protocol	Results
Thompson et al.	Male	Lean	Two intensities of cycling, high (68% VO_{2max} for 29 min) and low (35% VO_{2max} for 58 min). Control period of no exercise. Test meal 1 h post-exercise.	Brief suppression of subjective feeling of hunger. No reduction in energy intake.
Verger et al.	Male	Lean	Two treatments; 75 min continuous swimming and 75 min of rest. Test meal, 0, 30, 60 and 90 min post-exercise.	Increased hunger and food intake 1 h after exercise when compared with rest.
Verger et al.	Male	Lean	Two treatments; 2 h of variety of continuous athletic activities and 2-h rest period. Test meal 2-h post-exercise.	Energy intake increased after exercise.
King and Blundell	Male	Lean	Study 1: 4 conditions: 2 periods of rest, one followed by high-fat meal, other by low-fat meal. 2 periods of exercise (cycling), one followed by high-fat meal, other by low-fat meal.	Transitory suppression of hunger after exercise. Increase in energy intake during high-fat meal. No effect of exercise on food intake. Suppression of relative energy intake only if exercise followed by low-fat meal, which is reversed if followed by high-fat meal.
			Study 2: As Study 1, except cycling session replaced with treadmill running.	As above, i.e., no difference between the effects of cycling and running.
King et al.	Male	Lean	Study 1: 3 Treatment conditions: rest period, low-intensity exercise, and high-intensity exercise (cycling). Study 2: 3 Treatment conditions: rest period, high-intensity (short-duration), and high-intensity (long-duration) exercise (cycling).	Transitory suppression of subjective feeling of hunger with intense exercise only. No effect on energy intake. Transitory suppression of subjective feeling of hunger after exercise. No effect on energy intake. Suppression of relative energy intake.
Tremblay et al.	Male	Lean	Four treatments; 60 min treadmill (55-60% VO_{2max}) followed by low-fat diet, high-fat diet, and a mixed diet. One rest period followed by mixed diet.	Negative energy balance with exercise treatments followed by low-fat and mixed diet. Positive energy balance with exercise followed by high-fat diet.
Reger et al.	Female	Lean	Three treadmill running treatments: Long duration (60 min at 50% VO_{2max}), short-duration (30 min at 50% VO_{2max}) and mixed intensity (1 min at 70% VO_{2max} alternating with 3 min at 40% VO_{2max} for total of 30 min) and control treatment (no exercise). Test meal approx. 15 min post-exercise.	Brief suppression of subjective feeling of hunger. No effect on energy intake.
Jankowski and Foss	Male	Overweight	Three treatment periods: Running for 1 mile at 6.2 mph, running 440 yd at 6.2 mph and resting. Foods in house preweighed before study and 24 h later.	No difference in energy intakes.
Verger et al.	Male and female	Lean	Two treatments; 2 h of nonstop athletic activity and 2 h of rest. Test meal 0, 30, 60, and 120 min post-exercise.	Food intake and hunger increased 1 h after exercise compared with rest.
Kissileff et al.	Female	Lean + obese	Two intensities of cycling; high (40 min at 90 W) and low (40 min at 30 W). Control period of no exercise. Test meal 15 min post-exercise.	Reduction of food intake after intense exercise in lean but not obese individuals.

Abbreviation: VO_{2max}, maximum oxygen consumption.
(Courtesy of King NA, Tremblay A, Blundell JE: Effects of exercise on appetite control: Implications for energy balance. *Med Sci Sports Exerc* 29(8):1076-1089, 1997.)

Conclusions.—There is no compelling evidence that exercise-induced energy expenditure leads to a compensatory increase of energy intake. Rather, there appears to be a weak association between activity-induced energy expenditure and energy intake. However, physical activity can induce a negative energy balance and weight loss if the exercise regimen is followed and a judicious pattern of eating behavior is maintained.

▶ Popular opinion is that exercise cannot help the obese individual because it merely stimulates appetite. However, I have long held the view that given proper timing of a bout of activity, it can be an effective tactic in suppressing the pangs of hunger in an individual who is dieting. This review lists a number of recent papers showing that if exercise is performed immediately before a meal, appetite is indeed temporarily suppressed, although the long-term energy balance is unchanged. Various mechanisms might be invoked for this, including the secretion of catecholamines, with a resulting increase of blood sugar, the increase of core temperature, the secretion of tumor necrosing factor, and increased levels of exercise.

R.J. Shephard, M.D., Ph.D., D.P.E.

Physical Activity, Energy Expenditure and Fitness: An Evolutionary Perspective
Cordain L, Gotshall RW, Eaton SB, et al (Colorado State Univ, Fort Collins; Emory Univ, Atlanta, Ga; Marshall Univ, Huntington, W Va)
Int J Sports Med 19:328-335, 1998   6–2

Introduction.—For all mammals except *Homo sapiens*, food procurement depends upon energy expenditure. In affluent nations today, because food has become more affordable and accessible, and an energy surplus exists. An evolutionary perspective of physical activity, energy expenditure, and fitness, based on an extensive literature review using MEDLARS On-Line, Sport Discus, and Colorado Alliance Research Libraries and bibliographies of original articles, is reported.

Human Evolution.—The genetic composition of contemporary human beings has changed little over the last 40 millennia. The relationship among energy intake, energy expenditure, and specific motor activity remains equivalent to that experienced by Stone Age people who lived in a foraging environment. The amount of obligatory physical exertion necessary for hunting, gathering, carrying, digging, and escape from predators has been lessened with agriculture and industrialization. The result is an energy surplus, increased body mass, and distorted body composition, with an overabundance of adipose tissue relative to bone and muscle.

Energy Expenditure.—Resting metabolic rate (RMR) and total energy expenditure (TEE) expressed per kilogram of body weight probably remained consistent for 3.5 million years, until contemporary human beings became affluent and sedentary. Typical Westerners have TEE/kg/day values that barely equal the RMR/kg/day of recent hunter-gatherers and

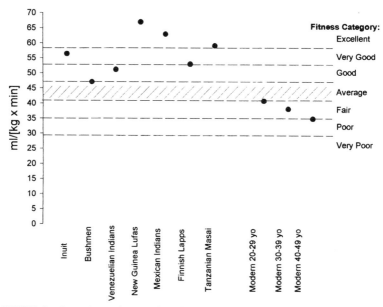

FIGURE 4.—Comparisons of maximal aerobic capacities (maximal oxygen consumption) between unacculturated and acculturated (industrialized) societies (adapted from [18]). Fitness categories based upon (51) for modern, acculturated societies. (Courtesy of Cordain L, Gotshall RW, Eaton SB, et al: Physical activity, energy expenditure and fitness: An evolutionary perspective. *Int J Sports Med* 19:328-335, 1998. Copyright Georg Thieme Verlag.)

the RMR/kg/day estimated for preagricultural humans. The RMR/kg/day decrease observed in modern human beings probably reflects altered body composition (more fat, less muscle) as a direct result of sedentary living. The TEE/kg/day of contemporary human beings is probably about 65% that of late Paleolithic Stone Agers.

Aerobic Fitness.—Hunter-gatherers and other traditional populations have aerobic fitness levels that range from good to excellent when plotted against fitness norms of contemporary North Americans (Fig 4). The limited physical activity of modern affluent human beings has resulted in mediocre aerobic fitness.

Guidelines for Fitness and Health.—The American College of Sports Medicine (ACSM) guidelines recommend participating in physical activity 3 to 5 days a week at 50% to 85% of maximum intensity continuously for 20 to 60 minutes to improve athletic performance and overall health. For health promotion, the ACSM recommends 30 minutes of physical activity for most days of the week. If ACSM recommendations for health promotion can be considered the minimum, what level is needed for optimizing health benefits? If the answer lies in the level of our ancestors, the optimal physical activity energy expenditure would be the equivalent of walking 406 kilometers (252 miles) per month, in addition to current physical activities.

Conclusion.—In the evolutionary perspective, it is the sedentary existence of today's affluent nations that is the extreme, not the lifestyle that prevailed before industrialization. The ACSM guidelines for daily energy expenditure amount to only 44% of the level expended among hunter-gatherers. The levels in these guidelines are almost certainly far below those of our preagricultural ancestors, and very likely beneath the level for which our genetically determined physiology and biochemistry have been programmed.

▶ In deciding upon the optimal pattern of physical activity, I have long been impressed by anthropological arguments. Human beings have adapted over many centuries to the life of the hunter-gatherer. In its traditional form, this existence required moderate intensities of exercise, continued for long periods and performed on several days during a typical week. However, there is little evidence that primitive human beings subjected themselves to anything resembling a triathlon or an ultramarathon race, and it is thus not surprising that when the current generation attempts to perform such feats, there are negative consequences for various body systems, ranging from a temporary decrease of cardiac output, muscle microtraumata and bone fractures to suppression of the immune system. The preventive value of traditional patterns of moderate but sustained physical activity has recently been highlighted by a natural experiment. The prevalence of both cardiac risk factors and actual cardiac disease has risen sharply among indigenous populations, as the populations have become acculturated to a "modern" lifestyle.[1] Cordain and associates pursue this theme through an extensive literature search, and make the point that recent technological developments have broken the link between the consumption of food and its pursuit. As daily energy expenditures have fallen from the anthropological optimum of 12–14 megajoule/day to around 8 megajoule/day, the adaptive capacity of the body has been surpassed. Various disorders of the cardiovascular system, the musculoskeletal system, and metabolism have resulted. It may be difficult for busy city-dwellers to get back to a regular energy expenditure of 14 megajoule/day, and there seems to be a need for time-saving ways to achieve a good balance between the intake and output of energy.

R.J. Shephard, M.D., Ph.D., D.P.E.

Reference

1. Shephard RJ: The Health Consequences of "Modernization." London, Cambridge University Press, 1996.

Long-term Maintenance of Weight Loss: Do People Who Lose Weight Through Various Weight Loss Methods Use Different Behaviors to Maintain Their Weight?

McGuire MT, Wing RR, Klem ML, et al (Univ of Pittsburgh, Pa; Univ of Colorado)
Int J Obes 22:572-577, 1998   6-3

Background.—A recent survey indicates that 72% of individuals who lost weight did so on their own. Twenty percent participated in a commercial weight-loss program, and 5% in a university-based program. The maintenance strategies of individuals who successfully lost weight on their own, who used organized weight-loss programs, and who used formal programs with liquid formula diets were compared.

Methods.—The study population consisted of 447 individuals who lost weight on their own, 313 who used organized programs, and 133 who used liquid formulas. All were members of the National Weight Control Registry. All had lost 15 kg or more and had kept the weight off for at least 1 year.

Findings.—Compared with the other 2 groups, liquid-diet users were more likely to be women, older, heavier, and to have a medical disorder before weight loss. The liquid-diet users reported greater use of dietary strategies and greater dietary restraint to maintain their weight loss. These participants also said that maintaining their weight was more difficult than losing weight, whereas participants who lost weight on their own said the reverse. Those who lost weight on their own reported expending a greater percentage of energy through activities such as running and weight-lifting. They also reported weighing themselves more often to maintain weight loss. All 3 groups maintain their weight loss by eating a low-energy diet and engaging in high levels of physical activity (Table 3).

Conclusions.—Though the participants in this study used different methods to lose weight, their strategies for maintaining weight loss were similar. Future studies are planned to determine whether method of weight loss is an independent factor in the long-term success of these participants.

▶ Many physicians and nutritionists regard the long-term control of obesity as a hopeless cause, and it is interesting to examine the case histories of a substantial group of individuals who have been successful in losing weight. Three facts stand out: the large majority of successful weight losers achieved the weight loss on their own, the contribution of physicians (except perhaps through some of the university programs) was negligible, and almost all participants who were successful combined a reduction of food intake with a vigorous exercise program.

The effectiveness of self-help is reminiscent of findings about smoking withdrawal: until an individual has decided to alter lifestyle, no program is of great value, and once the decision to alter lifestyle has been made, a program provides only a minor supporting role.

R.J. Shephard, M.D., Ph.D., D.P.E.

TABLE 3.—Energy Expenditure of Individuals Who Lost Weight Through Different Methods

	On Own (n = 447)	Organized Program (n = 313)	Liquid Formula (n = 133)	Significance
Energy expenditure per week[c] mean ± s.d.				
Total energy (kJ)	12996.6 ± 12992.8	10366.9 ± 10566.7	11468.5 ± 9809.5	NS
Energy expended in				
Strenuous activities (kJ)	4480.1 ± 7312.7	2488.3 ± 5091.2[a]	3134.9 ± 6269.4	P <0.03
Moderate activities (kJ)	7582.3 ± 9157.1	7076.4 ± 8762.3	7540.5 ± 7537.9	NS
Moderate activities (for example, aerobics, biking) (kJ)	2545.7 ± 4546.4	1776.3 ± 4372.7	2029.6 ± 4091.7	NS
Blocks walked (kJ)	4192.8 ± 7595.4	4604.1 ± 7338.9	4829.9 ± 6668.4	NS
Stairs climbed (kJ)	843.8 ± 872.9	695.9 ± 727.2	681.0 ± 795.0	NS
Light activities	934.2 ± 3144.8	802.2 ± 2899.1	792.9 ± 2176.8	NS

[a], differs from On Own
[b], differs from Organized Program.
[c], analyses controlled for age, gender, current body mass index (BMI), weight lost from maximum weight, and duration of years' weight loss; unadjusted means are shown.
Abbreviation: NS, not statistically significant.
(Courtesy of McGuire MT, Wing RR, Klem ML, et al: Long-term maintenance of weight loss: Do people who lose weight through various weight loss methods use different behaviors to maintain their weight? *Int J Obes Relat Metab Disord* 22:572-577, 1998.)

Fuel Metabolism in Men and Women During and After Long-Duration Exercise

Horton TJ, Pagliassotti MJ, Hobbs K, et al (Univ of Colorado, Denver)
J Appl Physiol 85:1823-1832, 1998   6–4

Objective.—Fuel oxidation during and after exercise was compared in men and women.

Methods.—Fuel consumption was measured on control days after subjects rested and on exercise days before and 2 hours after 2 hours on a cycle ergometer at 40% maximal oxygen intake. Circulating hormone and substrate levels were determined from blood samples obtained at baseline and every 30 minutes during exercise and every hour on control days. Dietary intake and body composition were also determined.

Results.—Although body fat mass was significantly greater in women than in men, activity levels, other aerobic activity, strength training, dietary intake, and body mass change were similar between the sexes. During exercise and recovery, energy expenditure was significantly greater in men than in women. Total carbohydrate and total protein oxidation, but not total fat oxidation, were significantly greater in men than in women (Table 4). Women burned significantly more fat for energy and men burned significantly more carbohydrate during exercise. Epinephrine and norepinephrine levels were significantly higher in men than in women during exercise.

Conclusion.—Men and women have different energy burning requirements during exercise. The reason why epinephrine and norepinephrine levels are greater in men than in women during exercise remains to be elucidated.

▶ The idea that men use more carbohydrate and women more fat during endurance exercise is a little contrary to expectation, because it seems more difficult to rid the body of surplus fat for women than for men.[1] As in so many physiologic studies, the samples of both men and women are small, particularly when divided between trained and untrained subgroups, and one immediately wonders whether they are representative of their gender. In this instance, matching was based on the self-reported volume and intensity of training, rather than maximal oxygen intake, which some find problematic. In 1 study, the trained men (137%) seem to have been somewhat less fit than the women (146%), relative to the general Toronto population.[2] This, in itself, might increase the relative fat use in the women.[3] However, the untrained groups (91% and 90% respectively) were quite well matched, as were the intakes of carbohydrate on control days. Unfortunately, the authors do not indicate whether gender differences varied between trained an untrained individuals. However, the higher levels of exercise-induced catecholamine secretion in men support the idea that they use a larger proportion of carbohydrate than women during vigorous physical activity.

R.J. Shephard, M.D., Ph.D., D.P.E.

TABLE 4.—Energy Expenditure and Fuel Oxidation

	n	EE, kJ/2 h	Absolute Fuel Oxidation, g/2 h			Relative Fuel Oxidation, % of Total EE		
			CHO	Fat	Protein	CHO	Fat	Protein
Cycling day								
Period 1								
Men	14	4,137 ± 252‡	125.4 ± 10‡	45.6 ± 3.5	6.2 ± 0.3†	53.1 ± 2.1†	43.7 ± 2.1*	3.1 ± 0.2
Women	13	2,821 ± 224	73.4 ± 6.3	36.3 ± 3.3	4.7 ± 0.4	45.7 ± 1.8	50.9 ± 1.8	3.4 ± 0.3
Period 2								
Men	14	739 ± 21‡ ¶	10.7 ± 0.8† ¶	10.8 ± 0.3† ¶	6.2 ± 0.3†	25.1 ± 1.3¶	58.3 ± 1.2¶	16.6 ± 0.7¶
Women	13	532 ± 24¶	6.9 ± 0.7¶	8.0 ± 0.5¶	4.7 ± 0.4	22.4 ± 1.8¶	59.6 ± 1.7∥	18.0 ± 1.6¶
Control day								
Period 1								
Men	14	638 ± 25‡‡	12.0 ± 0.8‡‡	7.7 ± 0.6‡‡	6.1 ± 0.3‡	33.1 ± 2.1‡‡	47.8 ± 2.8	18.9 ± 2.2‡‡
Women	13	514 ± 19‡‡	9.7 ± 1.0‡‡	6.6 ± 0.4‡‡	4.2 ± 0.3	32.8 ± 2.7‡‡	51.1 ± 2.6	16.1 ± 1.2‡‡
Period 2								
Men	14	647 ± 25‡‡	11.0 ± 0.9*∥	8.3 ± 0.5§‡‡	6.1 ± 0.3‡	32.0 ± 2.6**	50.7 ± 2.5††	17.2 ± 1.6
Women	13	518 ± 18	8.3 ± 0.7∥	7.3 ± 0.4¶	4.2 ± 0.3	27.9 ± 2.1∥	55.3 ± 2.5∥	16.0 ± 1.2

Note: Values are means ± SE. Period 1, rate of energy expenditure during first 2 hours of measurement (encompasses entire cycling period on cycling day); period 2, rate of energy expenditure during second 2 hours of measurement (encompasses postexercise recovery period on cycling day).

Significantly different from women: *P less than .02; †P less than .01; ‡P less than .001.

Significantly different from period 1 same day: §P less than .05; ∥P less than .01; ¶P less than .001.

Significantly different from same period cycling day: **P less than .05; ††P less than .01; ‡‡P less than .001.

(Courtesy of Horton TJ, Pagliassotti MJ, Hobbs K, et al: Fuel metabolism in men and women during and after long-duration exercise. *J Appl Physiol* 85:1823-1832, 1998).

References

1. Murray SJ, Shephard RJ, Greaves S, et al: Effects of cold stress and exercise on fat loss in females. *Eur J Appl Physiol* 55: 610-618, 1986.
2. Shephard RJ: *Aerobic Fitness and Health*. Champaign, Ill, Human Kinetics,
3. Hurley BF, Nemeth PM, Martin WH, et al: Muscle triglyceride utilization during exercise: Effect of training. *J Appl Physiol* 60: 562-567, 1986.

Nutritional Status of the Finnish Elite Ski Jumpers

Rankinen T, Lyytikäinen S, Vanninen E, et al (Univ of Kuopio, Finland)
Med Sci Sports Exerc 30:1592-1597, 1998   6–5

Background.—Major changes in ski jumping in the past decade have prompted skiers to try to control or lose body weight. The nutritional status of Finnish elite male ski jumpers was investigated.

Methods.—Twenty-one skiers and 20 age-matched control subjects were studied. Body composition was estimated using dual-energy x-ray absorptiometry. Dietary intake was evaluated using 4-day food records. Biochemical and hematologic indices were also analyzed.

Findings.—Although mean age and stature were comparable in the 2 groups, the ski jumpers had a lower mean body mass and body fat percentage. Amount of bone-free lean soft tissue and bone mineral content did not differ between groups. However, age and bone-free lean soft tissue–adjusted bone mineral density in the lumbar spine and proximal

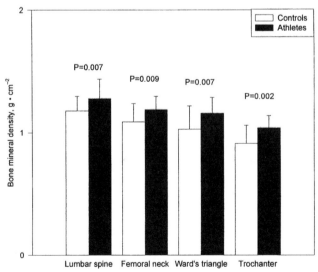

FIGURE 1.—Age and bone-free lean soft tissue adjusted bone mineral densities in lumbar spine, femoral neck, Ward's triangle, and trochanter in Finnish elite ski jumpers and nonathlete controls. (Courtesy of Rankinen T, Lyytikäinen S, Vanninen E, et al: Nutritional status of the Finnish elite ski jumpers. *Med Sci Sports Exerc* 30:1592-1597, 1998.)

femur was higher in the athletes. Mean energy intake was lower in the skiers than in control subjects, whereas the percentage of energy derived from carbohydrates was greater. The 2 groups were similar in their intake of thiamine, riboflavin, folate, vitamin C, calcium, and iron. Ski jumpers had lower intakes of vitamins D and E, magnesium, and zinc than control subjects. Neither group had abnormalities in biochemical or hematologic indices (Fig 1).

Conclusions.—This group of elite ski jumpers had lower body mass and energy intake than age-matched control subjects. However, the skiers' nutritional status was not compromised.

▶ Ski jumpers are here identified as 1 further category of athletes who deliberately embark on substantial weight-loss programs. The present group of competitors appears to have "got it right," achieving very low levels of body fat, apparently without incurring deficits in essential vitamins and trace elements, or decreases in lean tissue mass and bone density. Nevertheless, if weights 10 kg below the population average are being sought, nutritional status requires careful monitoring.

R.J. Shephard, M.D., Ph.D., D.P.E.

Energy Requirements of Middle-aged Men Are Modifiable by Physical Activity

Bunyard LB, Katzel LI, Busby-Whitehead MJ, et al (Baltimore Veterans Affairs Med Ctr, Md; Univ of Maryland, Baltimore; Johns Hopkins Bayview Med Institutions, Baltimore, Md)

Am J Clin Nutr 68:1136-1142, 1998   6–6

Background.—The energy requirements for maintaining weight decline with age. Many individuals gain body mass as they grow older because they do not reduce energy intake. The hypothesis that energy requirements for total daily mass maintenance in healthy, sedentary, middle-aged men will increase after regular aerobic exercise or aerobic exercise plus loss of body mass to levels similar to those in middle-age athletes was tested.

Methods.—Fourteen lean, sedentary men (group 1), 18 obese, sedentary men (group 2), and 10 male athletes were studied. Ages were comparable, with a mean of 58 years. Individuals were assessed at baseline and, in group 1, after 6 months of aerobic exercise or, in group 2, after 6 months of aerobic exercise plus weight loss. The athletes underwent 3 months of deconditioning.

Findings.—The interventions increased maximal oxygen intake by 15% in group 1 and by 13% in group 2. Maximal oxygen intake declined by 14% in group 3, eliminating the baseline differences among groups. Groups 1 and 2 had significant reductions in body fat. Fat-free mass declined in group 2. Mean daily energy requirements rose by 8% in group 1 and by 5% in group 2, reaching levels comparable to the baseline requirements of athletes. These values were correlated with maximal ox-

TABLE 2.—Energy Requirements for Weight Maintenance[1]

	Athletes ($n = 10$)	Lean, Sedentary Men ($n = 14$)	Obese, Sedentary Men ($n = 18$)
Energy requirements (J/d)			
Baseline	11832 ± 485^a	10037 ± 286^b	10606 ± 286^b
Postintervention	9816 ± 418^a	$10802 \pm 366^{a,b}$	11092 ± 291^b
Change	-2020 ± 490^2	770 ± 270^2	480 ± 240^3
$(J \cdot kg^{-1} \cdot d^{-1})$			
Baseline	172 ± 8^a	126 ± 4^b	110 ± 4^c
Postintervention	140 ± 7^a	138 ± 4^a	126 ± 4^a
Change	-32 ± 7^2	12 ± 3^2	15 ± 3^4
$(J \cdot kg\ FFM^{-1} \cdot d^{-1})$			
Baseline	201 ± 8^a	156 ± 4^b	159 ± 4^b
Postintervention	165 ± 7^a	169 ± 6^a	172 ± 4^a
Change	-36 ± 9^2	12 ± 4^3	12 ± 4^2

[1]$\bar{x} \pm$ SEM. Means within a row with different superscript letters are significantly different, $P < 0.05$ (analysis of variance [ANOVA]).
[2-4] Significant change (paired t test: [2]$P < 0.01$, [3]$P < 0.05$, [4]$P < 0.001$.
Abbreviation: FFM, fat-free mass.
(Courtesy of Bunyard LB, Katzel LI, Busby-Whitehead MJ, et al: Energy requirements of middle-aged men are modifiable by physical activity. *Am J Clin Nutr* 68:1136-1142. Copyright 1998, American Society of Clinical Nutrition.)

ygen intake and fat-free mass across the range of maximal oxygen intakes achieved by all participants (Table 2).

Conclusions.—Aerobic exercise eliminates the difference in energy requirements to maintain body mass between middle-aged sedentary and athletic men. Thus, regular physical exercise may modify the energy requirements of healthy, middle-aged men.

▶ The idea that habitual physical activity can augment resting metabolism[1,2] is an attractive one, particularly when dealing with mildly obese patients, because the potential benefits of a dietary regimen without exercise are often negated by a 10% to 15% reduction of resting metabolism. The effect seems to be exerted in part by a prolonged increase in resting metabolic rate after a given exercise bout, and partly by an increase in lean tissue mass. We have observed such a response in a small sample of moderately obese postcoronary patients who were followed up for 1 year. A regimen of progressive physical activity induced a 10% increase of resting metabolism, and this was sufficient to reduce body fat without special dietary treatment.[3]

R.J. Shephard, M.D., Ph.D., D.P.E.

References

1. Tremblay A, Fontaine E, Poehlman ET, et al: The effect of exercise training on resting metabolic rate in lean and moderately obese individuals. *Int J Obes* 10:511-517, 1986.
2. Poehlman ET, Danforth E: Endurance training increases resting metabolic rate and norepinephrine appearance into circulation in older individuals. *Am J Physiol* 261:E233-E239, 1991.
3. Mertens D, Kavanagh T, Campbell RB, et al: Exercise without dietary restriction as a means to long-term fat loss in the obese cardiac patient. *J Sports Med Phys Fitness* 38:310-316, 1998.

Effect of Exercise on the Proportion of Unsaturated Fatty Acids in Serum of Untrained Middle Aged Individuals

Mougios V, Kouidi E, Kyparos A, et al (Univ of Thessaloniki, Greece)

Br J Sports Med 32:58-62, 1998   6–7

Background.—A recent study of adolescent male athletes showed that prolonged exercise of variable intensity causes significant acute increases in the plasma ratio of unsaturated to saturated (U/S) fatty acids in the nonesterified fatty acid (NEFA) and triacylglycerol (TG) fractions. Whether prolonged moderate exercising by untrained middle-aged men and women affects the plasma ratio of U/S fatty acids in the NEFA and TG fractions was studied.

Methods.—Twenty-two healthy, untrained volunteers, aged 35-55, exercised on cycle ergometers at 50% to 55% maximal heart rate reserve for 1 hour. Blood samples obtained before and after exercise were analyzed for lactate, glucose, glycerol, individual NEFAs and TG acyl groups, cholesterol, high-density lipoprotein cholesterol, urea, cortisol, and testosterone. Adipose tissue biopsy specimens were analyzed for TG acyl group composition.

Findings.—In both sexes, serum total NEFAs significantly increased and total TG significantly decreased over the hour of exercise. Changes in individual fatty acids—in the NEFA and TG fractions—generally paralleled changes in the total pool, but were not proportionate. Consequently, U/S NEFAs rose in men and women, though nonsignificantly in men. The shift was in the direction of the adipose tissue TG. In addition, U/S acyl groups rose in both sexes, though nonsignificantly in women (Fig 1).

Conclusions.—In middle-aged men and women, prolonged moderate exercise increases the U/S ratio of serum NEFAs and TG. Given the protective role of unsaturated fatty acids against coronary heart disease, this finding may add to the known beneficial effects of exercise.

▶ Unsaturated fats do not all have the same significance for health. Simopoulos[1] argues that humans evolved with adaptation to an omega-6/omega-3 fatty acid ratio of around 1.0, and he suggests that cardiovascular health would be improved if there were an increased consumption of fish oils that are rich in omega-3 fatty acids. Circumpolar populations that consume large quantities of fish and the fat of marine mammals still have an omega-6/omega-3 ratio in this range.[2] However, modern diets give a much higher omega-6/omega-3 ratio, in the range of 5-10, and this contributes to the risk of atherosclerotic heart disease.

The present article suggests that if we are not willing to accept the flavor of cod liver oil, we can at least increase the proportion of unsaturated, nonesterified fatty acids in the blood by a training program that liberates fat from adipose tissue depots. Data is provided for 18-2 omega-6 fatty acids, but unfortunately not for the 20:5 and 22:6 omega-3 fatty acids that are derived from fish.

R.J. Shephard, M.D., Ph.D., D.P.E.

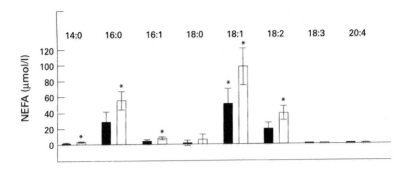

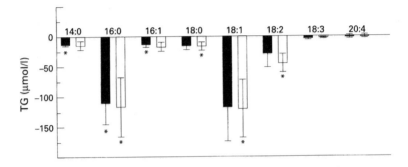

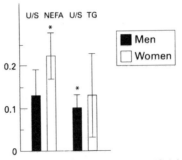

FIGURE 1.—Changes in concentration of individual serum nonesterified fatty acids (*NEFAs*) and triacylglycerol (*TG*) acyl groups, as well as in the unsaturated/saturated (*U/S*) ratio in men and women. *Asterisks* indicate significant changes. (Courtesy of Mougios V, Kouidi E, Kyparos A, et al: Effect of exercise on the proportion of unsaturated fatty acids in serum of untrained middle aged individuals. *Br J Sports Med* 32:58-62, 1998.)

References

1. Simopoulos, AP: Omega-3 fatty acids in health and disease in growth and development. *Am J Clin Nutr* 54:438-463, 1991.
2. Rode A, Shephard RJ, Vloshinsky PE, et al: Plasma fatty acid profiles of Canadian Inuit and Siberian nGanasan. *Arch Med Res* 54:10-20, 1995.

Effects of Diet and Exercise in Men and Postmenopausal Women With Low Levels of HDL Cholesterol and High Levels of LDL Cholesterol

Stefanick ML, Mackey S, Sheehan M, et al (Stanford Univ, Calif)
N Engl J Med 339:12-20, 1998   6–8

Background.—The National Cholesterol Education Program (NCEP) guidelines recommend exercise and weight loss to treat abnormalities in lipoprotein concentrations. However, the effects of exercise and the NCEP diet in persons with lipoprotein levels that put them at high risk for coronary heart disease (CHD) are unknown.

Methods.—Plasma lipoprotein levels were studied in 180 postmenopausal women, aged 45 to 64 years, and in 197 men, aged 30 to 64 years, with low high-density lipoprotein (HDL) and moderately increased low-density lipoprotein (LDL) cholesterol levels. The patients were assigned randomly to aerobic exercise, the NCEP Step 2 diet, which is moderately low in fat and cholesterol, diet plus exercise, or no intervention.

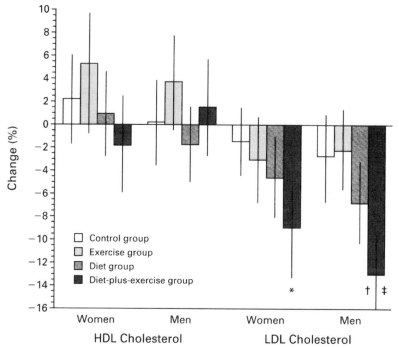

FIGURE 1.—Mean changes in plasma high-density lipoprotein HDL cholesterol and LDL cholesterol levels in the study groups at 1 year. The *vertical lines* represent 95% confidence intervals. Significance levels, after Bonferroni's adjustment for the 6 pairwise comparisons, are indicated as follows: *asterisk*, P less than .05 for the comparison with the control group; *dagger*, P less than .001 for the comparison with the control group; *double dagger*, P less than .001 for the comparison with the exercise group. (Reprinted by permission of *The New England Journal of Medicine*, from Stefanick ML, Mackey S, Sheehan M, et al: Effects of diet and exercise in men and postmenopausal women with low levels of HDL cholesterol and high levels of LDL cholesterol. *N Engl J Med* 339:12-20, 1998. Copyright Massachusetts Medical Society. All rights reserved.)

Findings.—During the 1-year study, dietary intake of fat and cholesterol declined as did body mass in women and men assigned to the NCEP diet, as compared with the control and exercise-only groups. The treatment groups did not differ significantly in changes in HDL cholesterol and triglyceride levels or in the ratio of total to HDL cholesterol levels. The serum LDL cholesterol level was significantly decreased among women and men in the diet-and-exercise group, as compared with the control group. Among men, the LDL cholesterol reduction in the diet-plus-exercise group was significant, as compared with the exercise group. Changes in LDL cholesterol levels were not significant in participants of either sex in the diet group, as compared with the control group (Fig 1).

Conclusions.—The NCEP Step 2 diet alone does not appear to lower LDL cholesterol levels in women or men with high-risk lipoprotein levels. Engaging in aerobic exercise is also necessary. These data underscore the importance of physical activity in the treatment of increased LDL cholesterol levels.

▶ Nutritionists often decry the value of exercise in the regulation of obesity. However, the present article by a well-respected group of investigators, based on a randomized controlled trial, shows that in men and women with high-risk lipoprotein levels, the traditional Step 2 diet failed to lower LDL cholesterol unless the patients also engaged in regular exercise. The target amount of exercise (walking 16 km a week) is not negligible, but for many people could be reached by walking to and from the commuter station each day. Not only is exercise a beneficial adjunct in terms of controlling plasma lipids, but it also confers many other health benefits that are not given by dieting alone.

R.J. Shephard, M.D., Ph.D., D.P.E.

A Moderate Glycemic Meal Before Endurance Exercise Can Enhance Performance

Kirwan JP, O'Gorman D, Evans WJ (Pennsylvania, State Univ, University Park)
J Appl Physiol 84:53-59, 1998   6–9

Introduction.—Carbohydrate intake before or during exercise may prolong the duration of aerobic exercise activities, but findings of previous studies have been inconsistent. To determine whether endurance exercise can be enhanced by a moderate glycemic meal, 6 women were studied who had eaten presweetened breakfast cereals before an exercise session.

Methods.—Participants, all of college age, were recreationally active. Forty-five minutes before semirecumbent cycle ergometer exercise to exhaustion, the women ate 75 g of available carbohydrate in the form of 2 breakfast cereals. During the exercise trial each participant drank at least

250 mL of water each half hour to ensure adequate hydration. A control trial consisted of 300 mL of water alone. Blood samples were obtained for measurements of glucose, free fatty acid (FFA), glycerol, insulin, epinephrine, and norepinephrine. Breath was sampled at 15-minute intervals after the meal and at 30-minute intervals during exercise. Muscle biopsy specimens obtained before the meal and immediately after exercise provided muscle glycogen concentrations.

Results.—Test meals consisted of sweetened whole-grain rolled oats (SROs) or sweetened whole-oat flour (SOF). During the SRO and SOF trials, plasma free fatty acid (FFA) concentrations were lower for the first 60 and 90 minutes of exercise, respectively, than during the control trial. Compared with the control trial, respiratory exchange ratios were higher at 90 and 120 minutes of exercise, respectively, for the SRO and SOF trials. Findings for glucose, insulin, FFA, glycerol, epinephrine, and norepinephrine concentrations and for the respiratory exchange ratio and muscle glycogen use were similar for all 3 trials when measured at exhaustion. Exercise time was similar for the SOF and control trials, but 16% longer in the SRO vs. the control trial.

Conclusions.—A moderate glycemic meal, ingested 45 minutes before cycle ergometer exercise, led to a significant improvement in exercise time. Metabolic responses, however, did not provide clear evidence for the mechanisms associated with improved performance.

▶ There have been fears that if carbohydrates are taken immediately before competition, a substantial secretion of insulin will be provoked, reducing blood glucose and impairing rather than enhancing performance. However, if the carbohydrate is well chosen, this is not necessarily the case. This study shows that a meal with a high-fiber content and a moderate glycemic index taken 45 minutes before exercise can enhance performance. The products tested (sweetened whole-grain rolled oats and sweetened whole oats flour) seem likely to appeal to the makers of proprietary foods, but also sound very similar to good old-fashioned porridge. Maybe the Scots were not too stupid to start the day with a good bowl of porridge!

R.J. Shephard, M.D., Ph.D., D.P.E.

Effect of Acute Plasma Volume Expression on Substrate Turnover During Prolonged Low-Intensity Exercise

Phillips SM, Green HJ, Grant SM, et al (Univ of Waterloo, Ont, Canada; McMaster Univ, Hamilton, Ont, Canada; Univ of Sydney, New South Wales, Australia)
Am J Physiol 273:E297-E304, 1997

6–10

Purpose.—The shift toward increased fat oxidation with exercise training has been associated with increases in mitochondrial content and in the potential for oxidative phosphorylation and β-oxidation. However, this cannot account for the alterations in substrate use observed during the

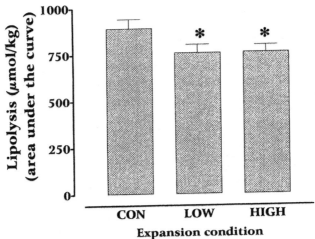

FIGURE 5.—Integrated lipolytic response during exercise with acute plasma volume expansion, expressed as area under glycerol R_a curve (μmol/kg). Values are means ± standard error (n = 8) for each condition. *Abbreviations*: CON, control; LOW, low plasma volume expansion; and HIGH, high plasma volume expansion. *Significantly less than CON (P less than 0.01). (Courtesy of Phillips SM, Green HJ, Grant SM, et al: Effect of acute plasma volume expansion on substrate turnover during prolonged low-intensity exercise. *Am J Physiol* 273:E297-E304, 1997. Copyright The American Physiological Society.)

initial days of training. An additional mechanism may be the increased plasma volume (PV) seen after increases in activity. To test this hypothesis, the authors studied the effects of increased PV on substrate turnover and oxidation in exercising volunteers.

Methods.—The study included 8 active but untrained men. The participants performed 3 2-hour bouts of cycle exercise at 46% of VO_{2peak}: 1 with 0% PV expansion, 1 after 14% PV expansion, and 1 after 21% PV expansion. These trials were performed in random order, with PV expansion achieved with the use of dextran. Primed continuous infusions of [6,6-$^2H_2$]glucose and [$^2H_5$]glycerol were used to assess glucose and glycerol turnover. Whole body lipolysis was assessed in terms of the glycerol rate of appearance (R_a).

Results.—Neither PV expansion condition altered glucose R_a or disappearance (R_d), at rest or during exercise. Both parameters approximately doubled at the start of exercise, and continued to increase thereafter, reaching more than 330% of resting levels by the end of the exercise period. As exercise progressed, glycerol R_a increased as well. The low PV expansion condition was associated with reduced total lipolysis during exercise. However, lipolysis was not further altered by the high PV expansion condition (Fig 5). Volume expansion had no effect on whole body fat or carbohydrate oxidation.

Conclusions.—Acute volume expansion, to levels equivalent to those observed during short-term training, reduces whole-body lipolysis. This effect may be related to reduced catecholamine secretion. Other adaptations may occur during the several days of training required for a full PV response to develop.

▶ One of the less appreciated benefits of endurance training is a shift from carbohydrate to fat metabolism. This shift has the effect of sparing glycogen during a long-distance event, so an individual can run farther before "hitting the wall." Muscle biopsies have shown a substantial increase of aerobic enzymes, and many physiologists have assumed that this was the main mechanism for the shift from carbohydrate to fat metabolism. However, the increase in tissue enzyme levels takes a week or more to develop, and training modifies metabolism more quickly than this. Increases in plasma volume are a more rapid response to training, and the present data provide valuable support for the idea that plasma volume expansion is the basis for at least early metabolic shifts.

R.J. Shephard, M.D., Ph.D., D.P.E.

Urine Osmolality and Conductivity As Indices of Hydration Status in Athletes in the Heat
Shirreffs SM, Maughan RJ (Univ Med School, Foresterhill, Aberdeen, Scotland)
Med Sci Sports Exerc 30:1598-1602, 1998   6–11

Background.—Dehydration levels likely to impair athletic performance are often reached before an athlete becomes thirsty. Thus, a simple, reliable index of hydration status would be useful.

Methods.—Three groups of individuals were studied. Osmolality was measured in the first urine sample of the day, obtained after waking but before breakfast. This standardized collection procedure enabled daily comparisons of individuals.

Findings.—According to laboratory measures, there was a difference in osmolality when individuals were dehydrated by a moderate degree compared with euhydration. The osmolality of the first morning urine sample of 11 control subjects averaged over 5 days was 675 mosmol·kg^{-1}. In 11

TABLE 2.—Manufacturer's Conductivity and Osmolality Ranges for Each Band of the Sparta 5 Conductivity Meter Plus the Measured Osmolality Range for Each Sparta 5 Reading From the Present Study

Sparta 5 Reading	Conductivity (μS·cm^{-1})	Osmolality (mosmol·kg^{-1})	Measured Osmolality (mosmol·kg^{-1})
1	<10	<341	184 (46-451)
2	10-15	341-510	480 (352-654)
3	15-21	510-716	708 (540-902)
4	21-25	716-852	805 (718-986)
5	>25	>852	984 (914-1112)

(Courtesy of Shirreffs SM, Maughan RJ: Urine osmolality and conductivity as indices of hydration status in athletes in the heat. *Med Sci Sports Exerc* 30:1598-1602, 1998.)

individuals hypohydrated by exercise followed by fluid restriction, morning urine osmolality was 924 mosmol·kg^{-1}. Measures from 29 athletes in warm-weather training demonstrated that, with appropriate feedback, athletes can maintain a satisfactory hydration status. Athletes in weight category sports tended to have a higher morning urine osmolality, reflecting attempts to dehydrate (Table 2).

Conclusions.—A hand-held portable conductivity device could provide athletes with reliable data on their hydration status from the measurement of the first morning urine. This would provide a quick, easy method for approximating hydration status from day to day.

▶ Dehydration may arise either acutely or chronically. The problem in acute dehydration is often that thirst provides an inadequate prompting to water replenishment.[1] When an athletic team must compete in a series of heats in a hot environment, there is also a real danger that cumulative dehydration may develop, in part caused by inadequate replacement of sodium ions lost in sweat. The 2 classic indications of dehydration are both very simple—a progressive decrease in body mass, and production of a dark, concentrated urine. Regular monitoring of body mass is an important preventive measure, but examination of the first urine sample of the day can also be helpful. The present data suggest that a simple portable indicator of conductivity correlate well with osmolality. It would be interesting to test the conductivity meter against the method used by a previous generation of physicians—the measurement of specific gravity.

R.J. Shephard, M.D., Ph.D., D.P.E.

Reference

1. Engell DB, Maller O, Sawka MN, et al: Thirst and fluid intake following graded hypohydration levels in humans. *Physiol Behav* 40:229-236, 1987.

Weight Loss Patterns and Success Rates in High School Wrestlers
Wroble RR, Moxley DP (Sports Medicine Grant, Columbus, Ohio)
Med Sci Sports Exerc 30:625-628, 1998   6–12

Background.—"Cutting weight"—the intentional loss of weight to compete in a lower weight class—is a common practice among wrestlers. However, there have been no direct measures of any performance advantage resulting from this practice. Weight loss patterns among high school varsity wrestlers and success rates associated with wrestling at a weight lower than recommended minimum wrestling weight (MWW) were analyzed.

Methods.—Skinfold thickness and percent body fat in 465 wrestlers at 16 schools were measured using the Lohman method. These boys voluntarily participated in an educational program, that explained the results, provided nutritional information on proper diet and methods of weight loss, and suggested a MWW corresponding to 5% body fat. The heavy-weight wrestlers were excluded from further analysis, leaving 159 varsity wrestlers in the study.

Findings.—Fifty-three wrestlers (33%) were wrestling below MWW. These boys' nonadherence to MWW ranged from 0% to 56% of all wrestlers. In the lightest 4 weight classes, 62% of participants wrestled below MWW, compared with 29% in the middle 4 classes and 6% in the heaviest 4 classes. Fifty-seven percent of the 53 wrestlers below MWW placed, compared with 33% of the 106 wrestling above MWW.

Conclusions.—A substantial percentage of wrestlers participating in a voluntary fat measurement and diet education program wrestled below recommended MWW, especially at lower weight classes. Wrestling below MWW resulted in greater success. However, MWW should not be based on wrestling performance effects.

▶ Old habits die hard: wrestlers do what wrestlers have done. In the fall of 1997, 3 collegiate wrestlers died within 33 days, largely because of unsafe weight-cutting practices. As a result, changes were made—notably in weight allowed and in timing of weigh-ins—that promise to make the sport safer. But the culture of a sport changes slowly. In 1995 we reported on weight loss beliefs and practices among high school wrestlers. That study showed that some high school wrestlers used extreme and bizarre meth-ods—not drinking, heavy sweating, vomiting, laxatives, diet pills, spitting, shivering—to cut weight and gain an edge.[1] This article continues that trend. One third of high school wrestlers in a voluntary body fat measurement and diet education program wrestled below their minimum wrestling weight. Those in the lower weight classes were especially likely to do this. Alas, wrestling below minimum weight was associated with greater wrestling success. We still have work to do.

E.R. Eichner, M.D.

Reference

1. Marquant LF, Sobal J: Weight loss beliefs, practices and support systems for high school wrestlers. *J Adolesc Health* 15:410-415, 1994. (1995 YEAR BOOK OF SPORTS MEDICINE.)

Effect of Carbohydrate Supplementation on Plasma Glutamine During Prolonged Exercise and Recovery
van Hall G, Saris WHM, Wagenmakers AJM (Univ of Maastricht, The Netherlands)
Int J Sports Med 19:82-86, 1998   6–13

Introduction.—Glutamine, the most abundant amino acid in human plasma and muscle, accounts for 71% of the amino acid release and 82% of the nitrogen release from muscle. Previous studies have suggested that muscle glycogen and glucose are carbon-chain precursors for glutamine

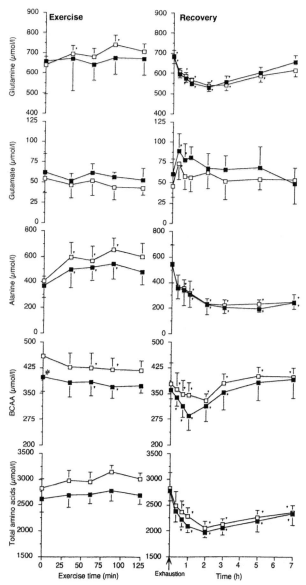

FIGURE 2.—Plasma amino acid concentration during exercise and recovery in 8 highly trained subjects during exercise and recovery. Values are means ± SEM obtained in the carbohydrate supplementation test (*closed squares*) and the control test (*open squares*). Values during exercise are of 8 subjects at 34 minutes, of 7 subjects at 61 minutes, of 5 subjects at 88 minutes, and of 2 subjects at 124 minutes. *Asterisk* indicates significant differences from the preexercise concentration during exercise as well as recovery. *Pound sign* indicates significant differences between the carbohydrate and control test. *Abbreviation:* BCAAs, brain-chain amino acids. (Courtesy of van Hall G, Saris WHM, Wagenmakers AJM: Effect of carbohydrate supplementation on plasma glutamine during prolonged exercise and recovery. *Int J Sports Med* 19:82-86, 1998. Copyright by Georg Thieme Verlag.)

synthesis in skeletal muscle. Eight trained cyclists were studied to determine whether carbohydrate supplementation affects plasma glutamine and other amino acids during exercise and recovery.

Methods.—Participants were 8 young men who had competed at national and international cycling events. They were studied while exercising on an electromagnetically braked cycle ergometer. On the 2 study occasions, the cyclists exercised to exhaustion, then had a 7-hour recovery period. They were provided with either water (control) or a carbohydrate (CHO) drink during the 59-140 minutes of exercise. Blood samples were obtained at intervals during the exercise and recovery periods.

Results.—Exercise did not appear to have an effect on plasma glutamine concentration, because significant increases were recorded only at some points during the control test. During the recovery period, however, there was a decrease in plasma glutamine activity from a mean of 682 μmol·L^{-1} at exhaustion to a mean of 552 μmol·L^{-1} after 2 hours of recovery for the control condition; the mean reduction for the CHO condition was from 685 to 534 μmol·L^{-1}. After 7 hours of recovery, there was a return of plasma glutamine concentrations to preexercise values. Both control and CHO exercise periods were accompanied by increases in alanine concentration. During recovery, concentrations of alanine and total amino acids decreased below the preexercise level (48% and 23%, respectively); decreases were still observed at 7 hours (Fig 2).

Conclusions.—The concentration of most plasma amino acids substantially decreases after moderate- to high-intensity exercise. Alanine and glutamine are also reduced in the postexercise period. The oral ingestion of carbohydrates before and during exercise had no effect on plasma glutamine or other amino acid concentrations, either during exercise or recovery.

▶ There has been considerable interest in recent years in the drop of plasma glutamine levels during and after exercise.[1] Although usually fairly small in magnitude, it has been argued that glutamine is an essential metabolite for the proliferation of lymphocytes, and the change is sufficient to account for the decrease in immune function that is observed in the first few hours after prolonged exercise.[2] The glutamine is being used as a substrate for hepatic gluconeogenesis, as muscle glycogen reserves are exhausted and blood glucose falls. It might thus be thought that carbohydrate supplements would counter the trend to a reduction in plasma glutamine, but in this study this was not the case. Possibly, the duration of exercise was too short for glycogen depletion; the authors suggest that under the conditions of their study, the decrease in plasma amino acids may be caused by synthesis of muscle protein, rather than gluconeogenesis.

R.J. Shephard, M.D., Ph.D., D.P.E.

References

1. Shephard RJ, Shek PN: Immunological hazards from nutritional imbalance in athletes. *Exerc Immunol Rev* 4:22-48, 1998.

2. Newsholme EA: Biochemical mechanisms to explain immunosuppression in well trained and overtrained athletes. *Int J Sports Med.* 15:142S-147S, 1994.

Carbohydrate Supplementation Improves Stroke Performance in Tennis

Vergauwen L, Brouns F, Hespel P (Katholieke Universiteit Leuven, Belgium; Sandoz Nutrition Research Centre, Maastricht, The Netherlands)
Med Sci Sports Exerc 30:1289-1295, 1998   6–14

Background.—Carbohydrate (CHO) administration before and during exercise substantially improves endurance exercise capacity. Caffeine has also been shown to postpone fatigue during prolonged steady-state exercise. The effects of CHO supplementation on the quality of stroke during prolonged simulated tennis match-play were determined.

Methods.—Thirteen well-trained Belgian tennis players participated in the study. On 3 separate occasions, the participants completed the Leuven Tennis Performance Test and shuttle run (SHR) before and after a strenuous, 2-hour training session. They received a placebo drink, a CHO solution, or CHO plus caffeine just before each training session, in a double-blind random order. Quality of stroke was assessed by measuring error rate, ball velocity, precision of ball placement, and a velocity-precision and velocity-precision-error index.

Findings.—In the placebo condition, stroke quality deteriorated for the first service and strokes during defensive rallies and for SHR performance. The CHO condition was associated with a lower increase in error rate and number of balls not reached in defensive rallies. Also, CHO attenuated the increase in error rate and reduction in velocity-precision and velocity-precision-error indices for the first service on fatigue. Administration of CHO improved posttest SHR performance. Stroke quality and SHR time were comparable in the CHO and the CHO-plus-caffeine condition (Table 2).

Conclusions.—Supplementation with CHO improves stroke quality in the final stages of prolonged tennis play. Carbohydrate ingestion may help tennis players maintain physical skill quality during long-lasting intermittent exercise to fatigue.

▶ Cerebral function depends on an adequate level of blood glucose. We have previously noted the potential impact of a low blood glucose on the choice of tactics in dinghy sailing[1], and others have noted that carbohydrate supplements have beneficial effects on soccer performance.[2] The development of effective methods of scoring tennis performance now demonstrates that tennis players benefit from carbohydrate supplements after 2 hours of training play against a well-matched opponent. The carbohydrate dose (0.7 g/kg body mass per hour) and fluid intake (400 mL/hour) used in these experiments were such that a total of about 100 g of carbohydrate was ingested in a 12% solution over the 2-hour session. It seems likely that a falling blood sugar contributed to the observed benefit of glucose, but this

TABLE 2.—The Effect of Carbohydrate Supplementation on Forehand and Backhand Quality in Defensive Situations

	Forehand				Backhand			
	Pretest	Placebo	Δ Fatigue CHO	CHO + CAF	Pretest	Placebo	Δ Fatigue CHO	CHO + CAF
Percentage of errors	40 ± 3	+6 ± 3	+3 ± 4	+4 ± 4	36 ± 3	+11 ± 3[a]	+1 ± 2[b]	+6 ± 4
Percentage of nonreached balls	11 ± 2	+4 ± 3	+3 ± 2	+2 ± 2[c]	9 ± 2	+8 ± 2[a]	+4 ± 2[a,b]	+8 ± 2[a,c]
Quality of nonerror shots								
Peak ball velocity (km·h^{-1})	104 ± 2	+3 ± 2	+3 ± 2	+2 ± 1[a]	97 ± 2	+2 ± 3	+5 ± 2[a]	+3 ± 2
Distance to sideline (cm)	141 ± 5	−4 ± 6	−4 ± 7	−4 ± 5	155 ± 8	−16 ± 11	+6 ± 10	+6 ± 7
Distance to baseline (cm)	338 ± 15	−37 ± 17[a]	−62 ± 15[a]	−17 ± 12[c]	367 ± 16	−25 ± 18	−27 ± 12[a]	+33 ± 19[b,c]
VP index	86 ± 3	+7 ± 4	+5 ± 4	+4 ± 2	72 ± 3	+2 ± 4	+5 ± 2[a]	+1 ± 3
VPE index	51 ± 3	+9 ± 4[a]	+5 ± 4	+5 ± 3	46 ± 3	+10 ± 3[a]	+4 ± 2	+4 ± 3[c]

Values are mean ± standard error of 13 observations. In defensive situations, 64 balls were projected close to either sideline and beyond the serviceline. For all variables studied, pretest values were similar (P greater than 0.05) during placebo and carbohydrate supplementation (CHO). Data were pooled and are presented as a single pretest score. Δ Fatigue represents pretest minus posttest score. For percentage of errors, percentage of nonreached balls, ball velocity, and the velocity-precision and velocity-precision-error indices, a positive Δ Fatigue corresponds with a decrease in posttest performance. For distance to the sideline and distance to the baseline, a decrease in performance is indicated by a negative value for Δ Fatigue.
[a]Significant (P less than 0.05) fatigue compared with pretest.
[b]Significant (P less than 0.05) difference compared with Δ Fatigue in placebo.
[c]Significant (P less than 0.05) difference compared with Δ Fatigue in CHO.
(Courtesy of Vergauwen L, Brouns F, Hespel P: Carbohydrate supplementation improves performance in tennis. *Med Sci Sports Exerc* 30:1289-1295, 1998.)

conclusion would have been strengthened had the investigators measured blood sugar levels. The authors suggest that correction of a decreasing explosive muscle strength was a further source of benefit.

R.J. Shephard, M.D., Ph.D., D.P.E.

References

1. Niinimaa VMJ, Wright G, Shephard RJ, et al: Characteristics of the successful dinghy sailor. *J Sports Med Phys Fitness* 17:83-96, 1977.
2. Muckle, DS: Glucose syrup ingestion and team performance in soccer. *Br J Sports Med* 7:340-343, 1973.

The Effect of Different Rehydration Drinks on Post-exercise Electrolyte Excretion in Trained Athletes

Brouns F, Kovacs EMR, Senden JMG (Maastricht Univ, The Netherlands)
Int J Sports Med 19:56-60, 1998   6–15

Background.—Athletes are generally not aware of how effective various drinks are in their rehydration and electrolyte replacement ability. The efficacy of postexercise ad libitum intake of commonly available rehydration drinks, including a hypertonic caffeinated soft drink (CC), a hypotonic mineral water (MW), and an isotonic carbohydrate-electrolyte solution (CES), on urinary electrolyte loss was determined.

Methods and Findings.—The study included 8 well-trained cyclists who dehydrated 3.2% of their body mass by cycling in the heat. In the first 2 hours of recovery, the cyclists randomly consumed ad libitum either a CC,

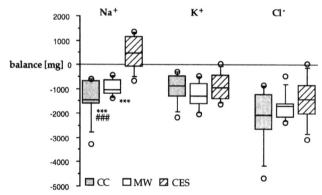

FIGURE 2.—Na^+, K^+ and Cl^- balance for each trial (median [P_{25}-P_{75} percentiles]) The results are expressed as box-and-whisker plots, in which the data are divided into 4 areas of equal frequency. The central box represents 50% of the data. The horizontal line inside the box is the median. The lower line of the box represents the 25% percentile and the upper line of the box represents the 75% percentile. The whiskers (*vertical lines*) extended to data points within 1.5 interquartile range. Separate circles are extreme values (beyond 1.5 interquartile range). *$P < .001$ vs. CES. †$P < .001$ versus MW. *Abbreviations:* CC, caffeinated soft drink; MW, mineral water; CES, isotonic carbohydrate-electrolyte solution. (Courtesy of Brouns F, Kovacs EMR, Senden JMG: The effect of different rehydration drinks on post-exercise electrolyte excretion in trained athletes. *Int J Sports Med* 19:56-60, 1998. Copyright 1998 by Georg Thieme Verlag.)

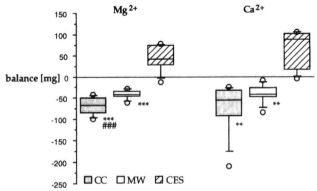

FIGURE 3.—Mg^{2+} and Ca^{2+} balance for each trial (median [P_{25}-P_{75} percentiles]) The results are expressed as box-and-whisker plots, in which the data are divided into 4 areas of equal frequency. The central box represents 50% of the data. The horizontal line inside the box is the median. The lower line of the box represents the 25% percentile and the upper line of the box represents the 75% percentile. The whiskers (vertical lines) extended to data points within 1.5 interquartile range. Separate circles are extreme values (beyond 1.5 interquartile range). *P less than .01 versus CES. † P less than .001 versus CES. ‡P less than .001 versus MW. *Abbreviations: CC*, caffeinated soft drink; *MW*, mineral water; *CES*, isotonic carbohydrate-electrolyte solution. (Courtesy of Brouns F, Kovacs EMR, Senden JMG: The effect of different rehydration drinks on post-exercise electrolyte excretion in trained athletes. *Int J Sports Med* 19:56-60, 1998. Copyright 1998 by Georg Thieme Verlag.)

MW, or CES. Fluid intake and urine loss were 2.77 and 1 kg, respectively, with CC; 2.15 and 0.96 kg with MW; and 2.86 and 1.1 kg with CES. Electrolyte retention was determined by electrolyte intake with the drink and loss with the urine. Intake of the CC and MW, which were low in electrolytes, resulted in a marked loss of Na^+, K^+, CL^-, Mg^{2+}, and Ca^{2+}. Intake of CES resulted in retention of Na^+, Mg^{2+}, and Ca^{2+}, whereas K^+ and Cl^- loss were unaffected. The higher electrolyte content of CES compared with CC and MW accounted for the significantly lower Na^+, Mg^{2+}, and Ca^{2+} loss with CES. In addition, CC potentiated urinary Mg^{2+} and Ca^{2+} excretion (Figs 2 and 3).

Conclusions.—Postexercise MW or CC consumption results in a negative electrolyte balance. Drinks that contain caffeine potentiate the excretion of Mg^{2+} and Ca^{2+}. Intake of CES with moderate amounts of Na^+, Mg^{2+}, and Ca^{2+} results in sufficient replacement to compensate for urinary losses.

▶ Athletic teams often practice twice a day in conditions of high heat and humidity. Athletes should be discouraged from drinking mineral water or caffeine-containing drinks between practice sessions. Mineral water may effect electrolyte balance and caffeine containing drinks may potentiate Mg^{2+} and Ca^{2+} excretion. The authors recommend drinking a carbohydrate-electrolyte solution containing moderate amounts of Na^+, Mg^{2+}, and Ca^{2+} to compensate for urinary losses.

F.J. George A.T.C., P.T

Effect of Hypohydration on Gastric Emptying and Intestinal Absorption During Exercise

Ryan AJ, Lambert GP, Shi X, et al (Univ of Iowa, Iowa City)
J Appl Physiol 84:1581-1588, 1998   6–16

Objective.—Exercise-induced dehydration can impair gastric emptying. To determine the effect of dehydration and hyperthermia on intestinal water flux, gastric emptying, and intestinal absorption were examined during repeated ingestion of a dilute (7%) carbohydrate-electrolyte solution (CES). The effects of moderate (3%) body mass hypohydration on gastric emptying and intestinal absorption of a water placebo (WP) were studied. Also studied was the efficacy of 3 different CES in terms of gastric emptying, intestinal absorption, and plasma volume changes while volunteers exercised in a hypohydrated state.

Methods.—Seven healthy volunteers (2 women), with an average age of 26.7, completed 5 cycling exercise experiments for 85 minutes at 65% maximal oxygen uptake, with at least 7 days between each experiment. Subjects repeatedly drank either WP or a 6%, 8%, or 9% CES the morning after hypohydration. Gastric emptying and intestinal absorption were determined through a nasogastric tube advanced into the gastric antrum and a multilumen tube placed in the duodenum and first 0.25 cm of jejunum. Hypohydration was induced 12–16 hours before each experiment by undertaking low-intensity exercise on a treadmill in a hot, humid

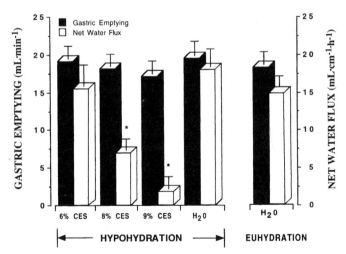

FIGURE 1.—Gastric emptying rate and net intestinal water flux during 5 different 85-minute bouts of cycling exercise (65% maximal oxygen consumption) in a cool (22 ± 2°C) environment. Exercise was performed after a hypohydration. (approximately 2.7% body weight) or euhydration protocol. Subjects (N = 7) ingested either water placebo (WP) or 1 of 3 carbohydrate-electrolyte solutions (CES) as a large bolus (4.6 mL/kg body wt) before exercise and as small serial feedings (2.3 mL/kg body wt) at every 10 minutes during exercise. Intestinal test segment spanned the proximal (50 cm) small intestine. Values are means ± standard error. *Asterisk* indicates values significantly different from 6% CES and WP at *P* less than 0.05. (Courtesy of Ryan AJ, Lambert GP, Shi X, et al: Effect of hypohydration on gastric emptying and intestinal absorption during exercise. *J Appl Physiol* 84:1581-1588, 1998).

room. Volunteers also participated in a euhydration protocol in which they did not exercise but ate small meals every 10 minutes and drank approximately 2 L fluids as a bolus 5 minutes before exercising.

Results.—Gastric emptying rates were similar during the 5 experiments. Hypohydration did not alter the gastric emptying rate of WP or intestinal water absorption (Fig 1). During exercise after hypohydration, intestinal water absorption was significantly greater when WP and 6% CES were used than when 8% or 9% CES was used (18.3 and 16.5 mL/cm/hour, respectively, vs. 6.9 and 1.8 mL/cm/hour). During hypohydration, drinking 6% CES resulted in net sodium ion absorption, whereas drinking 8% or 9% CES led to net sodium ion secretion. Core temperature, heart rate, and plasma volume changes were similar for all 5 experiments.

Conclusion.—Whereas gastric emptying and intestinal absorption were not adversely affected ny hypohydration to approximately 3% of body mass while drinking WP during exercise, consumption of 8% or 9% CES decreased intestinal water absorption.

▶ There have been suggestions that dehydration exceeding a 4% decrease in body mass can impair gastric emptying, thus limiting the opportunity for rehydration.[1,2] In the earlier experiments, fluid was provided as a single large drink of 400 mL, and this may have altered gastric function; the optimal pattern of fluid ingestion when exercising in the heat is to take a small volume of fluid (for example, 150 mL) every 15 minutes. Also, the extent of dehydration was greater than in the study abstracted here (a 4% or 5% decrease in body mass), and this also could explain the discrepant findings.

We have argued that the water associated with glycogen and other resources allow a marathon runner to lose up to 3% of body mass before any substantial dehydration occurs.[3] This article gives some support to this view, because the exercise-induced change in plasma volume is no greater than that when exercising during euhydration. Activation of sympathetic and renin-angiotensin systems by severe dehydration may actually inhibit fluid absorption and promote the secretion of water.[4] If water loss can be reversed at 3% decrease in body mass, but not at 4%, this is a further reason for monitoring fluid balance closely under warm conditions.

R.J. Shephard, M.D., Ph.D., D.P.E.

References

1. Neufer PD, Young AJ, Sawka MN: Gastric emptying during exercise: Effects of heat stress and hypohydration. *Eur J Appl Physiol* 58:433-439, 1989.
2. Rehrer NJ, Beckers EJ, Brouns F, et al: Effects of dehydration on gastric emptying and gastrointestinal distress while running. *Med Sci Sports Exerc* 22:790-795, 1990.
3. Kavanagh T, Shephard RJ: On the choice of fluid for the hydration of middle-aged marathon runners. *Br J Sports Med* 11:26-35, 1977.
4. Levens NR. Control of intestinal absorption by the renin-angiotensin system. *Am J Physiol* 249:G3-G15, 1985.

Effect of Beverage Osmolality on Intestinal Fluid Absorption During Exercise

Gisolfi CV, Summers RW, Lambert GP, et al (Univ of Iowa, Iowa City)
J Appl Physiol 85:1941-1948, 1998   6–17

Objective.—The effects of osmolality on intestinal fluid absorption were studied after exercise using water and 3 rehydration beverages.

Methods.—A water placebo and three 6% carbohydrate-electrolyte (CHO-E) solutions containing 2 or 3 forms of CHO, with mean osmolalities of 197, 295, or 414mOsm/kg H_2O, were ingested by 7 healthy individuals during 85 minutes of cycle exercise corresponding to 60% to 65% peak oxygen intake. Experiments were performed a week apart with an 8-hour fast. Gastric emptying and intestinal absorption were measured by using a multilumen tube attached to a nasogastric tube. On an empty stomach, individuals drank 20% of the total volume to be ingested (based on 23 mL/kg body mass), began exercising 5 minutes later, and consumed 10% of the volume every 10 minutes thereafter. Plasma volume, osmolality, Na+, K+, and glucose levels were measured every 20 minutes, heart rate every 15 minutes, and rectal temperature, body mass, and urine volume after exercise.

Results.—One person did not complete the study. In the remaining subjects, the gastric emptying rate of the hypertonic solution was delayed, resulting in a significantly higher gastric volume compared with water, the isotonic solution, or the hypotonic solution. After equilibration, average gastric emptying times were similar for all beverages, but mean gastric volume was significantly greater for the hypertonic beverage than for the other beverages. After the equilibration period, there were no differences between beverages in gastric volume or gastric emptying over time. Water was absorbed significantly faster in the jejunum than in the duodenum. Gastric emptying and total fluid absorption rates were similar for all solutions. Changes in plasma volume over time and plasma K+ and Na+ concentrations were similar for all solutions. Urine production was similar for all beverages.

Conclusion.—Beverage osmolality does not affect intestinal fluid absorption during exercise, and total fluid absorption of such beverages is similar to that of water.

▶ There has been growing acceptance of the idea that fluid ingestion and maintenance of body weight under hot conditions are similar for the ingestion of water and proprietary preparations. However, a gain in weight is not quite the same thing as absorption of water, since the fluid may merely be sitting in the stomach. There have remained suggestions that the presence of small amounts of glucose or salt in the fluid helps absorption from the intestine. The present data indicate that if the fluid is taken orally, rather than by intestinal intubation, at least in the first 0.5 m of the duodenum and jejunum there is no difference in fluid absorption between water and glucose/salt preparations; indeed, the volume that is absorbed tends to be largest for pure water. Thus, only argument for the proprietary preparations remains flavor; if people enjoy what they are drinking, they may be tempted to ingest more.

R.J. Shephard, M.D., Ph.D., D.P.E.

Influence of Fluid Intake Pattern on Short-term Recovery From Prolonged, Submaximal Running and Subsequent Exercise Capacity

Wong SH, Williams C, Simpson M, et al (Loughborough Univ, UK; Kyushu Univ, Kasuga, Japan)
J Sports Sci 16:143-152, 1998   6–18

Background.—The main causes of fatigue during prolonged, exhaustive exercise are the depletion of endogenous carbohydrate stores and dehydration. The efficacy of a carbohydrate-electrolyte solution during 4 hours of recovery from prolonged, submaximal running on subsequent endurance capacity were investigated.

Methods.—Seven well-trained female and male athletes, mean age 20 years, ran on a level treadmill for 90 minutes or until volitional fatigue (T1) on 2 occasions 7 to 10 days apart. Four hours later, the subjects ran at the same speed for as long as possible (T2) to measure endurance capacity. During the 4-hour recovery period on 1 occasion, the subjects were permitted to drink a carbohydrate-electrolyte solution ad libitum. On the other occasion, the volume of the same fluid was prescribed on the basis of body mass loss calculations during T1.

Findings.—Exercise time to exhaustion was 16% longer during T2 in the prescribed intake trial than in the ad libitum trial. Although total volume ingested did not differ between conditions, the volume of carbohydrate-electrolyte solution consumed in the fourth hour of the rehydration recovery period was greater in the prescribed intake trial than in the ad libitum trial. The amount of glucose consumed in this period during the prescribed intake trial was also higher than in the ad libitum trial. Blood lactate concentration was greater at the beginning of T2 in the prescribed intake trial than in the ad libitum trial. Blood glucose, plasma insulin, free fatty acid concentrations, and urine volume did not differ between trials.

Conclusions.—Drinking a prescribed volume of a carbohydrate-electrolyte solution to replace body fluid losses after prolonged exercise restores endurance capacity more efficiently than ad libitum rehydration during 4 hours of recovery. The prescribed volume approach is superior to ad libitum rehydration even when the total volumes ingested are the same.

▶ The results of this study indicate that fluid replacement should be at a prescribed rate to enhance short-term recovery. This may be especially important for athletes practicing twice a day in hot, humid weather. The author emphasizes the importance of ingesting 50 g of carbohydrate within 15 minutes after exercise to hasten recovery of muscle glycogen.

F.J. George, ATC, PT

Effect of a Carbohydrate-Electrolyte Drink on Endurance Capacity During Prolonged Intermittent High Intensity Running

Nassis GP, Williams C, Chisnall P (Loughborough Univ, England)
Br J Sports Med 32:248-252, 1998   6–19

Objective.—Fatigue, associated with exercise and resulting in reductions in muscle glycogen and blood glucose, can be delayed by ingesting carbohydrates. The influence on endurance capacity of drinking a carbohydrate-electrolyte solution was investigated during prolonged, intermittent, high-intensity running in a double-blind, randomized, placebo-controlled trial.

Methods.—Nine endurance trained athletes (1 woman) completed a 16-minute continuous submaximal running test to exhaustion on a motorized uphill treadmill to determine the relationship between running speed and oxygen cost. Maximal oxygen uptake (VO_2 MAX) was determined. After fasting overnight, participants then ran to exhaustion on 2 days, separated by at least 10 days, while drinking either a water placebo or a 6.9% carbohydrate-electrolyte solution (CHO) before and at 20-minute intervals during the run. After warming up, runners performed 15 second bouts of fast running separated by 10 seconds of slow running for the first hour (equivalent to 80% VO_2 MAX), for from 60 to 100 minutes (equivalent to 85% VO_2 MAX), and for from 100 minutes to fatigue (equivalent to 90% VO_2 MAX). Determinations were made of glucose and lactate in capillary blood at baseline and at 20-minute intervals during exercise. Sweat rate and carbohydrate oxidation rate were also determined.

Results.—Performance times for both the placebo and CHO trials were similar. Heart rate and perceived rate of exertion were significantly higher only at 40 minutes of exercise in the CHO trial. Oxygen uptake, rate of carbohydrate oxidation, sweat rate, and blood glucose concentrations were similar for both trials. Lactate concentration differed significantly only at exhaustion.

Conclusion.—Drinking a 6.9% CHO solution during prolonged intermittent running does not forestall onset of fatigue.

▶ The authors of this study concluded that there was no improvement in performance of the subjects who drank a 6.9% CHO, compared with those who drank a placebo during repeated bouts of high-intensity running. The testing procedure is stated to be similar to demands placed on an athlete participating in soccer. The subjects fasted for 10 to 12 hours prior to the test and did not use a "carbohydrate loading" technique, which is very common among high-level soccer athletes.

F.J. George, ATC, PT

Fluid and Carbohydrate Replacement During Intermittent Exercise

Shi X, Gisolfi CV (The Gatorade Company, Barrington, Ill; Univ of Iowa, Iowa City)
Sports Med 25:157-172, 1998   6–20

Background.—Drinking a carbohydrate-electrolyte solution during prolonged exercise has been found to help maintain blood volume, assist in thermoregulation, reduce the risk of heat injury, provide exogenous energy, and enhance performance. However, appropriate fluid replacement during intermittent exercise has not been investigated widely. These authors review pertinent studies on fluid replacement for intermittent exercise.

Review.—The available evidence suggests that, because of high exercise intensity, sweat loss and glycogen depletion during intermittent exercise are comparable to that during continuous exercise for a similar period. Thus, fluid replacement may be even more important during intermittent exercise than during continuous exercise to maintain a high level of performance and to help prevent thermal injury in a warm environment. Evidence also suggests that the volume of ingested fluid is essential for rapid gastric emptying and complete rehydration. Osmolality (250-370 mOsm/kg), carbohydrate concentration (5% to 7%), and carbohydrate type (multiple transportable carbohydrates) need to be considered when selecting an appropriate beverage for rehydration and carbohydrate supplementation during intermittent exercise.

Concentration.—Fluid replacement is very important for intermittent exercise, though it has not been studied extensively. More research would be useful to increase coaches' and athletes' appreciation of the need for fluid balance and carbohydrate supplementation during intermittent exercise.

▶ The importance of fluid replacement for athletes in sports such as soccer, football, basketball, and hockey is stressed in this article. The authors indicate that water absorption is enhanced by a great number of transport mechanisms. Different types of carbohydrates activate different transport mechanisms, which increase the overall absorption rate.

Gone are the days when fluid replacement was withheld from athletes. Athletes in hot and humid conditions should be forced to drink before the activity, during the activity, and after the activity. Sport drinks may enhance performance, but because of expense not all athletic programs may be able to afford them. Drinking enough water before and during an activity will prevent many of the heat-related emergencies that were common in the past.

F.J. George, ATC, PT

Hypohydration Effects on Skeletal Muscle Performance and Metabolism: A ³¹P-MRS Study

Montain SJ, Smith SA, Mattot RP, et al (United State Army Research Inst of Environmental Medicine, Natick, Mass; Boston Univ; Harvard Med School, Boston)

J Appl Physiol 84:1889-1894, 1998
6–21

Objective.—The effects of hypohydration on skeletal muscle performance and metabolism are not well understood. ³¹P-MRS was used to measure high-energy phosphates and pH during exhaustive single-leg, knee-extension exercise when subjects were euhydrated and hypohydrated to determine whether hypohydration reduces skeletal muscle performance and whether increased H^+ and P_i concentrations might contribute to performance degradation.

Methods.—This study obtained 1.5-T whole body magnetic resonance spectroscopy images from 10 healthy, physically active volunteers (5 men), aged 21 to 40, during supine single-leg, knee-extension exercise to exhaustion when euhydrated and when hypohydrated (drinking restricted to produce a 4% decrease in body mass). ³¹P spectra were collected at rest and during exercise using hard-pulse 25.85 MHz excitation signals. Volunteers performed exercises in a hot room (40°C, 20% relative humidity).

Results.—Hypohydration decreased endurance time and mean endurance (Fig 2). Hypohydration did not affect muscle strength. Hydration did not change P_i/β-ATP, pH, and ratio of P_i to $PCr(P_i/PCr)$.

Conclusion.—Whereas hypohydration decreases muscle endurance and endurance time, it does not affect muscle strength or $H+$ or P_i concentrations.

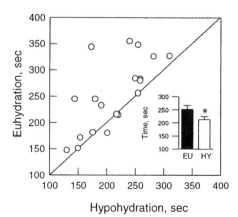

Hypohydration, sec

FIGURE 2.—Individual (O) and group mean (solid line) results for time to fatigue for subjects euhydrated (EU) and hypohydrated (HY) by 4% of initial body weight. *Inset*: hypohydration less than euhydration, *P less than 0.05. (Courtesy of Montain SJ, Smith SA, Mattot RP, et al: Hypohydration effects on skeletal muscle performance and metabolism: A ³¹P-MRS study. *J Appl Physiol* 84:1889-1894, 1998).

▶ Despite the best advice of sports physicians, many athletes still reduce their body mass by several kilograms in an attempt to make a specific weight category. This study confirms previous research in showing that such behavior reduces muscular endurance by a substantial 15%. The evidence is more convincing than in many previous trials, since a crossover design allowed control for previous exercise and heat exposure. The mechanism limiting muscular endurance remains unclear; in this study, magnetic resonance spectroscopy showed that a greater change in hydrogen ion and phosphate concentrations was not responsible. Possibilities include an alteration in Ca2+ release or uptake, or some central nervous consequence of dehydration, such as an increased perception of effort.

R.J. Shephard, M.D., Ph.D., D.P.E.

Human Thermoregulatory Responses During Serial Cold-Water Immersions
Castellani JW, Young AJ, Sawka MN, et al (US Army Research Inst of Environmental Medicine, Natick, Mass)
J Appl Physiol 85:204-209, 1998   6–22

Objective.—Fatigue of shivering and vasoconstriction may indicate thermoregulatory system fatigue. Whether cold-water immersions repeated several times in 1 day would lead to thermoregulatory fatigue, and whether second and third serial immersions, would blunt shivering thermogenesis, reduce peripheral vasoconstriction, and result in a greater fall in core temperature were tested during serial cold-water immersions.

Methods.—Eight healthy men with an average age of 24.4 years were quickly immersed to the shoulders in 20°C water for 120 minutes on 3 separate days at 7 AM, 11 AM, and 6 PM (control period) and then at the same hours on 1 day (test period). Pre- and post-immersion rectal temperature, mean weighted skin temperature, mean weighted heat flow, oxygen uptake, and body heat storage were recorded. Plasma glucose and norepinephrine determinations were made at pre-immersion and at 30, 60, 90, and 120 minutes.

Results.—Rectal temperatures were significantly lower after the 1-day repeat immersions than after initial immersion. Heat debt was significantly higher and heat production was significantly lower after the 1-day repeat immersions than after initial immersion. Metabolic heat production was significantly lower after the 1-day repeat immersions.

Conclusion.—Serial cold water immersions appear to affect the body's ability to thermoregulate and increase the risk of hypothermia as a result of attenuation of the metabolic heat response.

▶ The authors have successfully proven the hypothesis that serial cold-water immersions repeated over a short period would lead to the inability of the body to thermoregulate effectively, thus increasing a person's risk of hypothermia. However, the question of whether this phenomena is caused by an attenuation of metabolic heat response to cold or the early development of cold habituation is not answered. Presumably, the clinical relevance of this observed thermoregulatory system fatigue pertains to extended periods of outdoor activity in cold weather for athletes, the military, and emergency rescue teams.

J.S. Torg, M.D.

A Physiological Strain Index to Evaluate Heat Stress

Moran DS, Shitzer A, Pandolf KB (United States Army Research Inst of Environmental Medicine, Natick, Mass; Heller Inst of Med Research, Tel Hashomer, Israel; Technion, Haifa, Israel)
Am J Physiol 75:25:R129-R134, 1998   6–23

Objective.—Heat strain is the inability to maintain body core temperature within the appropriate range. Existing indices have difficulty discriminating between metabolic rates and different clothing. A simple phys-

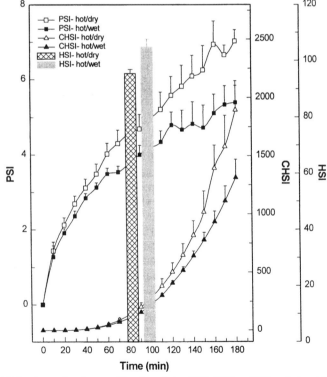

FIGURE 4.—Comparison between Heat Stress Index (HSI), CHSI, and PSI applied on Montain et al. (20) database. Note that HSI rated the hot-wet climate as the higher strain, in contradiction to CHSI and PSI, which rated the hot-dry climate as the higher strain. (Courtesy of Moran DS, Shitzer, Pandolf KB: A physiological strain index to evaluate heat stress. *Am J Physiol* 275:R129-R134, 1998. Copyright The American Philosophical Society.)

iological strain index (PSI) was developed for use in hot environments. It indicates heat strain online, is applicable to analyzing databases, and is sensitive enough to differentiate between similar exposures that differ in 1 variable, such as clothing, metabolic rate, and climate.

Methods.—After a medical examination, 100 healthy males at different levels of fitness and heat acclimation, exercised in a hot-dry climatic condition of 40°C and 40% relative humidity for 120 per manuscript minutes. After resting 10 minutes, volunteers walked on a treadmill at 1.34 m/s at a 2% grade. Heart rate and rectal temperature were monitored continuously, and cold water was supplied ad libitum. Maximal rectal temperature and heart rate increase defining hyperthermia were set at 3°C and 120 beats/min, respectively.

Results.—The normalized PSI was defined as: $PSI = 5(T_{ret}-T_{re0})/(39.5-T_{re0})$ + $5(HR_t-HR_0)/(180-HR_0)$ where T_{ret} and HR_t are rectal temperature and heart rate measured at any time and T_{re0} and HR_0 are baseline measurements. Validity testing of the index was conducted using data from 7 men who wore protective clothing and exercised in both hot and dry and in hot and wet conditions. Whereas the cumulative heat strain index (CHSI) and PSI found higher physiological strain in hot-dry climate, heat strain index (HSI) found the hot-wet climate more physiologically stressful. The PSI for the 2 climates was significantly different (Fig 4).

Conclusion.—The new PSI index based only on heart rate and rectal temperature could effectively distinguish between heat stress in hot-wet vs. hot-dry climates. Whether this index is applicable to women and other age groups remains to be investigated.

▶ The thermal strain imposed on athletes by a hot environment is commonly evaluated by an environmental index originally developed by Minard,[1] the wet bulb globe temperature (WBGT): $WBGT = 0.7 (T_W) + 0.2 (T_G) + 0.1 (T_D)$. T_W is the wet bulb temperature, T_G is the globe temperature, and T_D is the dry bulb temperature. This equation works well in providing a good idea of the thermal load imposed by a given environment, but it also helps to allow for inter-individual differences in heat tolerance, using a personal index of the resulting heat stress. The method described in the report of Moran et al, allows a simple combination of 2 indicators of heat stress—the increases in rectal temperature and heart rate into a single measure. To date, the index has been applied to soldiers exercising at a military pace. A need to evaluate how well the index performs at the more intensive exercise rates found in athletic competition now exists.

R.J. Shephard, M.D., Ph.D., D.P.E.

Reference

1. Minard D: Prevention of heat casualties in Marine Corps recruits. Period of 1955-1960, with comparative incidence rates and climatic heat stresses in other training categories. *Mil Med* 126: 261-272, 1961.

Double-Blind Intervention Trial on Modulation of Ozone Effects on Pulmonary Function by Antioxidant Supplements

Grievink L, Zijlstra AG, Ke X, et al (Wageningen Agricultural Univ, The Netherlands)

Am J Epidemiol 149:306-314, 1999   6–24

Purpose.—Exposure to ozone during exercise causes an acute decline in lung function. Ozone exposure is also associated with increased levels of inflammatory mediators, such as neutrophils and prostaglandins, in bronchoalveolar lavage. Antioxidants such as vitamin C and E may protect against acute effects of ozone exposure. This placebo-controlled trial examined the impact of antioxidant vitamin supplementation on the acute pulmonary effects of ozone.

Methods.—Thirty-eight Dutch bicyclists underwent lung function studies before and after training sessions on an average of 10 occasions each. One group of subjects received 15 weeks of antioxidant vitamin supplementation, consisting of vitamin E 100 mg/day, and vitamin C, 500 mg/day; the other group received placebo. The effects of ambient ozone exposure on lung function with and without vitamin supplementation were analyzed.

Results.—The average ozone concentration on the test days was 77 µg/m³. In response to a 100 µg/m³–difference in ozone exposure, forced expiratory volume in 1 second decreased 1 mL in the vitamin group vs. 95 mL in the placebo group. The reduction in forced vital capacity was 42 vs. 12 mL. The significant differences between groups became more apparent after exclusion of noncompliant subjects (Fig 2).

Conclusion.—Supplementation with the antioxidant vitamins C and E appears to lessen the acute pulmonary function effects of ozone exposure during exercise. Given a 100 µg/m³ difference in ozone exposure, vitamin supplementation might protect against a 2% reduction in forced expiratory volume in 1 second and a 1.5% reduction in forced vital capacity.

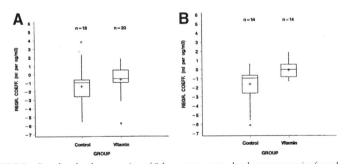

FIGURE 2.—Boxplots for the regression of 8-hour mean ozone level on postexercise forced expiratory volume in 1 second (milliliters per microgram per meter³) in vitamin-using cyclists and control cyclists, The Netherlands, 1996. Shown are the median value (*center line in box*), the mean value (+), the 25th and 75th percentiles, that is, the interquartile range (*borders of the box*), the range of values (*vertical lines*) and outliers. A, All subjects; B, Good compliers only. (Courtesy of Grievink L, Zijlstra AG, Ke X, et al: Double-blind intervention trial on modulation of ozone effects on pulmonary function by antioxidant supplements. *Am J Epidemiol* 149:306-314, 1999.)

► There is growing recognition that even quite low concentrations of ozone can have adverse effects on health. Negative effects on lung function in cyclists have been demonstrated at levels of less than 120 µg/m³.[1] Moreover, this seems to be evidence of lung damage rather than simply a reaction to respiratory discomfort, as bronchoalveolar lavage shows the presence of inflammatory mediators.[2] The main source of the ozone is a chemical reaction on automotive exhaust induced by bright sunlight. One possible remedy for the athlete is, thus, to avoid exercising at times of the day when there is bright sunlight. However, this may not always be possible, and the administration of antioxidant vitamins seems a simple and relatively harmless chemotherapeutic approach.

R.J. Shephard, M.D., Ph.D., D.P.E.

References

1. Brunekreef B, Hoek G, Breugelmans O, et al: Respiratory effects of low-level photochemical air pollution in amateur cyclists. *Am J Respir Crit Care Med* 150:962-966, 1994.
2. Devlin RB, McDonnell WF, Becker S, et al: Time-dependent changes of inflammatory mediators in the lungs of humans exposed to 0.4 ppm ozone for 2 hr: A comparison of mediators found in bronchoalveolar lavage fluid 1 and 18 hr after exposure. *Toxicol Appl Pharmacol* 138:176-185, 1996.

Individual Variation in Response to Altitude Training
Chapman RF, Stray-Gundersen J, Levine BD (Presbyterian Hosp of Dallas; Univ of Texas, Dallas)
J Appl Physiol 85:1448-1456, 1998   6–25

Objective.—Even after high-altitude training, some competitive endurance athletes do not improve sea level performance because of iron deficiency, despite high-dose iron supplementation. In studies, mean maximal oxygen uptake improved despite large individual variation. This variability was investigated retrospectively in collegiate runners retrospectively divided into responders and nonresponders to altitude training.

Methods.—Collegiate distance runners (27 men, 12 women; average age, 21.6 years) trained at sea level for 6 weeks, lived at a moderate altitude (2,500 m) for 28 days, and trained either at low or moderate altitude. Time to run 5,000 meters at sea level was measured at baseline and after the study. Erythropoietin (Epo) and hemoglobin concentrations were determined before and after acclimatization and compared with values obtained from 22 elite distance runners who had had 4 weeks of altitude training.

Results.—Responders had a significantly greater increase than nonresponders in Epo (6.5 vs . 4.7 U/mL) (Fig 3). Responders had a significantly larger increase than nonresponders in the total red cell volume (8% vs. 0%) and maximal oxygen uptake (69.2 vs. 64.4 mL/min/kg after 4 weeks at altitude. Whereas interval training at altitude declined significantly by

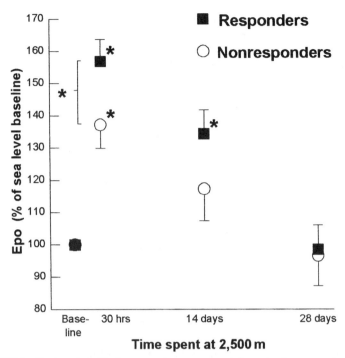

FIGURE 3.—Erythropoietin (*Epo*) concentration measures at 4 time points in retrospective group of responders and nonresponders to altitude training. Baseline and 28-day blood samples were drawn at sea level; 30-hour and 14-day blood samples were drawn at 2,500 m. Values are means ± SE. Statistical comparisons are within groups versus baseline time point, unless indicated by *open bracket*. Asterisk indicates P of .05 or less. (Courtesy of Chapman RF, Stray-Gundersen J, Levine BD: Individual variation in response to altitude training. *J Appl Physiol* 85:1448-1456, 1998).

9% in nonresponders, it was essentially unchanged in responders. Variability to altitude training can be explained by an altitude-acclimatization effect and a training effect. Variability in the magnitude of the Epo response can be accounted for by individual differences in hypoxic ventilation drive, oxygen half-saturation pressure of hemoglobin, or sensitivity to hypoxia at the point of Epo release. Despite the fact that all athletes received oral iron supplements, the difference in cell volume was not explained by iron deficiency. Epo release from the kidney appears to vary, with nonresponders requiring a greater hypoxic stimulus to induce sufficient release.

Conclusion.—Hypoxic exercise tolerance appears to vary with the individual. Epo screening and training velocity response measured shortly after arrival at altitude may predict which athletes will respond to altitude training and which will not.

▶ Last year we covered a benchmark study by this group.[1] It found that both "living high and training high"and "living high and training low" increased aerobic power, but living high and training low better improved track performance at sea level. That is, those who lived high and trained low improved 5-km run time by a mean of 13 seconds, or about 1.5%. Despite this small mean improvement, the range of 5-km run times was wide. In fact, 15 of 39 runners ("nonresponders") failed to improve run time, whereas 17 others ("responders") improved by more than 14 seconds.

This study explores differences between nonresponders and responders. In general, responders had a larger acute increase in erythropoietin level, total red cell volume, and maximal aerobic capacity and were better able to train hard at altitude. The mechanisms of these differences remain unclear, but this analysis offers the possibility of screening athletes and tailoring altitude training.

E.R. Eichner, M.D.

Reference

1. Levine BD, Stray-Gundersen J: "Living high-training low": Effect of moderate-altitude acclimatization with low-altitude training on performance. *J Appl Physiol* 83:102-112, 1997. (1998 Year Book of Sports Medicine, pp 242-244.)

7 Biomechanics

Muscle Activation Differences Between Eccentric and Concentric Isokinetic Exercise
Kellis E, Baltzopoulos V (Univ of Northumbria, Newcastle upon Tyne, England; Manchester Metropolitan Univ, England)
Med Sci Sports Exerc 30:1616-1623, 1998   7–1

Objective.—Neuromuscular activity of knee muscles was compared under isometric and isotonic conditions.

Methods.—Electromyographic (EMG) activity during knee flexion and extension was recorded for 12 women, average age 20.5, by using a dynamometer to measure submaximal and maximal eccentric and concentric repetitions at 4 angular velocities (30, 90, 120, and 150 degrees/sec) and at 65 and 30 degrees of knee flexion. EMG activities of the vastus lateralis, rectus femoris, vastus medialis, and hamstrings were recorded. Maximum moments for each type of action and angular velocity were determined. Three-factor ANOVA was used to assess differences between maximum normalized activities for eccentric and concentric moments.

Results.—Normalized eccentric moments were significantly greater than concentric moments during both extension and flexion (Fig 1). Integrated concentric EMG activity was significantly greater than integrated eccentric EMG activity during knee extension and flexion. Whereas EMG activity increased with faster concentric speeds, force decreased with increasing angular velocity.

Conclusion.—Neuromuscular activity in the knee was greater in the eccentric than in the concentric mode and increased with angular velocity.

▶ It has been consistently reported that maximum eccentric moments produced during isokinetic testing are greater than concentric moments. However, maximum isokinetic performance also varies as a function of angular velocity. This study reported that the maximum eccentric knee extension moments exceeded the concentric moments by 22.5% at 30 degrees/sec and by 107% at 150 degrees/sec, while the flexor moments were 3% and 46% higher compared with the concentric moments at 30 and 150 degrees/sec, respectively. There was also found to be lower EMG output during eccentric contraction than during concentric contractions, likely due to the activation of the elastic components to assist with force production during eccentric contractions. Increased EMG activity was also

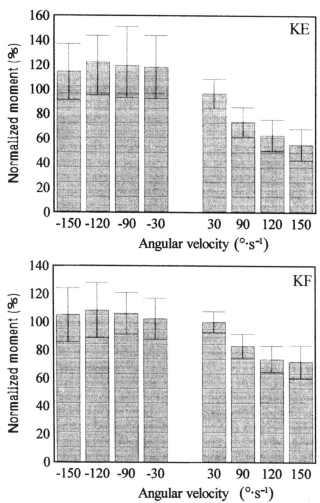

FIGURE 1.—Maximum knee extension (*KE*) and flexion (*KF*) resultant joint moment at different concentric (positive) and eccentric (negative) angular velocities. (Courtesy of Kellis E, Baltzopoulos V: Muscle activation differences between eccentric and concentric isokinetic exercise. *Med Sci Sports Exerc* 30:1616-1623, 1998.)

seen at faster speeds, even though the moment significantly decreases. The enhanced understanding of eccentric contractions during isokinetic exercise will be useful for those professionals who use this technique for training and rehabilitation of muscles.

M.J.L. Alexander, Ph.D.

Muscle Performance and Enzymatic Adaptations to Sprint Interval Training

MacDougall JD, Hicks AL, MacDonald JR, et al (McMaster Univ, Hamilton, Ont, Canada)

J Appl Physiol 84:2138-2142, 1998   7–2

Objective.—The effect of sprint exercise training on glycolytic enzyme activity is controversial. Glycolytic and oxidative enzyme activity was investigated in a group of healthy, physically fit young adults before and after they underwent a program of fitness sprint interval training.

Methods.—Twelve healthy male students, average age 22.7 years, trained on a cycle ergometer using 30-second maximum-effort intervals 3 times a week on alternate days for 7 weeks. During week 1, they had 4 intervals with 4 minutes of recovery that progressed to 10 intervals with 2.5 minutes of recovery at week 7. Maximum power output, total work over the 30-second intervals, and maximal oxygen consumption were measured before and after the program. Hexokinase, total glycogen phosphorylase, phosphofructokinase, lactate dehydrogenase, citrate synthase, succinate dehydrogenase, malate dehydrogenase, and 3-hydroxyacyl-CoA dehydrogenase activities were assessed using percutaneous needle biopsy specimens taken from the vastus lateralis.

Results.—Peak power output and total work increased significantly from before to after training. Maximal oxygen consumption increased significantly from 3.73 to 4.01 L/min, and maximal oxygen consumption relative to body mass also increased significantly from 51 to 54.5 mL/kg/min. Hexokinase, lactate dehydrogenase, and 3-hydroxyacyl-CoA dehydrogenase activities increased significantly from before training (5.10, 35.17, and 2.99 mol/kg protein/h, respectively) to after training (5.58, 37.65, and 4.15 mol/kg protein/h, respectively). Citrate synthase, malate dehydrogenase, and succinate dehydrogenase activities increased significantly by 36%, 29%, and 65%, respectively. 3-Hydroxyacyl-CoA dehydrogenase activity increased by a nonsignificant 39%.

Conclusion.—Intense sprint interval training increases glycolytic and oxidative muscle enzyme activity, peak power output, and oxygen consumption.

▶ There is some controversy regarding the effects of sprint training on glycolytic and mitochondrial enzymes. This study used a protocol of intensive 30-second maximum sprint training on a cycle ergometer, and found significant changes in the enzyme profile after training. As expected, they found increases in the maximal enzyme activity of the glycolytic enzymes after the training program. In addition, they found increases in oxidative enzyme activity, as well as in maximal oxygen uptake after anaerobic training. The authors noted that training at an intensity that exceeds $\dot{V}O_{2\ max}$ may be a more important component than the volume of training to stimulate an increase in muscle oxidative potential. This finding has some implications for increasing the intensity of training of aerobic athletes such as cyclists and distance runners.

M.J.L. Alexander, Ph.D.

Pre-flight Characteristics of Hecht Vaults

Yeadon MR, King MA, Sprigings EJ (Loughborough Univ, UK; Univ of Saskatchewan, Saskatoon, Canada)
J Sports Sci 16:349-356, 1998   7–3

Objective.—The Hecht vault is a counterrotation vault in which the preflight direction of rotation is reversed during contact, with the opposite direction of rotation in postflight provided by the horse. Most studies of the mechanics of vaulting have focused on continuous rotation vaults; only theoretical studies of the Hecht vault have been reported. The technique of the Hecht vault was studied to determine how the preflight characteristics affect postflight performance.

Methods.—The analysis included all Hecht vaults performed by 27 elite gymnasts at a Canadian national competition. The vaults were videotaped and analyzed using the direct linear transformation technique. In addition to analyzing the effects of preflight characteristics on postflight performance, the investigators compared the techniques of the Hecht vault with previously reported data on the handspring somersault vault.

Results.—Vertical velocity of the mass center and body angle at horse contact were significantly correlated with the maximum height of the mass center during postflight. The shoulder angle at horse contact was significantly related to backwards body rotation during postflight. Variables significantly related to score in the competition were body angle at horse

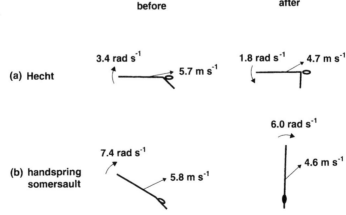

FIGURE 1.—Mean conditions just before and after contact with the horse in **A**, the Hecht vault (this study) and **B**, the handspring somersault (Takei Y, Kim EJ: Techniques used in performing the handspring and salto forward tucked vault at the 1988 Olympic Games. *Int J Sport Biomech* 6:111-138, 1990) (Courtesy of Yeadon MR, King MA, Sprigings EJ: Pre-flight characteristics of Hecht vaults. *J Sports Sci* 16:349-356, 1998. Published by Taylor & Francis, Ltd. at http: www.tandf.cc.uk/journals/jsp.htm.)

contact and maximum height of the mass center during postflight. Comparison with the handspring somersault vault suggested that the Hecht vault was associated with a longer, lower, and faster preflight, and with slower rotation at horse contact (Fig 1).

Conclusion.—For gymnasts performing the Hecht vault, height, distance, and correct rotation during postflight depend on the proper combination of variables during preflight. The technique of the Hecht vault differs in several significant ways from that of the handspring somersault vault. As experience is gained with this vault, techniques will improve for achieving greater body angles at horse contact.

▶ The Hecht vault is a difficult counter rotation vault in gymnastics in which the direction of rotation in preflight is reversed during contact, with the vaulting horse producing the opposite direction of rotation in postflight. Computer simulations of the Hecht vault have suggested that it requires a longer preflight time, a low flight path, and near zero vertical velocity at horse contact, as compared with a conventional vault. Film analysis of 27 elite gymnasts performing the Hecht suggested that successful performance is related to a high horizontal velocity at horse contact, which produces a greater displacement after horse contact. Greater body and shoulder angles at horse contact are also related to a longer flight time and greater distance travelled. This type of analysis is important for coaches in preparing gymnasts for high-level competition in the vault.

M.J.L. Alexander, Ph.D.

Muscle Coordination in Cycling: Effect of Surface Incline and Posture
Li L, Caldwell GE (Univ of Massachusetts, Amherst)
J Appl Physiol 85:927-934, 1998   7–4

Objective.—Most cycling studies involve riding on a level surface. Lower extremity neuromuscular changes were evaluated during incline riding and during standing on the pedals.

Methods.—Electromyographic data from 6 left lower extremity muscles of 8 experienced healthy male cyclists, average age 24, and videos were obtained while individuals were pedaling on a level surface while seated (LS), up an 8% grade while seated (US), and up an 8% grade while standing (ST)—each at a constant work rate (250 W).

Results.—Muscle activity patterns differed for different muscles (Fig 2). Mean peak electromyographic findings during ST were significantly higher for the gluteus maximus (GM), rectus femoris (RF), and tibialis anterior (TA) muscles than for other muscle groups. Electromyographic activities for the biceps femoris (BF), gastrocnemius (GC), and vastus lateralis (VL) were similar under different conditions. Neuromuscular coordination was not significantly affected by changing the grade. Muscle activity of hip and knee extensors was significantly increased during standing posture com-

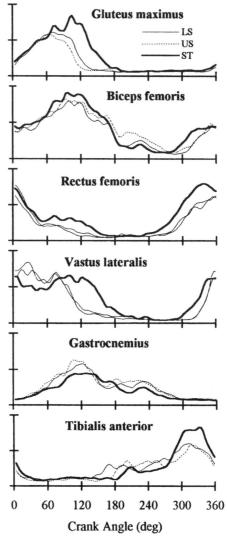

FIGURE 2.—Ensemble curves of linear envelope electromyography for 6 muscles for all conditions. *LS*, level seated; *US*, uphill seated; *ST*, uphill standing. All curves in 1 panel here used same arbitrary units on vertical axes. Scales of vertical axes used in different panels may be different. Horizontal axes are labeled by corresponding crank angle (in degrees). One complete cycle = top dead center from 0° to 360°. (Courtesy of Li L, Caldwell GE: Muscle coordination in cycling: Effect of surface incline and posture. *J Appl Physiol* 85:927-934, 1998.)

pared with sitting posture. Duration of GM, RF, and VL activity was extended over a greater portion of the crank cycle in the ST condition.

Conclusion.—Whereas changing the cycling grade does not significantly affect lower extremity neuromuscular coordination in cycling, changing from a sitting to a standing posture increases muscle activity of the GM and RF muscles significantly. Increases in the activity of the GM and VL muscles were larger and lasted longer in the standing position.

▶ This study compared the activity of the pedaling muscles while pedaling an ergometer on the level while seated, pedaling at 8% uphill while seated, and pedaling at 8% uphill while standing. The change of cycling grade from 0% to 8% did not change the pattern of muscular activity in cycling. Major increases in muscular activity level were seen in gluteus maximus and rectus femoris when standing on the pedals. They noted that biarticular muscles exhibited greater modifications in activity than the monoarticular muscles. This article suggests that cycling training should be modified for hilly race courses in which the athletes spend more time in the standing position on the pedals, due to the differences in muscular activity.

M.J.L. Alexander, Ph.D.

Comparisons of the Ski Turn Techniques of Experienced and Intermediate Skiers
Müller E, Bartlett R, Raschner C, et al (Universität Salzburg, Austria; Staffordshire Univ, Stoke-on-Trent, England)
J Sports Sci 16:545-559, 1998   7–5

Background.—Few studies have addressed the biomechanics of alpine skiing, partially because of the difficulty of analyzing 3-dimensional movements taking place over large areas. Differences in the performance of various ski turns between intermediate and advanced skiers were assessed.

Methods.—The analysis included 5 experienced ski instructors and 5 intermediate skiers, all male. The subjects were videotaped on a specially prepared ski slope while performing 4 different turns: the upstem turn, the downstem turn, the parallel turn, and the parallel step turn. For data analysis, each turn was divided into an initiation phase and first and second steering phases. Three-dimensional analyses were performed to compare turn performance between the 2 groups (Fig 1).

Results.—Most of the significant differences between the intermediate and advanced skiers occurred during the initiation phase of each turn. For the upstem turn, this involved differences in the hip axis-hand axis angle and the edging angle of the uphill ski. Differences in the initiation phase of the downstem turn were noted in the hip axis-hand axis angle, the shoulder axis-fall line angle, and the edging angle of the uphill ski. For this turn, the 2 groups also differed in the standard deviation of the distance between the ski tips during the second steering phase.

At the start of the initiation phase of the parallel step turn, there were significant differences in the edging angle of the downhill ski and the downhill ski to movement direction angle. This turn was also associated with differences in the edging angle of the downhill ski in the middle of the second steering phase and in the shoulder axis to movement direction angle at the end of the second steering phase. For the parallel turn,

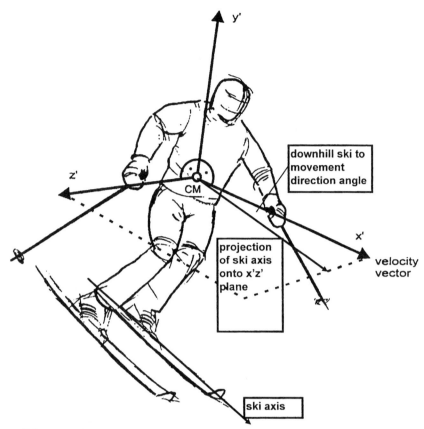

FIGURE 1.—The coordinate system of the angles to the movement direction. (Courtesy of Müller E, Bartlett R, Raschner C, et al: Comparisons of the ski turn techniques of experienced and intermediate skiers. *J Sports Sci* 16:545-549, 1998. Published by Taylor & Francis, Ltd. at http:www.tandf.cc.uk/ journals/jsp.htm.)

differences in the initiation phase included the time at which the ski pole was set, the uphill knee angle at the start of the initiation phase, and the range of the knee angle of the uphill leg from the start to the finish of the initiation phase. Also noted were differences in the edging angle of the downhill ski in the middle of the second steering phase and the shoulder axis to movement direction angle at the end of the same phase. For all turns, the intermediate skiers showed much greater variability than the advanced skiers.

Conclusion.—The major differences in turn performance between intermediate and advanced alpine skiers are found in the initiation phase of the turns. For intermediate skiers, it is difficult to achieve the correct edging angle for the up-unweighting push-off and to control upper body movement through this phase. These differences are most pronounced during the parallel and parallel-step turns, which are the more difficult turns.

▶ There is a scarcity of published biomechanics literature describing the techniques of alpine ski turns. This is because of the difficulty in collecting 3-dimensional biomechanical film data in an alpine environment during a high-speed race. In this study, there were significant differences between groups in several important turning variables, including shoulder angle, edging angle, and angle between the skis.

The major differences between the 2 groups were found in the initiation phase of each of the turns analyzed, especially in the correct edging angle for the unweighting and in the control of the movement of the upper body during this phase. This study provides an important early step in the description of the key aspects of ski turning which should be emphasized to intermediate skiers to improve their skill and safety during racing.

M.J.L. Alexander, Ph.D.

Electromyographic Analysis of Grand-Plié in Ballet and Modern Dancers
Trepman E, Gellman RE, Micheli LJ, et al (Boston Univ; New England Baptist Hosp, Boston; Harvard Med School, Boston)
Med Sci Sports Exerc 30:1708-1720, 1998   7–6

Introduction.—Only recently has electromyography (EMG) been applied to the movements of dance. This new source of information may have important implications for injury rehabilitation or preparation for performance in dancers. The plié is a basic dance movement in which the dancer maintains the torso, spine, and pelvis in stable condition while lowering with coordinated hip and knee flexion, and then returning to starting position with hip and knee extension. The grand plié, performed by supporting the entire body on the metatarsal head region and toes, is deeper and more difficult than the demi-plié, in which the foot remains flat on the floor. There is ongoing debate over the risks and benefits of the grand-plié in dance training. An EMG study of lower extremity muscle activity in the grand-plié was performed.

Methods.—EMG studies were performed in 12 female professional dancers: 5 ballet dancers and 7 modern dancers. All dancers were studied while they were performing the grand-plié in classical first position (Fig 1). The data were analyzed to test the hypothesis that the grand-plié was fundamentally different from the demi-plié in terms of muscle use. The muscles used by the 2 different types of dancers were compared as well.

Results.—During grand-plié, the tibialis anterior muscle showed continuous EMG activity from heel-off during the lowering phase, through midcycle, and ending at heel-on during the rising phase. In addition, most of the ballerinas showed continued tibialis anterior activity at the end of the rising phase. The vastus lateralis and vastus medialis showed peak activity during the lowering phase, with a decrease at midcyle and another peak during the rising phase. Ballet dancers showed increased vastus lateralis and medialis activity at the end of the rising phase, though modern dancers did not. Adductor muscle activity peaked during the lowering

GRAND-PLIE

◄──── LOWERING ──►◄──── RISING ────►
PHASE | PHASE

START   HEEL-OFF   MIDCYCLE   HEEL-ON   END

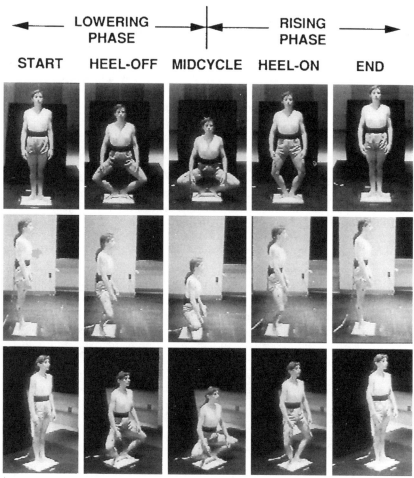

FIGURE 1.—Ballet dancer performing grand-plié in classical first position (turned out), as seen from front (**top row**), side (**middle row**), and oblique (**bottom row**) views. The dancer is positioned upright just before the start of the grand-plié (**first column**), proceeds through the lowering phase heel-off (**second column**) to midcycle (**third column**), and then through rising phase heel-off (**fourth column**) to completion of the movement at the end of rising phase (**fifth column**). (Courtesy of Trepman E, Gellman RE, Micheli LJ, et al: Electromyographic analysis of grand-plié in ballet and modern dancers. *Med Sci Sports Exerc* 30:1708-1720, 1998.)

phase from heel-off to midcyle, with a reduction at midcycle and another peak in the early rising phase. Ballet dancers had a lower midcycle reduction and a subsequent higher peak in adductor activity than the modern dancers. The lateral and medial gastrocnemius, gluteus maximus, and hamstring muscles showed variable EMG activity.

Conclusions.—This EMG study of professional dancers identifies 3 major types of lower extremity muscle movement. The characteristic activity required to perform the grand-plié is accompanied by variations related to the discipline of dance training and also by personal variations related to factors such as balance, habit, and individual training. Ballet and modern dancers varied in vastus lateralis and medialis activity in the midcycle reducing during grand-plié, despite the lack of difference in knee flexion. The data suggest that patellofemoral joint reaction force at midcyle is lower in ballet dancers than in modern dancers.

▶ This study examined the EMG activity of the muscles of the lower extremity involved in the grand-plié of both ballet and modern dancers. This movement consists of lowering the body downward to a position of full knee flexion with the toes turned outward, then rising to a full stand. The heels are raised from the floor during this movement. The movement is very difficult for all but trained dancers, as it requires considerable strength and balance to perform skillfully. The authors determined that eccentric muscle contraction controlled the lowering phase, whereas concentric contractions produced the return to stand. The tibialis anterior was active throughout the movement to stabilize the ankle joint in plantarflexion, and the abductors were active throughout the movement to assist with maintenance of turn-out. Quadriceps muscle activity was greater in modern dancers than in ballet dancers, likely due to lack of use of the movement in modern dance and extensive use in the training of ballet dancers. There are very few studies in the literature describing EMG activity during dance movements, but this topic is important in rehabilitation of dance injuries.

M.J.L. Alexander, Ph.D.

Static Versus Dynamic Predictions of Protective Stepping Following Waist–Pull Perturbations in Young and Older Adults
Pai Y-C, Rogers MW, Patton J, et al (Northwestern Univ, Chicago; Geriatric Medicine Associates, Denver; Marianjoy Rehabilitation Hosp, Wheaton, Ill)
J Biomech 31:1111-1118, 1998   7–7

Objective.—Older individuals are more likely to fall, possibly because these individuals may not effectively initiate and execute protective stepping to prevent loss of balance. The extent to which individuals of different ages and fall status would execute steps to recover balance as a function of different magnitudes of waist-pull disturbances of stance was determined, and the model predictions based on critical center of mass (COM) displacement-velocity values were compared with the predictions made solely on the COM displacement against experimentally recorded conditions of induced stepping.

Methods.—Thirteen young subjects, 18 older nonfallers, and 18 older fallers stood on 2 separate platforms and were told to react naturally to waist pulls at 3 levels of forward waist-pulls applied at low, medium, and high levels of displacement, ramp velocities, and peak accelerations. Reactions were recorded with a video camera used to record position of

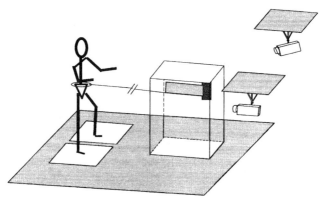

FIGURE 2.—Schematic sketch of the experimental setup: a subject standing on the force platforms facing motion capture cameras while waiting for a waist-pull perturbation. The safety harness is not shown. (Reprinted from the Journal of Biomechanics, Volume 31, Pai Y-C, Rogers MW, Patton J, et al: Static versus dynamic predictions of protective stepping following waist–pull perturbations in young and older adults, pages 1111-1118, Copyright 1998, with kind permission from Elsevier Science Ltd, The Boulevard, Langford Lane, Kidlington OX5 1GB UK.)

2-dimensional reflective markers (Fig 2). COM phase trajectories were calculated from motion analysis.

Results.—Older individuals stepped significantly more often than younger individuals at the low perturbation level. All individuals except 4 stepped at most trials at the middle-perturbations levels. All individuals stepped at every trial at the high-perturbation level. Fallers stepped in 52% of low-perturbation trials, nonfallers stepped in 17.3% of trials, and young individuals stepped in 2.7% of trials. The static model predicted 5% of stepping trials, whereas the dynamic model predicted 65%. The dynamic model also predicted when a step would occur.

Conclusion.—Fallers are more likely than nonfallers to step in response to perturbations. The dynamic model predicted stepping in 65% of trials.

▶ Protective stepping is a common response for balance recovery in the normal environment. Steps may occur in anticipation of an impending collision or fall, or in reaction to imposed horizontal movement of the body COM, which was the protocol used in this study. Elderly persons who have experienced falls may be using unskilled stepping patterns to prevent loss of balance, such as taking a protective step to increase the base of support when it was not required. This study confirmed that older fallers would initiate steps more frequently and at lower levels of perturbation intensity than younger subjects. The fear of falling was likely greater for the elderly, so they adopted a safer movement strategy by stepping when the COM reached within 10% of the boundary of the base. The authors concluded that their waist-pull protocol may be useful in predicting risk of falls in older adults.

M.J.L. Alexander, Ph.D.

1997 Volvo Award Winner in Biomechanical Studies: Kinematic Behavior of the Porcine Lumbar Spine: A Chronic Lesion Model

Kaigle AM, Holm SH, Hansson TH (Sahlgrenska Univ Hosp, Göteborg, Sweden)

Spine 22:2796-2806, 1997   7–8

Introduction.—Injuries to the passive structures of spinal motion segments adversely affect segmental kinematics. Stimulation of the surrounding musculature may stabilize the motion segment. However, no dynamic, in vivo studies have measured the in vivo kinematics of degenerated lumbar motion segments or the stabilizing function of the surrounding musculature. This study used a pig model of intervertebral disc and facet joint degeneration in the lumbar spine.

Methods.—Six types of chronic lesions were created in the lumbar spines of 44 pigs: sham, disc anulus, disc nucleus, facet capsule, facet joint slit, and facet joint wedge. After 3 months, the pigs were instrumented for measurement of sagittal kinematics in the L3-L4 motion segment (Fig 2). Measurements were made during flexion-extension, with and without stimulation of the lumbar paraspinal muscles. The pattern of motion analysis included the flexion-extension end point, the maximum range of motion, and hysteresis.

Results.—The results showed significant kinematic changes resulting from chronic lumbar spinal lesions. The changes were especially apparent on analysis of maximum range of motion and comparison of changes in axial translation. On stimulation of the paraspinal muscles, hysteresis was reduced in segments with sham, facet capsule, and disc nucleus lesions, but

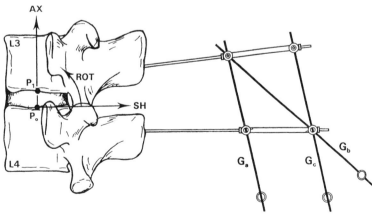

FIGURE 2.—Schematic diagram of intervertebral motion device attached to L3-L4 motion segment. *Ga, Gb,* and *Gc* indicate locations of 3 displacement transducers. Sliding linkage allows displacement of transducers between intraosseous pins. Sagittal rotation (*ROT*), axial translation (*AX*), and anteroposterior shear translation (*SH*) were computed for P_1 rotative to P_0. (Courtesy of Kaigle AM, Holm SH, Hansson TH: 1997 Volvo award winner in biomechanical studies: Kinematic behavior of the porcine lumbar spine: A chronic lesion model. *Spine* 22:2796-2806, 1997.)

increased in those with disc anulus, facet slit joint, and facet joint wedge lesions.

Conclusions.—This in vivo model documents the development of chronic degenerative changes in the lumbar spine with time after the creation of surgical lesions. Dynamic measurements of maximum range of motion during flexion-extension provide a sensitive indicator of changes in segmental kinetics resulting from chronic lesions. Axial translation is the most significant kinematic variable for assessing ranges of motion during flexion extension. The lumbar paraspinal muscles offer less stability during flexion-extension in segments with intervertebral disc or facet joint lesions.

▶ Chronic lesions of the spinal segments often produce altered segment kinematics, so there is an abnormal type and range of motion between the segments. The spines of pigs were injured by producing chronic lesions resembling those in human disc degeneration and facet hypertrophy. A unique intervertebral motion device determined the 3 dimensional motion characteristics of the injured spines. The authors were able to determine the effects of each type of lesion on the intersegment motion at the level of the lesion. They determined that axial translation was the motion variable most affected by the lesions. Spinal injury also results in less efficient stabilization from the lumbar extensor muscles, because of decreased feedback from the injured segment. This study provides an insightful summary of some of the most important effects of chronic injury to the lumbar spine.

M.J.L. Alexander, Ph.D.

Comparison Between Two Dynamic Methods to Estimate Triaxial Net Reaction Moments at the L5/S1 Joint During Lifting

Larivière C, Gagnon D (Université de Sherbrooke, Québec)
Clin Biomech 13:36-47, 1998   7–9

Purpose.—Validated, dynamic 3-dimensional (3D) models demonstrating spinal loading are needed to assess the risks associated with manual materials handling (MMH) tasks. The upward model, designed for gait analysis, is based on measured external forces at the feet. Downward models are more practical for assessing MMH activities, but several challenges remain to be addressed. This study examined the validity of the upward and downward 3D biomechanical dynamic multisegment models.

Methods.—One young male subject was studied using 4 video cameras and 2 force platforms to derive data from 66 static and 108 dynamic trials (Fig 1). The upward and downward model were compared according to the criterion of net moments at the L5/S1 joint. Both models were used to calculate axial rotation, lateral bending, and flexion/extension. Peak L5/S1 net joint moments for different task parameters were subjected to sensitivity analysis. The effects of different regression equations and of the L5/S1 joint center location were evaluated, as were various techniques of estimating the shoulder joint center.

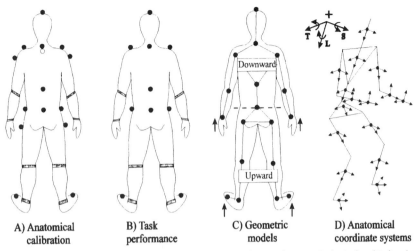

| A) Anatomical | B) Task | C) Geometric | D) Anatomical |
| calibration | performance | models | coordinate systems |

FIGURE 1.—Positions of the 23 and 18 anatomic markers (spheres and elastic bands) for the anatomical calibration (A) and the task performance (B), respectively. These markers configurations were needed to build the 2 geometric models (C). The orientation of anatomical coordinate systems and the positive signs of moments are shown (D). (Courtesy of Larivière C, Gagnon D: Comparison between two dynamic methods to estimate triaxial net reaction moments at the L5/S1 joint during lifting. *Clin Biomech* 13:36-47, 1998 with permission from Elsevier Science.)

Results.—For static tasks, the 2 models showed good agreement in terms of net moments at the L5/S1 joint. However, the models showed greater disagreement for moments of the dynamic tasks, with differences of up to 78 Nm in an extension task. Both the upward and downward models were sensitive to various task parameters, including movement or load asymmetry, movement rate, and load magnitude.

Conclusions.—These 3D biomechanical dynamic multisegment models show good agreement in estimating triaxial net moments for static tasks, less so for dynamic tests. Both models are sensitive to various controlled task parameters affecting net joint moments. Future studies should include direct measurement of the external forces at each hand and validation in a larger number of subjects.

▶ Low back problems often arise in the workplace from improper MMH. There have been numerous attempts to develop and validate 3-dimensional dynamic models that can quantify the loads on the spine, but these models have many sources of error because of their complexity. Some of the sources of error include estimation of the acceleration and anthropometric parameters of the segments, the location of joint centers, and the location of the external forces and torques. The models compared were the upward model that used the measured external forces at the feet and the downward model that used an estimation of the forces on the hands. The models were tested using a single subject performing numerous MMH tasks, which was a limitation of the study. They concluded that the upward model was more accurate for predicting lumbar forces and torques, because the downward model used only estimates of the forces on the hands. They recommended the use of a load cell to measure forces on the hands if the downward model is used, as well as better estimations of the accelerations of the upper segments.

M.J.L. Alexander, Ph.D.

The Morphology and Biomechanics of Latissimus Dorsi

Bogduk N, Johnson G, Spalding D (Univ of Newcastle, Australia; Univ of Newcastle upon Tyne, England)
Clin Biomech 13:377-385, 1998   7–10

Purpose.—In addition to its role as a shoulder adductor and extensor, the latissimus dorsi may act on the lumbar spine and sacroiliac joint. Although the anatomy of the latissimus dorsi has been well described, these studies are not sufficient to explain its action. Its action on the lumbar spine and sacroiliac joint may have been overstated. An anatomical study was performed to investigate the actions of the latissimus dorsi on these 3 sites.

Methods.—Latissimus dorsi dissection was performed in 5 adult cadavers. Fascicular anatomy was studied by determining the size, attachment, and orientation of each fascicle. Based on physiologic cross-sectional area, each fascicle's maximum force was estimated by application of a force coefficient. The forces and moments of each fascicle were then added to determine the maximal force exerted for latissimus dorsi action on the shoulder, lumbar spine, and sacroiliac joint.

Results.—The latissimus dorsi fascicles demonstrated segmental attachments to the spinous processes of the lower 6 thoracic and the upper 2 lumbar vertebrae, the lateral raphe of the thoracolumbar fascia, the iliac crest, and the lower 3 ribs (Fig 2). The size of the fascicles was uniform across a given muscle but variable between specimens. Estimates of maximal total force on the shoulder ranged from 162 to 529 newtons. However, considering the muscle attachments, only a fraction of that force could act on the lumbar spine. Maximal extensor moment on the lumbar spine was 6.3 newton meters, and maximum force across the sacroiliac joint was 30 newtons.

Conclusions.—The findings clarify the actions of the latissimus dorsi in the shoulder, lumbar spine, and sacroiliac joint. Its major functions are to move the upper limb or raise the entire trunk in brachiation. In contrast to previous anatomical reports, it appears to make little contribution to extension of the lumbar spine or bracing of the sacroiliac joint. Future models of the latissimus dorsi should focus on the shoulder, not the lumbar spine.

▶ The latissimus dorsi has been attributed a significant role by several investigators in providing an extensor moment to help support lumbar loads. Because of the latissimus dorsi's attachment to the thoracolumbar fascia, it

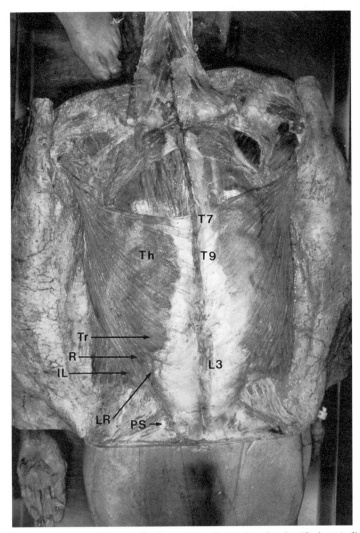

FIGURE 2.—A dissection of the latissimus dorsi bilaterally. *LR*, lateral raphe; *Th*, thoracic fibres; *Tr*, transitional fibres; *R*, raphe fibres; *IL*, iliac fibres; *PS*, posterior superior iliac spine. Costal fibres are not evident in this posterior view for they lie deep to the iliac fibres. The numbers mark the spinous processes. (Courtesy of Bogduk N, Johnson G, Spalding D: The morphology and biomechanics of latissimus dorsi. *Clin Biomech* 13:377-385, 1998. Reprinted from *Clinical Biomechanics*, vol. 13, pp 377-385, copyright 1998, with kind permission from Elsevier Science Ltd, The Boulevard, Langford Land, Kidlington OX5 1GB UK.)

has been suggested that contraction of the muscle can pull on the posterior lumbar spine, as well as providing support for the sacroiliac joint. This study provides an extensive anatomical study of the latissimus dorsi of 5 adult cadavers, in which the muscle was dissected fascicle by fascicle to determine the muscle structure and cross-sectional area. The authors concluded that the muscle has no significant effect on the lumbar spine or the sacroiliac joint, and that its role is primarily in forceful adduction and medial rotation of the humerus. This study provides some useful and persuasive evidence regarding the role of this muscle.

M.J.L. Alexander, Ph.D.

Velocity Effects on the Scapulo-humeral Rhythm
de Groot JH, Valstar ER, Arwert HJ (Delft Univ, The Netherlands; Univ Hosp Leiden, The Netherlands)
Clin Biomech 13:593-602, 1998   7–11

Introduction.—Accurate measures of shoulder kinematics are possible only through invasive methods: placement of percutaneous pins in the bones or biplanar radiograph photogrammetry of marker implants. An alternative, noninvasive method is palpation and subsequent recording of the 3-dimensional position of skeletal landmarks. This method is simple, but static. Motions are modelled using interpolation of the subsequent position recordings. This method has yet to be validated and was examined to determine whether stationary measurements of scapulo-humeral posture can be used for the description of the kinematics of the shoulder mechanism during movements in the scapular plane.

Methods.—Seven healthy participants (1 woman), aged 21 to 25, performed an alternating abduction-adduction motion of the arm in a plane 30° forward-rotated with respect to the frontal plane. This was done at 3 submaximal frequencies: 0.04 Hz, 0.25 Hz, and 0.50 Hz. Humeral and scapular motions were recorded using a 2-dimensional radiograph video

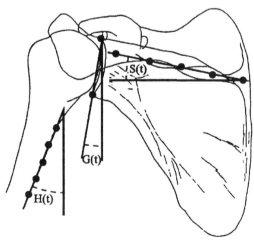

FIGURE 2.—Schematic projection of the right shoulder at time (*t*). The *Dots*, digitized positions on the humerus (*H*), the glenoid (*G*), and the scapular spine (*S*). Angles *H(t)* and *G(t)* were determined with respect of the vertical frame axis; *S(t)* was determined with respect to the horizontal frame axis. (Reprinted from de Groot JH, Valstar ER, Arwert HJ: Velocity effects on the scapulo-humeral rhythm. *Clin Biomech* 13:593-602, copyright 1998, with kind permission from Elsevier Science Ltd, The Boulevard, Langford Land, Kidlington OX5 1GB UK.)

system. Angles were used to define the motions of the humerus, scapular spine, and glenoid ridge (Fig 2). The sinusoidal motion curves were depicted by the offset, amplitude, and phase of the motions.

Results.—A significant effect of arm motion on the phase and amplitude of the scapular motion was detected using repeated measurements multivariate analysis of variance. Magnitude of the effects was negligible for these applications at submaximal arm motion velocities.

Conclusion.—The 3-dimensional motions of the shoulder are a consequence of the kinetic restraints of the skeletal system and the coordinated muscle forces; they are 1 of the few properties that can be quantified. These motions contain pertinent information essential to assessment of clinical interventions and physiotherapy, to analysis of ergonomic and biomechanical problems, and to the analysis of clinical disorders, including subacromial disorders and glenohumeral subluxation.

▶ This study employed a new technique of measuring shoulder motions: a 2-dimensional x-ray video system. This technique enabled exact measurement of the positions of the scapula and humerus during abduction/adduction of the shoulder joint at varying speeds. The authors determined that the scapulo-humeral rhythm changed significantly during movement velocity changes. The motions of both the scapular spine and the glenoid fossa decreased with increasing speed of motion. However, the amount of motion discrepancy (6°) was small enough that stationary recordings could be used to describe the kinematics of the shoulder motions at submaximal velocities. This finding is important in the clinical evaluation of shoulder disorders such as shoulder impingement and subluxation, which can then be evaluated by standard stationary X rays.

M.J.L. Alexander, Ph.D.

Comparison of Two Methods for Computing Abduction Moment Arms of the Rotator Cuff
Hughes RE, Niebur G, Liu J, et al (Mayo Clinic and Mayo Found, Rochester, Minn)
J Biomech 31:157-160, 1998   7–12

Objective.—Any model to predict rotator cuff muscle forces must include information on the muscle moment arms in the glenohumeral joint. In some models, these moment arms are estimated using an idealized minimum distance path from the origin to the insertion, passing around the bony geometry. Others calculate moment arms from data on tendon excursion and joint angles. This study compared estimates of abduction moment arms for the supraspinatus, infraspinatus, and subscapularis calculated by the origin-insertion and tendon excursion methods (Fig 1).

Methods.—Ten fresh frozen cadaver shoulders were mounted for testing in a custom-designed experimental setup. Abduction moment arms were subsequently estimated by evaluating the slope of tendon excursion vs. the

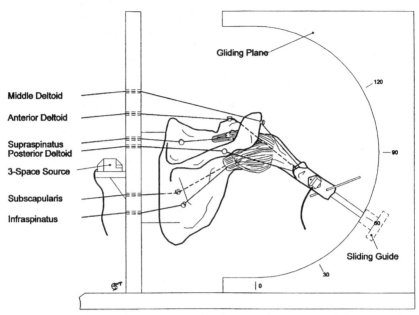

FIGURE 1.—Experimental setup. (Courtesy of Hughes RE, Niebur G, Liu J, et al: Comparison of two methods for computing abduction moment arms of the rotator cuff. *J Biomech* 31:157-160, 1998 with kind permission from Elsevier Science Ltd, The Boulevard, Langford Lane, Kidlington OX5 16B UK.)

joint angle relationship, and by using an idealized origin-insertion model of the musculoskeletal system.

Results.—Estimated abduction moment arms were larger with the tendon excursion method than with the origin-insertion method, particularly for the infraspinatus and subscapularis muscles at low abduction angles. The average difference was 3.1 mm for the supraspinatus muscle, 3.9 mm for the subscapularis, and 7.2 mm for the infraspinatus. The differences were apparent near the beginning of motion for the infraspinatus and subscapularis, and in the midrange of motion for the supraspinatus.

Conclusions.—Estimates of abduction moment arms in the rotator cuff vary significantly depending on the model used. The origin-insertion method obtains higher muscle force estimates than the tendon excursion method. The differences are most apparent for the subscapularis and infraspinatus muscles.

▶ Rotator cuff tears are 1 of the most common shoulder injuries that occur in an older adult population. Surgical repair of the torn rotator cuff muscles requires knowledge of the muscle moment arms for these muscles. The purpose of this study was to compare abduction moment arms of the supraspinatus, infraspinatus, and subscapularis muscles computed by 2 different methods using 10 cadaver specimens. One method used to estimate abduction moment arm was to find the slope of the tendon excursion vs. joint angle relationship and model the relationship using polynomial regression. The second method modeled the glenohumeral joint as a sphere with the muscle lines of pull from origin to insertion of the muscle wrapped around the head of the humerus. The origin insertion method of computing moment arms produces higher values and may give higher muscle force estimates. Sources of error with such models include humeral head translation and modeling the humeral head as a perfect sphere.

M.J.L. Alexander, Ph.D.

Biomechanical Response of the Passive Human Knee Joint Under Anterior-Posterior Forces
Bendjaballah MZ, Shirazi-Adl A, Zukor DJ (Ecole Polytechnique, Montréal; McGill Univ, Montréal)
Clin Biomech 13:625-633, 1998   7–13

Introduction.—Many studies have examined the mechanics of the knee joint, with particular attention to mechanics under drawer forces. However, many details of the biomechanics of the knee, including the role of boundary conditions, load transmission through the menisci and articular cartilage, and coupling between the menisci and cruciate ligaments, remain uncertain. The authors have created a nonlinear, 3-dimensional model of the human tibiofemoral joint to examine the biomechanics of the joint in full extension under anterior/posterior drawer forces up to 400 N.

Methods.—The model was created using computer-assisted tomography and finite element mesh generation with direct digitation techniques (Fig 1). In nonlinear elastostatic analyses, the tibiofemoral joint was considered in full extension under anterior and posterior loads, of up to 400 N, applied to the tibial or femoral shaft. The effects of various boundary conditions, anterior or posterior cruciate ligament deficiency, and total unilateral medial or lateral meniscectomy were also examined.

Results.—Total primary anterior-posterior motion in response to forces of ±400 N was about 9 mm. In addition, coupled external tibial rotation of about 9 degrees was calculated in response to femoral posterior forces of 400 N; rotation in response to anterior forces of the same magnitude was about 10 degrees. The type of loading and the boundary conditions had an important impact on the response. The anterior cruciate ligament served as the main restraint to femoral posterior forces, and the posterior cruciate ligament to anterior drawer forces. When either cruciate ligament was cut, anterior-posterior motion increased significantly. Without cruciate ligaments, the primary restraint in anterior-posterior forces was the collateral ligaments. Compressive forces on the tibial plateau—particularly the medial tibial plateau in anterior cruciate ligament-deficient joints—were subject to much greater compressive forces. Medial meniscectomy resulted in increased joint primary anterior-posterior laxity, as well as increased coupled tibial external rotation, increased lateral plateau forces, and increased stress on the articular cartilage of the lateral plateau.

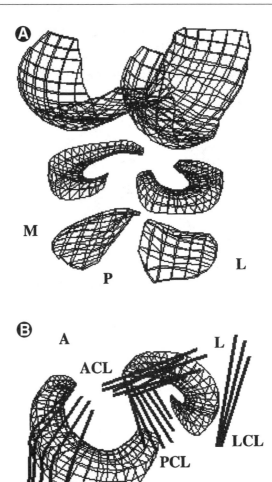

FIGURE 1.—Finite element model of the tibiofemoral joint. The bony structures are modeled as rigid bodies and are not shown. **A,** typical posterolateral view of the model showing the cartilage layers and menisci. There are 6 contact regions: femoral cartilage against exposed tibial cartilage, femoral cartilage against proximal meniscal surface, and distal meniscal surface against covered cartilage; all 3 at both medial and lateral compartments. **B,** model of menisci and ligaments. The major ligaments are: the anteromedial/posterolateral bundles of the posterior cruciate ligament (PCL), the lateral collateral ligament (LCL), and the medial collateral ligament (MCL). Each ligament bundle is represented by a 2-node axial element; also shown is the attachment of the MCL to the periphery of the medial meniscus. The MCL also wraps around the proximal medial bony edge of the tibia (not shown here). *Abbreviations:* M, medial; L, lateral; A, anterior; P, posterior. The bony structures are not shown. (Reprinted from Bendjaballah MZ, Shirazi-Adl S, Zukor DJ: Biomechanical response of the passive human knee joint under anterior-posterior forces. *Clin Biomech* 13:625-633, 1998, with permission from Elsevier Science Ltd, The Boulevard, Langford Lane, Kidlington OX5 1GB UK.)

Conclusions.—This 3-dimensional model of the passive human tibio-femoral joint suggests that the medial meniscus takes on an important role in the anterior cruciate ligament-deficient knee. The effect of medial meniscectomy is much greater than that of lateral meniscectomy. In knees undergoing anterior cruciate ligament replacement or meniscal transplantation to restore joint stability, avoidance of stress on the articular cartilage requires coupling between the anterior cruciate ligament and medial meniscus. If any of these structures is missing, the response of the joint will be dramatically different.

▶ This study used a complex finite element model to examine the response of the injured knee joint to anterior-posterior forces. The model enabled the investigators to cut each of the knee joint ligaments in turn, to determine its effect on the laxity in the knee joint. As others have reported, the authors found the anterior and posterior cruciate ligaments to be the primary restraints to anterior-posterior translation. When the cruciates were cut, the medial and lateral collateral ligaments became the primary restraints. The medial tibial plateau experienced much higher compressive forces when the anterior cruciate was cut, emphasizing the importance of the medial meniscus in resisting these forces. This study emphasizes the importance of each of the structures of the knee joint complex. Injury to any one of the structures produces increased stresses on the articular cartilage and may lead to early degenerative arthritis.

M.J.L. Alexander, Ph.D.

Biomechanical Study of Tibialis Anterior Tendon Transfer
Hui JHP, Goh JCH, Lee EH (Natl Univ Hosp, Singapore)
Clin Orthop 349:249-255, 1998   7–14

Background.—The tibialis anterior muscle is a dorsiflexor and inverter of the foot. Tibialis anterior tendon transfer is a commonly used operation for patients with recurrent congenital clubfoot or paralytic equinovarus foot deformity in cerebral palsy. However, there are no biomechanical data to identify the ideal route and site of transfer. A cadaver study was performed to determine the optimal site of tibialis anterior tendon insertion for ankle and foot motion. In addition, the effects of split and total tendon transfer were compared.

Methods.—The study used 10 fresh normal anatomical lower-leg specimens. After being freed from its insertion on the navicular, the lateral half of the tibialis anterior tendon was passed beneath the extensor retinaculum and anchored to the appropriate tarsal bone using a barbed staple. Ankle and foot motion in response to tension were measured using strain-gauged flexible goniometers (Fig 1). The tendon was anchored first along the axis of the second metatarsal, then in serial fashion to the axes of the third through fifth metatarsals. Further experiments were performed using the

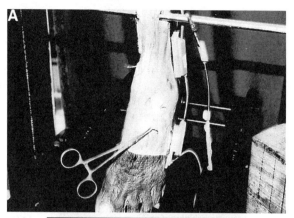

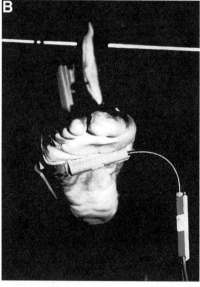

FIGURE 1.—Two strain-gauged flexible electrogoniometers were used to monitor the ankle and foot motion: **A**, plantar and dorsiflexion, and **B**, pronation and supination. (Courtesy of Hui JHP, Goh JCH, Lee EH: Biomechanical study of tibialis anterior tendon transfer. *Clin Orthop* 349:249-255, 1998.)

whole tibialis anterior tendon, and the effects of split and total tendon transfer were compared.

Results.—The ideal insertion point for split tendon transfer appeared to be the fourth metatarsal axis. This site resulted in maximal dorsiflexion with minimal supination and pronation. The third metatarsal axis was the ideal insertion site for whole tendon transfer. Split tendon transfer offered a somewhat greater average maximum dorsiflexion than whole tendon transfer; however, the difference was not significant. The foot became more inverted with insertion lateral to the optimal axis, and more inverted with insertion medial to the optimal axis.

Conclusion.—This cadaver study suggests that the optimal insertion site for split tibialis anterior tendon transfer is along the fourth metatarsal axis, whereas that for total tendon transfer is the third axis. These insertion points provide maximal dorsiflexion with minimal supination and pronation. This biomechanical study provides a somewhat objective view of tibialis anterior tendon transfer; it finds little difference in the effects of split vs. total tendon transfer.

▶ The tibialis anterior is the main muscle producing dorsiflexion of the foot during normal gait. In foot deformities in cerebral palsy, the foot remains in a position of plantarflexion and eversion, with the eversion being aided by the tibialis anterior. A treatment of this condition consists of transferring the anterior tibial tendon to the lateral border of the foot to restore the balance in foot function.

This study determined the optimum site of anterior tibial tendon transfer and compared the split tendon to the whole tendon transfer. The optimal site for the split tendon transfer was found to be insertion on the fourth metatarsal axis; whereas for the whole tendon, the optimal site was the third metatarsal axis. However, because this study was performed using cadaver feet attached to a strain gauge apparatus, it is unclear whether this procedure is equally effective on an actual patient.

M.J.L. Alexander, Ph.D.

Inhibition of the Quadriceps Muscles in Elite Male Volleyball Players
Huber A, Suter E, Herzog W (Univ of Calgary, Alberta, Canada)
J Sports Sci 16:281-289, 1998   7–15

Background.—Muscle inhibition, usually assessed with the interpolated twitch technique, refers to the inability to fully recruit all motor units of a muscle. The interpolated twitch technique applys an electrical stimulus applied to the contracted quadriceps muscle to estimate the number of motor units not fully activated. Healthy, untrained subjects show near-complete activation of their quadriceps muscles—ie, low muscle inhibition. It has been suggested that, because of training effects, elite volleyball players may have lower quadriceps muscle inhibition than untrained subjects. Quadriceps muscle inhibition and knee extensor moments were assessed in elite male volleyball players.

Methods.—The interpolated twitch technique was used to evaluate quadriceps muscle inhibition in 13 members of the Canadian men's national volleyball team. The measurements were obtained during isometric quadriceps contractions at knee angles of 30 and 60 degrees from full extension; knee extensor moments were measured at the same angles. Associations between muscle inhibition, knee extensor moment, and previous knee surgery or knee pain were examined.

Results.—Both knee extensor moments and muscle inhibition were greater at a knee angle of 60 degrees than at 30 degrees. At both angles, the volleyball players showed greater knee extensor moments than a previously studied group of healthy, untrained subjects. However, muscle inhibition was similar for athletes and controls. Knee extensor moments were no different for athletes with a history of knee injury, but muscle inhibition was significantly lower in legs with a history of injury. Muscle inhibition was unaffected by knee pain, but knee extensor moments were significantly reduced.

Conclusions.—In elite volleyball players, knee injury has no effect on knee extensor moment, but knee pain decreases knee extensor moment. Knee injury reduces muscle inhibition, but pain does not. The effect of pain on knee extensor moment may be related to quadriceps muscle atrophy resulted from disruption of training. If the pain becomes chronic, muscle inhibition is reduced, probably because muscle activation is improved by intense rehabilitation. Athletes with a history of knee injury can recruit available motor units more completely, thus allowing them to produce the same knee extensor moments as uninjured athletes. This additional recruitment may offset the loss of muscle mass incurred during injury and detraining.

▶ Volleyball players are required to produce high muscle forces in a short period of time in their jumping muscles, which include the hip extensors, knee extensors and plantarflexors. The contribution of the knee extensors to jumping height has been estimated at 56%. Elite volleyball players also suffer a high incidence of knee injury and pain, which has been found to inhibit activation of the quadriceps, reducing the knee extensor moments. This inability to recruit all the motor units of a muscle has been termed "muscle inhibition," which can be studied by the interpolated twitch technique. This study concluded that muscle inhibition in legs with previous injuries was lower than in legs with no previous injury, likely because of the intense rehabilitation program that athletes undergo following injury. The rehabilitation program enables athletes to recruit available motor units more completely and maintain quadriceps strength in a previously injured knee. This study provides some interesting insight into the processes possibly associated with knee joint injury in elite athletes.

M.J.L. Alexander, Ph.D.

Kinematics of Valgus Bracing for Medial Gonarthrosis: Technical Report
Davidson PL, Sanderson DJ, Loomer RL (School of Human Kinetics, BC, Canada; Univ of British Columbia, Canada)
Clin Biomech 13:414-419, 1998   7–16

Purpose.—In addition to cartilage breakdown, patients with medial compartment gonarthrosis of the knee may have medial joint space narrowing and excessive varus alignment of the tibia relative to the femur, the result of abnormal force loading within the joint. The concept supporting valgus bracing for medial gonarthrosis is to correct the varus deformity

Mid-Stance

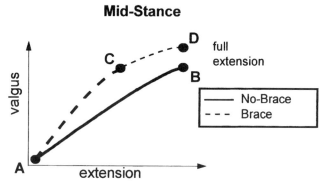

FIGURE 3.—Polar diagram of data from knee flexion angle (horizonal axis) and shank coronal angle (vertical axis) during mid-stance for brace (solid line) and no-brace (dotted line) conditions. Knee extends from point A (maximum flexion) to points B and C (minimum flexion). Hypothetical extension with brace shown from point C to D. (Courtesy of Davidson PL, Sanderson DJ, Loomer RL: Kinematics of valgus bracing for medial gonarthrosis: Technical report. *Clin Biomech* 13:414-419, 1998 with permission from Elsevier Science.)

and to shift joint contact force toward the lateral compartment. This study examined the effects of valgus knee bracing on joint kinematics during gait, focusing on alignment of the shank and thigh segments, in patients with medial gonarthrosis.

Methods.—The study included 12 men, mean age 55, who wore a valgus knee brace for medial gonarthrosis. Kinematic analysis was performed using 2 gen-blocked digital video cameras with the subjects walking on a treadmill at speeds of 1.5 and 2.1 m/s. Reflective markers on the braced leg provided kinematic data, which were used to calculate flexion, coronal, and axial rotation angles of the thigh and shank segments in a global co-ordinate system. Data calibration was performed based on the patient standing, without the brace, and averaged more than 5 step cycles at 4 specific intervals during the stance phase.

Results.—Valgus bracing did not alter the thigh coronal angle. However, shank coronal angle at toe-off was significantly reduced in the brace condition. Bracing resisted valgus forces in the coronal plane transmitted through the helical strap of the brace, thus significantly preventing full extension (Fig 3). The helical strap also produced axial forces resulting in significant external rotation of the thigh axial angle throughout the stance phase, as well as internal rotation of the shank axial angle during knee extension at heel strike and mid-stance. Analysis revealed unexpected external rotation of the shank axial angle during knee flexion, perhaps related to the brace hinge.

Conclusions.—In patients with medial gonarthrosis of the knee, valgus bracing apparently alters joint kinematics in the flexion, coronal, and axial planes, transmitting forces from 1 place to another. The contribution of these kinematic effects to pain relief remain unclear. The analysis suggests that the interaction between the patient and brace is more complicated than previously thought.

▶ Knee osteoarthritis often affects the medial compartment of the knee joint, and the cartilage breakdown is often accompanied by medial joint space narrowing and excessive varus alignment of the tibia with respect to the femur. This condition is often treated with a valgus brace, which attempts to realign the knee joint surfaces and move the tibia and femur to a more vertical alignment. This study examined the effects of such bracing on the gait biomechanics of 12 subjects with knee osteoarthritis. There were no significant effects of the brace on coronal angles of the leg segments except on the shank at toe-off. The brace did restrict full extension, which unloaded the knee joint somewhat, as well as the brace strap forces created significant external rotation of the thigh, which may have assisted in unloading the medial compartment. The authors suggest that further research is required to investigate the role of axial motion in knee joint force distributions.

M.J.L. Alexander, Ph.D.

In Vivo **Measurement of the Series Elasticity Release Curve of Human Triceps Surae Muscle**
Hof AL (Univ of Groningen, The Netherlands)
J Biomech 31:793-800, 1998   7–17

Introduction.—The act of running has been compared to the bouncing of a ball. The hypothesis is that potential and kinetic energy of the trunk are stored briefly as elastic energy in the leg extensor muscles during the first half of stance, then released in the second half. This hypothesis is problematic because only indirect estimates are available for the elastic properties of human muscle. Two elastic components can be distinguished in a single muscle-tendon complex: the serial-elastic component in series with the contractile component, and the parallel elastic component parallel to the contractile component (Fig 1). An antagonist muscle group is always present. Even when passive, the force caused by its parallel elastic component is still present. Measurements of the elasticity curves of the human triceps surae muscle group, the primary plantarflexor of the foot were obtained by quick-release experiments on a specifically developed ergometer.

Results.—The force-extension characteristics of the series-elastic component of the triceps surae muscle were measured in vivo using a hydraulic controlled-release ergometer in 12 participants. A linear relation was observed between muscle moment and extension, with a stiffness K_1, preceded by a quadratic toe region at low moments. Stiffness K_1 rose with the level of activation of the muscle. Values ranged between 250 and 400 N m rad^{-1} at an ankle moment of 100 nm. Elastic stretch corresponded to around 30 degrees, a substantial amount compared with the total ankle movement range. The elastic energy stored in the serial-elastic component

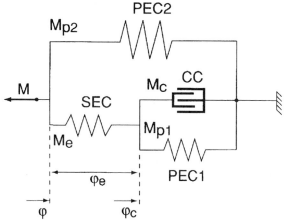

FIGURE 1.—Model of the elastic and contractile components in a muscle-tendon complex, with an inactive antagonist. Moment around and angle of the joint are given to represent muscle force and length. ø, ankle angle (neutral position is 1.57 rad = 90); $ø_e$, equivalent length of SEC in angular units; $ø_c$, equivalent length of CC. *Abbreviations*: M, total moment; M_e, moment acting on SEC; M_{p1} and M_{p2}, moments resulting from PEC1 and PEC2, respectively; *SEC*, series-elastic component; *CC*, contractile component; *PEC1*, parallel elastic component of agonist; *PEC2*, parallel elastic component of antagonist. (Reprinted from Hof AL: *In vivo* measurement of the series elasticity release curve of human triceps surae muscle. *J Biomech* 31:793-800, copyright 1998, with kind permission from Elsevier Science Ltd, The Boulevard, Langford Lane, Kidlington OX5 1GB UK.)

was 23 to 37 at a moment of 150 nm and 31 to 37 at a moment of 180 nm. These values correspond to the peak moments in walking and running, respectively.

Conclusion.—These energy values enable the conservation of negative (eccentric) work into a subsequent phase of positive (concentric) work in both walking and running.

▶ During running, the serial-elastic component of the leg muscles stores elastic energy during the first half of stance and releases that energy during the takeoff phase. This study attempted to measure the elastic properties of the plantarflexors of the ankle joint by means of a hydraulic ergometer. The author found that the amount of stretch in the human triceps surae was considerable: the length change in the average muscle was 8% during peak walking speed. The amount of stretch decreased with increasing running speed and increasing tendon force, because of increasing stiffness due to the viscoelastic properties of tendon and connective tissue. The author concludes that he successfully measured elastic energy in the plantarflexor muscle group, and that energy saving by elastic energy is a likely mechanism in human locomotion. However, the results are based on the ability of the ergometer to accurately measure the serial-elastic component of muscle, and that ability is as yet unverified.

M.J.L. Alexander, Ph.D.

Effects of Patellar Tendon Adhesion to the Anterior Tibia on Knee Mechanics

Ahmad CS, Kwak SD, Ateshian GA, et al (Columbia Univ, New York; Steadman-Hawkins Clinic, Vail, Colo)
Am J Sports Med 26:715-724, 1998   7–18

Objective.—Patella infera, the most common cause of pain after anterior cruciate ligament (ACL) reconstruction, is associated with patellar tendon adhesion to the anterior tibia. The effects of patellar adhesion have not been quantified. An accurate model for patellar tendon adhesion was developed, the relationship between patellar tendon adhesion and patella infera were characterized, the effect of adhesion on both patellofemoral

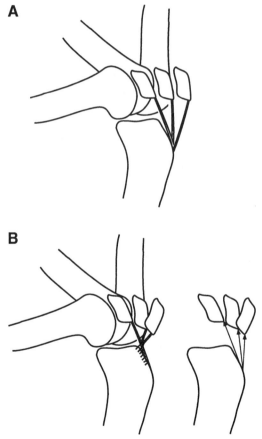

FIGURE 9.—Patellar tendon insertion on the tibia. **A**, normal knee flexion. **B**, knee flexion with patellar tendon shortening, which increased knee extension. (Courtesy of Ahmad CS, Kwak SD, Ateshian GA, et al: Effects of patellar tendon adhesion to the anterior tibia on knee mechanics. *Am J Sports Med* 26:715-724, 1998.)

and tibiofemoral kinematics and contact were determined, and the effect of adhesion on the knee extensor mechanism was elucidated.

Methods.—Five cadaveric knees were loaded in an open kinematic chain configuration. Partial and full patellar tendon adhesion to the anterior tibia was simulated by compressing a metal plate against the tendon. Position and orientation of each bone in the knee joint was tested at various flexion angles before and after knee dissection. Translation and rotation data were recorded at different flexion angles.

Results.—Patellar tendon adhesions resulted in medial and distal translations that were greatest at full extension and rotation in the sagittal plane that was maximal at full extension. Whereas the magnitude of patellofemoral contact remained unchanged, patellar and femoral surface contacts were shifted distally. Patellar tendon adhesions shifted the tibia laterally, anteriorly, and distally particularly at 30 to 60 degrees of flexion and increased internal rotation and rotation in the sagittal plane. Resultant posterior shifts in contact areas of the tibiofemoral joint were greatest at 60 degrees of flexion in both medial and lateral plateaus. The medial and anterior lateral condyle shift on the femoral side was maximal at 30 degrees of flexion. Patellar tendon length and knee extension force were significantly decreased by adhesions particularly at full extension (Fig 9).

Conclusion.—Patellar tendon adhesion leads to patella infera that interferes with patellofemoral and tibiofemoral kinematics and probably causes the pain after ACL.

▶ Anterior knee pain is a common complication after knee injuries and surgeries, especially after ACL reconstructions, and it has been related to patellar tendon adhesion to the anterior tibia and patella infera. This problem occurs after patellar tendon harvest for use as an ACL replacement. Patellar tendon adhesion caused significant alterations in both patellofemoral and tibiofemoral kinematics and reduced knee extension force. This tendon adhesion effectively decrease the length of the patellar tendon, and the shorter tendon decreases patellar mobility. This shorter tendon also alters patellar cartilage stresses, which may produce anterior knee pain after ACL surgery. Several surgical procedures to correct patellar tendon adhesion are described, but the key to treatment of this surgical complication is early diagnosis.

M.J.L. Alexander, Ph.D.

Mechanical Output and Electromyographic Parameters in Males and Females During Fatiguing Knee-Extensions
Wretling ML, Henriksson-Larsén K (Univ of Umeå, Sweden; Natl Inst for Working Life, Umeå, Sweden)
Int J Sports Med 19:401-407, 1998   7–19

Objective.—Changes in mechanical output and electromyographic (EMG) variables are commonly used as indicators of muscle strength and

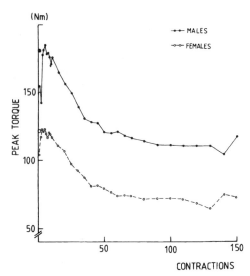

FIGURE 1.—Absolute changes in peak torque (Nm) in relation to contraction and number in male and female participants. Reference contractions are denoted by *larger symbols*. (Courtesy of Wretling ML, Henriksson-Larsén K: Mechanical output and electromyographic parameters in males and females during fatiguing knee-extensions. *Int J Sports Med* 19:401-407, 1998. Georg Thieme Verlag.)

fatigue. Such studies generally assume that participants can activate all motor units during initial trials and that relative changes can be calculated thereafter. However, this approach overlooks the possible contributions of participant training and experience. This study assessed changes in mechanical and EMG output, from initial to subsequent muscular contractions, in untrained male and female participants.

Methods.—Sixteen untrained young adults, 8 men and 8 women, were studied while performing voluntary maximum knee extensions on a Cybex II isokinetic dynamometer. During a series of single maximum contractions and a series of repetitive maximum contractions, EMG activity in the vastus lateralis, vastus medialis, and rectus femoris muscles was recorded. Muscle activation during the first and subsequent contractions was compared, and possible differences between the sexes were assessed.

Results.—In each trial, the participants could not perform with maximum effort during the initial repetitions. Mechanical output and EMG variables both increased during the first 4 to 10 repetitions (Fig 1). Mechanical output peaked within 10 contractions in both sexes. Output then decreased gradually before reaching a plateau. Mean power frequency decreased during the first 10 to 70 contractions, until the participants reached an endurance level. Men had larger mean power frequency values than women. Unlike previous investigators, the authors found a relative decline in the rise in signal amplitude between the reference contraction and the plateau. Men and women were similar in terms of mechanical output, EMG parameters, and subjective experience of fatigue.

Conclusions.—In untrained men and women performing isokinetic knee extensions to fatigue, mechanical output and EMG values both increase through the first 4 to 10 repetitions. The use of initial contractions as the reference value could therefore affect the results of muscle fatigue studies. The best reference might be a maximum contraction performed before the fatigue trial. The reduction in repetitive motion syndrome, observed between the reference contraction and the fatigue level, may be explained by a dropout of type 2 muscle fibers.

▶ In most earlier studies of muscular fatigue that have measured mechanical or EMG output, the first trial has been used as the criterion. This study determined that there are increases in both force output and EMG during 4 to 10 maximal trials, in both sexes. This finding suggests that untrained subjects are unable to show a synchronized activation of all motor units early in a trial and that the criterion should be the top trial out of the first 10. Both sexes replicated the previously reported 2-phase pattern in mean power frequency after the 10 initial contractions, with a gradual decrease through 70 contractions, and then a maintenance level. There were no differences, in mechanical output or EMG activity during these fatiguing contractions, between males and females, but there was a relatively low number of subjects. There were also no differences in perception of pain, discomfort, or fatigue (using Borg's scale) between males and females. It would be interesting to see this study replicated with a larger number of subjects, to determine if the lack of significant differences between sexes persists.

M.J.L. Alexander, Ph.D.

Individual Muscle Contributions to the In Vivo Achilles Tendon Force
Arndt AN, Komi PV, Brüggemann G-P, et al (German Sport Univ, Cologne, Germany; Univ of Jyväskylä, Finland)
Clin Biomech 13:532-541, 1998
7–20

Background.—Research on the etiology of Achilles' tendon injury has implicated the occurrence of nonuniform stress over the cross-sectional area, which may influence function. However, this has not been demonstrated empirically. Individual muscle contributions to the in vivo Achilles' tendon force were investigated.

Methods.—In vivo Achilles' tendon forces were measured using an optic fiber method during isometric plantarflexions at systematically varied knee angles and contraction intensities. A comparison to the plantar force determined underneath the metatarsal heads enabled the calculation of the contribution of the Achilles tendon to plantarflexion moment. The Achilles' tendon force was differentiated into gastrocnemius and soleus contributions, and individual muscle patterns were noted.

Findings.—The mean Achilles' tendon contribution to the resultant moment was 67.4%, varying at different knee angles and contraction intensities. A force discrepancy of 967 newtons was recorded between

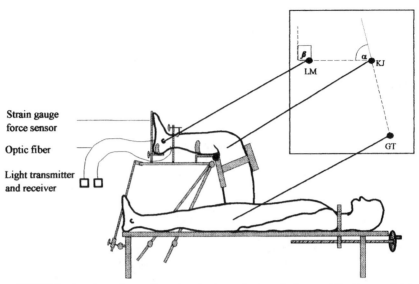

FIGURE 2.—Experimental setup. Execution of an isometric plantarflexion at a defined knee angle (α). The ankle angle (β) was set at 90 degrees. *Abbreviations:* LM, lateral maleolus; *KJ,* knee joint center; *GT,* greater trochanter. (Reprinted from *Clinical Biomechanics* courtesy of Arndt AN, Komi PV, Brüggemann G-P, et al: Individual muscle contributions to the in vivo Achilles tendon force. *Clin Biomech* 13:532-541, copyright 1998, with kind permission from Elsevier Science Ltd, The Boulevard, Langford Lane, Kidlington OX5 1GB UK.)

gastrocnemius and soleus over a gastrocnemius length of change of 2.67 cm, which corresponded to a 21 newton/mm²–stress discrepancy over the tendon cross-sectional area. Individual activation patterns were evident in separate muscles (Fig 2).

Conclusion.—Nonuniform stress has been implicated in the etiology of Achilles tendon injury. Such loading appears to result from discrepancies in individual muscle forces.

▶ The clinical relevance of this article is 2-fold. It indicates 2 important factors in tendon injury etiology: (1) load concentration within the tendon and (2) frictional forces between individual collagen fibers. Presumably, both mechanisms subject the tendon to localized fiber damage, subsequent inflammation and partial and possibly total rupture. The article also implies that nonuniform forces produced by the triceps surae may lead to different effects on the achilles tendon-calcaneous junction.

J.S. Torg, M.D.

Gender Difference in Joint Biomechanics During Walking: Normative Study in Young Adults

Kerrigan DC, Todd MK, Croce UD (Harvard Med School, Boston; Università di Sassari, Italy, Rome)
Am J Phys Med Rehabil 77:2-7, 1998   7–21

Introduction.—Although it is generally agreed that men and women walk differently, there are few data on specific differences in gait biomechanics between the sexes. A quantitative analysis was performed to examine joint biomechanical differences during gait in healthy, young men and women.

Methods.—The study included 99 able-bodied young adults, aged 20 to 40 years. Gait analyses were performed using an optoelectronic motion analysis and force platform system. Sagittal kinematic and kinetic data—representing joint motion and joint torque and power, respectively—were compared between males and females. All kinetic data were normalized for height and weight.

Results.—Women had a greater cadence than men. Although women's stride length was less than in men, it was greater after normalization for height. Compared with men, gait analysis of women showed significantly greater hip flexion, less knee extension before initial contact, greater knee flexion moment in pre-swing, and greater peak mechanical joint power absorption at the knee in pre-swing. Women also showed trends toward greater peak knee flexion, ankle plantar flexion, hip power generation in loading response, knee extension moment at initial contact, and greater ankle power generation in pre-swing, but these were not significant after accounting for multiple comparisons (Table 2).

Conclusions.—This study demonstrates some significant differences in joint biomechanics during gait in healthy young men and women. The data will provide a useful biomechanical reference for clinical and research purposes, although each gait laboratory should develop its own sex-specific reference databases. The clinical implications of the sex differences noted remain to be determined.

▶ It is generally agreed that most males and females walk differently and that most observers can determine gender in a darkened setting by the pattern of lighted joint movements. Comparisons of biomechanical movement differences between genders have not been previously reported for a large sample study such as the 100 subjects compared here. Significant differences were found between genders in several gait variables: females had significantly greater hip flexion and less knee extension before initial contact, greater knee flexion moment in pre-swing, and greater knee power absorption in pre-swing. The greater power values may be related to the higher cadences in females. Although several of the gait variables were found different between genders, the clinical relevance of these differences requires future study.

M.J.L. Alexander, Ph.D.

TABLE 2.—Female vs. Male Biomechanical Gait Values

	Females			Males			P Values
	Mean	Intersubject (SD)	Total (SD)	Mean	Intersubject (SD)	Total (SD)	
Hip flexion moment stance (N · m/Kg · m)	0.44	(0.10)	(0.12)	0.40	(0.09)	(0.11)	0.073
Hip extension moment (N · m/Kg · m)	0.57	(0.15)	(0.17)	0.56	(0.14)	(0.15)	0.700
Hip flexion moment swing (N · m/Kg · m)	0.11	(0.05)	(0.06)	0.12	(0.04)	(0.05)	0.426
Hip power generation loading response (W/kg · m)	0.57	(0.30)	(0.34)	0.43	(0.21)	(0.26)	0.008*
Hip power absorption (W/kg · m)	0.45	(0.19)	(0.23)	0.44	(0.16)	(0.20)	0.636
Hip power generation pre-swing (W/kg · m)	0.94	(0.26)	(0.31)	0.88	(0.26)	(0.32)	0.221
Knee extension moment initial contact (N · m/Kg · m)	0.09	(0.03)	(0.05)	0.11	(0.03)	(0.05)	0.010*
Knee flexion moment loading response (N · m/Kg · m)	0.37	(0.13)	(0.15)	0.34	(0.14)	(0.16)	0.236
Knee extension moment terminal stance (N · m/Kg · m)	0.14	(0.06)	(0.08)	0.16	(0.07)	(0.09)	0.156
Knee flexion moment pre-swing (N · m/Kg · m)	0.29	(0.07)	(0.09)	0.23	(0.08)	(0.09)	<0.001†
Knee power absorption loading response (W/kg · m)	0.35	(0.20)	(0.26)	0.33	(0.21)	(0.24)	0.662
Knee power generation mid stance (W/kg · m)	0.46	(0.25)	(0.29)	0.41	(0.16)	(0.19)	0.196
Knee power absorption pre-swing (W/kg · m)	1.43	(0.46)	(0.54)	1.12	(0.43)	(0.51)	0.001†
Ankle plantar flexion moment (N · m/Kg · m)	0.09	(0.03)	(0.04)	0.08	(0.03)	(0.04)	0.062
Ankle dorsiflexion moment (N · m/Kg · m)	0.78	(0.07)	(0.08)	0.80	(0.07)	(0.09)	0.126
Ankle power absorption (W/kg · m)	0.38	(0.12)	(0.18)	0.36	(0.09)	(0.15)	0.417
Ankle power generation pre-swing (W/kg · m)	2.19	(0.48)	(0.58)	1.96	(0.32)	(0.43)	0.005*

*Statistically significant difference at P <0.05/27 = 0.0019.
†Near significant difference at 0.0019 < P < 0.05.
(Courtesy of Kerrigan DC, Todd MK, Croce UD: Gender difference in joint biomechanics during walking: Normative study in young adults. Am J Phys Med Rehabil 77:2-7, 1998.)

Gait Biomechanics Are Not Normal After Anterior Cruciate Ligament Reconstruction and Accelerated Rehabilitation

Devita P, Hortobagyi T, Barrier J (East Carolina Univ, Greenville, NC)
Med Sci Sports Exerc 30:1481-1488, 1998   7–22

Objective.—Accelerated rehabilitation after anterior cruciate ligament (ACL) reconstruction is designed to return patients to athletic activities within 6 months. Such patients may regain normal peak torque at the knee between 10 and 22 months after surgery, but there are no data indicating that knee, hip, and ankle muscle function returns to normal during gait. Lower extremity joint kinematics, kinetics, and energetics were compared between healthy individuals and individuals having undergone ACL reconstruction and accelerated rehabilitation.

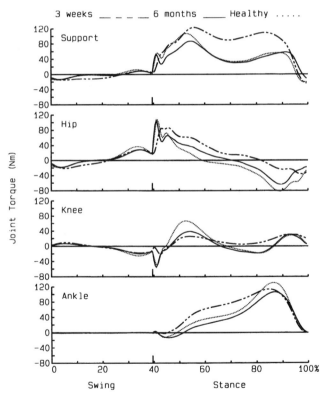

FIGURE 2.—Joint torque curves from the three groups. Positive values indicate extensor or plantarflexor torque. At 3 weeks after surgery, there were large extensor (plantarflexor) torques at the hip and ankle and a low extensor torque at the knee during stance. The total support torque, the sum of the joint torques, was highly extensor and was necessary to support the injured subjects who were more flexed than healthy individuals. The joint torques improved after rehabilitation but only the ankle torque returned to a normal value. The extensor torques at the hip and knee were still larger than and smaller than normal at the 6-month test. (Courtesy of Devita P, Hortobagyi T, Barrier J: Gait mechanics are not normal after anterior cruciate ligament reconstruction and accelerated rehabilitation. *Med Sci Sports Exerc* 30:1481-1488, 1998.)

Methods.—Sagittal plane torque and power were calculated for 22 healthy individuals and for 8 patients with repair of complete rupture of the ACL 3 weeks and 6 months after injury. Force during normal stride and angular position for the hip, knee, and ankle joints were calculated.

Results.—For the injured group, range of motion during swing was 10% smaller at the hip, 39% larger at the knee, and 32% larger at the ankle at 6 months compared with 3 weeks; the average position of the hip, knee, and ankle joints was 48%, 35%, and 63% less flexed; the extensor angular impulse at the hip and plantarflexor angular impulse at the ankle was 38% and 35% smaller; and extensor angular impulse at the knee during the first half of stance was 20% larger (Fig 2). Kinematic variables were similar for both groups. In the injured group at 6 months, the extensor angular impulse at the hip was 37% larger than the control group, the extensor angular impulse at the knee during the first half of stance was 57% of the control group impulse, positive work at the hip during the first half of stance was only 44%, and negative and positive work increased significantly by 250% and 267%, respectively. In the injured group, work at the hip was 77% of that in the control group, negative work at the knee was 53% of that in the control group, and positive work at the knee was only 44% of that in the control group.

Conclusion.—After ACL reconstruction and accelerated rehabilitation, patients have a normal gait but a larger extensor torque at the hip making more work and a smaller extensor torque at the knee that results in less work. These altered kinetics could result in knee symptoms later on.

▶ It is known that injury to the ACL causes neuromuscular adaptations to the entire lower extremity, and these may affect gait mechanics. Gait kinematics returned to normal following 6 months of rehabilitation in ACL-injured subjects; however, joint torques did not return to normal levels. Subjects had a decrement in the magnitude of the extensor torque and angular impulse compared with healthy controls, likely due to the loss of the central one third of the patellar tendon as a ligament replacement. Hip torques increased following rehabilitation, likely because injured subjects maintained forward progression with a greater reliance on the hip extensors compared with controls. These adaptations in gait may provide increased protection for the repaired and rehabilitated knee but may eventually produce an increased rate of knee symptoms in this population.

M.J.L. Alexander, Ph.D.

Comparison of Vertical Ground Reaction Forces During Overground and Treadmill Walking
White SC, Yack HJ, Tucker CA, et al (State Univ of New York, Buffalo; Univ of Iowa, Iowa City)
Med Sci Sports Exerc 30:1537-1542, 1998   7–23

Objective.—Individuals do not walk the same way overground as they do on a treadmill. Vertical foot-ground reaction forces for overground walking were compared with vertical foot-belt reaction forces at 3 speeds and at comparable cadences and stride lengths.

Methods.—Healthy active volunteers (n = 24, 11 males) participated in treadmill walking trials at 3 speeds and 3- to 5-minute walking over a 12-m walkway. Vertical force curves were constructed and compared. Cadence, stride-length, and walking speed were calculated for each trial and each walking speed for both walking modes.

Results.—Walking speed, cadence, and stride length were not significantly different between the 2 walking modes (Fig 1). Force magnitude during mid-stance was significantly different for normal and fast walking speeds and in late stance for normal and fast walking speeds. Force patterns were similar, however, and changes in force magnitude were consistent for each person.

Conclusion.—Treadmill and overground walking force patterns are different. Differences in peak force magnitudes appear to be dependent on walking speed.

▶ Treadmill walking is often used rather than overground walking in clinical locomotion research due to the ability to control speed and to easily film numerous strides. However, there may be some significant differences in gait parameters, such as stride length or stride frequency, when walking on a treadmill. Comparison of gait parameters for 24 subjects revealed no significant differences in stride length or cadence between the two conditions. There were found to be some differences between the vertical ground reaction forces in overground and treadmill walking in certain phases of gait, but these were very small. Treadmill walking can be generalized to overground walking for research purposes for a group of average subjects.

M.J.L. Alexander, Ph.D.

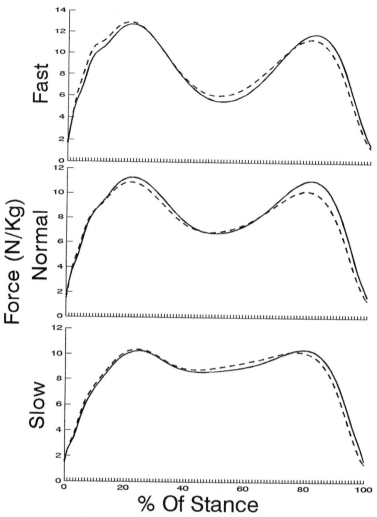

FIGURE 1.—Mean ensemble averaged vertical foot-ground reaction force curves for 24 subjects. Curves were normalized to 100% of stance time (initial foot contact to toe-off of same limb), and forces were normalized by subject mass (N/kg). Group average force-time (% stance) curves are presented at each of 3 different walking speeds overground (*solid line*) and on a treadmill (*dashed line*). (Courtesy of White SC, Yack HJ, Tucker CA, et al: Comparison of vertical ground reaction forces during overground and treadmill walking. *Med Sci Sports Exerc* 30:1537-1542, 1998.)

Running Injuries: A Biomechanical Approach

Novacheck TF (East Univ, St Paul, Minn)
J Bone Joint Surg Am 80-A:1220-1233, 1998   7–24

Objective.—Each year, running injuries change the performance or practice of 25% to 50% of runners. Treatment or prevention of these injuries requires knowledge of how they occur. Gait analysis has generated new biomechanical information about the physiology and pathophysiology of the musculoskeletal system.

Biomechanics of Forward Human Locomotion.—Walking changes to running when double support is eliminated and replaced with double float. As speed increases and the point of initial contact changes from the hindfoot to the forefoot, running has progressed to sprinting. Studies of the gait cycle have demonstrated that whereas potential and kinetic energy are out of phase during walking, the 2 types of energy are in phase during running, causing the body to change the way it maintains energy efficiency. The kinematics and kinetics of the gait cycle provide descriptions of movement, the forces that are responsible for that movement, and the effect of those forces on muscles, joints, tendons, and ligaments. Learning the biomechanical stresses that cause common injuries can aid in the design of specific exercises that can counter the forces that lead to those injuries.

Biomechanics, Physiology, and Pathophysiology of Tendons: Insights Into Mechanisms of Injury.—The tendon responds to injury either regeneratively, or degeneratively, producing new tissue that is structurally and functionally normal or that is more vulnerable to injury, respectively. Continued abusive sports activity, along with such factors as hypoxia, poor nutrition, hypovascularity, hormonal changes, chronic inflammation, and aging, results in increased matrix degeneration or inadequate matrix synthesis.

Soft-Tissue Stresses for Specific Musculotendinous Units.—Anterior knee pain is commonly caused by periarticular soft-tissue degeneration and inflammation or by excessive stress on knee cartilage. Iliotibial-band syndrome results from friction between the iliotibial band and the lateral femoral condyle. Achilles tendinopathy results from active muscle forces that occur during midstance rather than from shoe wear or running surface. Plantar fasciitis results from stress in the plantar fascia that occurs during weight transference from the hindfoot to the ball of the foot. The condition is exacerbated by excessive pronation.

Conclusion.—Studies of the biomechanics of running activities can provide descriptive information about potential areas of injury. Understanding what is normal aids in the understanding of what can go wrong and provides insight into treatment plans and training modifications.

▶ This article is a comprehensive review of the biomechanics of forward human motion and of the biomechanics, physiology, and pathophysiology of tendon injury. The original article is recommended reading for the interested practitioner.

J.S. Torg, M.D.

▶ This review provides a thorough and insightful discussion of basic running mechanics and of how these mechanics are related to running injuries. The review includes a discussion of anterior knee pain, plantar fasciitis, Achilles' tendinitis and iliotibial band friction syndrome, all of which are common running injuries. Each of these injuries has been related to one of the kinematic or kinetic phases of the running cycle. For example, plantar fasciitis is caused by excessive stretch on the plantar fascia during the time of mid stance, when stress in the tissue can be as high as 3 times body weight. Excessive pronation increases the force along the medial part of the fascia, predisposing it to strain-related injury. This information is a valuable resource for health care professionals who work with injured runners.

M.J.L. Alexander, Ph.D.

Evaluation of a Bone's *In Vivo* 24-hour Loading History for Physical Exercise Compared With Background Loading
Konieczynski DD, Truty MJ, Biewener AA (Univ of Chicago)
J Orthop Res 16:29-37, 1998   7–25

Purpose.—Several different approaches have been used to study the response of bone to mechanical loading. The identification of factors underlying osteoregulation is important to understanding these charges. Previous studies of osteoregulation in response to exercise have given conflicting results, possibly because of the impact of background loading during nonexercise periods. This study evaluated the impact of physical exercise vs. background activity on the loading of bone in vivo during a 24-hour study.

Methods.—The investigators placed strain gauges on the tibiotarsus of White Leghorn chickens, at a late stage of skeletal growth, to evaluate cortical strains in vivo. The animals performed treadmill exercise 15 minutes per day, at 60% maximum speed, while carrying external weights of 20% body mass. During nonexercise periods, background strains were measured. The 24-hour loading history was compiled, and the osteogenic stimulus potential of brief exercise vs. background activity was evaluated. In addition, the daily effective strain stimulus was calculated and related to the loading history of the exercise program.

Results.—Analysis of the 24-hour loading history showed significant differences between background and exercise activity. Exercise was associated with a higher magnitude and number of cyclic strain events—more than 500 microstains and 2,500 cycles per day—than background activity—less than 500 microstrains, with a mean of 775 cycles per day (Fig 2). More than 97% of daily effective strain stimulus for bone adaptation was linked to exercise strain, even though only 1% of the day was spent in exercise. Calculated daily effective strain stimulus was comparable to that generated by artificial loading of isolated avian ulnae. This level was sufficient either to maintain bone mass or to produce a 15% increase in cortical cross-sectional area.

Conclusions.—Short bouts of exercise and daily background activity act differently as osteogenic stimuli in adaptive bone modeling. Treadmill exercise can produce increased cyclic bone strain distinct from that related to sedentary background activity. The daily effective strain stimulus ap-

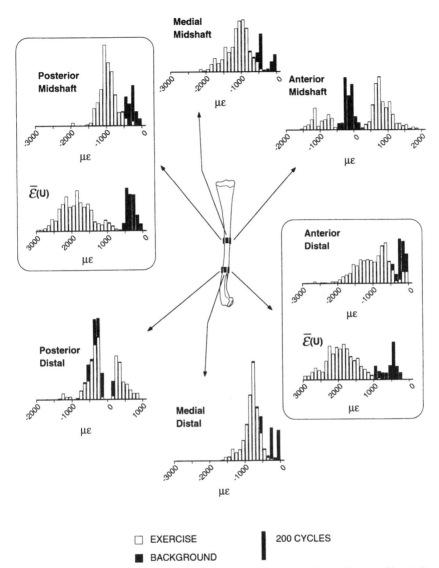

FIGURE 2.—Frequency distributions describing the combined 24-hour loading histories of longitudinal strain for all animals. Also shown are the combined 24-hour loading histories of energy-equivalent strain, for all animals, at the posterior midshaft and anterior distal sites. Populations of strain were statistically different (P less than 0.0001) for exercise and background activity at all sites. *Abbreviations*: $\mu\epsilon$, microstrain; $\epsilon(U)$, energy equivalent strain. (Courtesy of Konieczynski DD, Truty MJ, Biewener AA: Evaluation of a bone's *in vivo* 24-hour loading history for physical exercise compared with background loading. *J Orthop Res* 16:29-37, 1998.)

pears useful for measuring skeletal loading histories for different types of exercise. The relative contributions of other mechanical and nonmechanical factors to this index remain to be determined.

▶ It has been previously reported that bone formation in animals is most responsive to dynamic rather than static components of loading. However, dynamic loading can occur either through an exercise regimen or through intermittent background exercise activity, such as handling or being startled. This comparison of bone strain levels during exercise and background activities showed that both the magnitude and number of cyclic strain events are greater during exercise, even though exercise made up less than 1% of the time in a day (15 minutes). The amount of strain to the bone during background activity is insufficient to maintain or increase bone mass. As seen in previous studies examining the response of bone to mechanical loading, increased loading levels lead to increased bone formation, and decreased loading levels lead to reduced bone formation. Older adults should attempt to perform daily exercise at a strain rate high enough to stress the bone to increase bone formation.

M.J.L. Alexander, Ph.D.

The Mechanical Properties of Human Alar and Transverse Ligaments at Slow and Fast Extension Rates
Panjabi MM, Crisco JJ III, Lydon C, et al (Yale Univ, New Haven, Conn; Schulthess Klinik, Zurich, Switzerland)
Clin Biomech 13:112-120, 1998   7–26

Introduction.—The alar and transverse ligaments are key to the stability of the craniocervical joint. Biomechanical studies of these ligaments have been performed but have used relatively slow extension rates, compared with the fast extension rates at which real-life trauma occurs. This cadaver study evaluated the biomechanics of the alar and transverse ligaments at both slow and fast extension rates.

Methods.—Nineteen alar and 11 transverse ligaments were mounted for study on a specialized testing machine. Each ligament was tested at a slow extension rate of 0.1 mm/sec, then at a fast rate of 920 mm/sec. Force and elongation curves and other biomechanical parameters were compared. Stretching at the slow extension rate proceeded up to 70 N for the alar ligament and 140 N for the transverse ligament. Then, the ligaments were stretched to failure at the fast extension rate. The study hypothesized that the 2 ligaments would show similar behavior at the fast extension rate.

Results.—Before testing, average length was 11.2 mm for the alar ligament versus 18.0 mm for the transverse ligament. During testing at the slow extension rate, average strain on the alar ligament decreased from 16.4% to 0.3%, whereas stiffness increased from 80 to 2,316 N/mm and absorbed energy decreased from 47.4 to 1.3 Nmm, as extension rate increased from slow to fast. By the failure point, average strain was 3.1%,

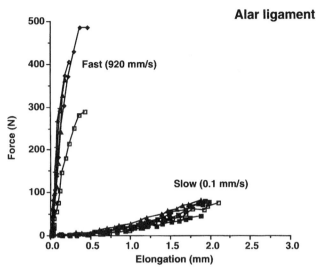

FIGURE 4.—Dens-alar ligament-occiput complex force-elongation curves at slow (0.1 mm/sec) and fast (920 mm/sec) extension rates. (Reprinted from Panjabi MM, Crisco JJ III, Lydon C, et al: The mechanical properties of human alar and transverse ligaments at slow and fast extension rates. *Clin Biomech* 13:112-120, copyright 1998 with kind permission from Elsevier Science Ltd, The Boulevard, Langford Lane, Kidlington OX5 1GB UK.)

force was 367 N, and energy absorbed was 123 Nmm (Fig 4). Strain on the transverse ligament at 140 N decreased from 12.5% to 0.6%, with stiffness increasing from 141 to 1,472 N/mm, and absorbed energy decreasing from 96.1 to 7.6 Nmm as the extension rate increased from slow to fast. At the failure point for the transverse ligament, strain was 2.3%, force was 436 N, and absorbed energy was 101 Nmm.

Conclusion.—For both the alar and transverse ligaments, the extension rate has a significant impact on strain, stiffness, and energy absorbed at subinjury loads. At an increasing extension rate, strain and absorbed energy decrease to less than one tenth, whereas stiffness increases to greater than 10 times. The alar ligament is weaker than the transverse ligament; however, it has higher failure strain, leading to greater absorbed energy when strained at a fast extension rate. These biomechanical findings suggest that real ligamentous injuries may result from much smaller ligament deformations than previously thought.

▶ The alar and transverse ligaments are the 2 major stabilizers of the upper cervical spine and may be injured during high-speed collisions, such as seen in football or in automobile accidents. The alar ligaments act to limit head-axis axial rotation and are paired structures connecting the dens to the occipital condyles on either side. The transverse ligament is the strongest ligament of the upper cervical spine and acts to restrict flexion and anterior displacement of the atlas. The ligament runs horizontally across the anterior arch of the atlas and keeps the dens in place.

The ligament strain and energy absorbed to failure was much greater at slow strain rates than at faster strain rates, while stiffness increased dramatically at faster strain rates. There were differences in the responses of each ligament to the different strain rates; for example, the alar ligament was 30 times stiffer under fast loading conditions, while the transverse ligament was 10 times stiffer. The authors note that much smaller ligament deformations than previously thought produced ligamentous injuries.

M.J.L. Alexander, Ph.D.

8 Muscle Training and Rehabilitation

Resistance Training and Elite Athletes: Adaptations and Program Considerations
Kraemer WJ, Duncan ND, Volek JS (Pennsylvania State Univ, University Park)
J Orthop Sports Phys Ther 28:110-119, 1998   8–1

Objective.—There are still ignorance and misinformation about the benefits of resistance training to elite athletes. The scientific aspects of the benefits, physiological adaptations, and weight training principles and program guidelines are reviewed.

Benefits.—Increasing muscular strength results in an increase in the maximal force production. The almost immediate rapid improvement in strength indicates a recruitment of motor units, ranging in size from small to large, that result in a continuum of force production capabilities. Resistance training can reduce the incidence of, or moderate, injuries.

Morphological Adaptations.—Resistance training can produce cardiovascular benefits, growth of muscle tissue, and augmentation of hormone production, and can increase the lactate threshold, and increase or decrease acute and chronic endocrine responses.

Weight Training.—Periodized programs are strategically individualized to an athlete's peak training cycle and divided over the training year, with specific objectives and goals for each period. The 3- to 6-set workout (multiple set) program provides superior results to the single-set protocol. The most important variable controlling the rate and quality of development of a particular feature of muscular performance is intensity, which can be determined by using repetition maximums. Duration of rest periods needs to be individualized to the athlete and the type of exercise to maximize physiological adaptations to training. Muscular strengthening and power adaptation exercises must be specific for each muscle group, and should simulate the types of muscular actions used in the sport, at the same velocity. Increasing power output requires improving both the force and velocity components of muscle activation.

Conclusion.—Although strength training improves athletic performance, resistance exercises must be tailored to the individual athlete and should mimic as closely as possible the type and velocity of muscular movement involved in the chosen sport, while they also minimize the risk of injury.

▶ The need for strength training has been accepted by most athletic training programs and there has been a significant increase in the number of strength and conditioning coaches used by these programs. The authors stress the need for specificity of training, which should include consideration of not only the type of resistance training but also the velocity of movement. (Please see Abstract 4–11.)

F.J. George, A.T.C., P.T.

Strength Training: Single Versus Multiple Sets
Carpinelli RN, Otto RM (Adelphi Univ, Garden City, NY)
Sports Med 26:73-84, 1998

8–2

Background.—The number of sets needed in a training program to increase muscular strength and hypertrophy continues to be unclear. The value of single vs. multiple sets was discussed in a literature review.

Discussion.—Though trainers commonly believe that at least 3 sets of each exercise are needed to elicit the best results in strength and hypertrophy, most studies comparing the outcomes of training with single and multiple sets do not support this belief. Most evidence suggests that, for a 4- to 25-week training, single sets do not lead to significant differences in strength or hypertrophy. Though design limitations in previous studies make such conclusions tentative, there is little scientific evidence and no theoretical basis for the belief that a greater volume of exercise produces greater increases in strength or hypertrophy. Athletes and other fitness enthusiasts should engage in the minimal volume of exercise to attain the desired response.

▶ The authors recommend a minimal volume of exercise, rather than the highest tolerable volume, to attain the benefits of resistance exercise. A number of studies have compared different amounts of repetitions and found no difference in strength gain resulting from 1 set or multiple sets of a resistance exercise. (Please read Abstract 4–9.)

F.J. George, A.T.C., P.T.

Quantification of Elastic Resistance Knee Rehabilitation Exercises

Hintermeister RA, Bey MJ, Lange GW, et al (Steadman-Hawkins Sports Medicine Found, Vail, Colo; Univ of Michigan, Ann Arbor; Santa Rosa Outpatient Ctr for Children and Adults, San Antonio, Tex; et al)

J Orthop Sports Phys Ther 28:40-50, 1998   8–3

Objective.—There have been no formal studies validating the benefit of elastic resistance exercises for knee rehabilitation. Muscle activation levels, knee joint angles, and applied force were measured during 5 classic resistance knee rehabilitation exercises.

Methods.—Twelve volunteers (6 women), average age 30, with no history of knee problems performed double knee dips, hamstring pulls, leg presses, single knee dips, and side-to-side jump exercises. Joint ranges of motion, elastic resistance, and electromyogram activity of the vastus medialis, vastus lateralis, rectus femoris, medial hamstrings, biceps femoris, tibialis anterior, and gluteus maximus were measured.

Results.—Measurements demonstrated that these 5 exercises strengthened muscles, increased endurance, and, in the range of motion used, did not compromise the injured knee. Exercises can progress through increased muscle activity or through increased resistance (Table 3).

Conclusion.—These 5 exercises can be adjusted to individual patients and can provide a continuum of rehabilitation for a variety of knee injuries.

▶ The authors present good evidence for using elastic resistance in knee rehabilitation programs. The potential for patellofemoral joint complications does exist when the patient is using these exercises. Elastic resistance appears to be an inexpensive method of providing patients with an effective home program for rehabilitating knee injuries.

F.J. George, A.T.C., P.T.

TABLE 3.—General Rehabilitation Exercise Timelines

Exercise	Nonoperative Injury	Injury Continuum Debridement/ Menisectomy	ACL Reconstruction
Double knee dip	ASAP	ASAP	ASAP
Hamstring pull	ASAP	ASAP	ASAP
Leg press	ASAP	ASAP	ASAP
Single knee dip	4-6 weeks*	6 weeks*	6 weeks
Side-to-side jump	6-8 weeks*	6-8 weeks*	12 weeks

*Possibly sooner, depending on the severity of the initial injury and the patient's preexisting fitness level.

Abbreviations: ASAP, as soon as possible; *ACL,* anterior cruciate ligament.

(Courtesy of Hintermeister RA, Bey MJ, Lange GW, et al: Quantification of elastic resistance knee rehabilitation exercise. *J Orthop Sports Phys Ther* 28:40-50, 1998).

An Electromyographical Analysis of the Scapular Stabilizing Synergists During a Push-up Progression

Lear LJ, Gross MT (Univ of North Carolina, Chapel Hill)
J Orthop Sports Phys Ther 28:146-157, 1998   8–4

Objective.—There is little information on the effect of closed kinetic chain exercises on the scapular rotators. The influence of difficulty level and alteration of the base of support for the push-up with a plus on

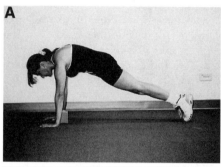

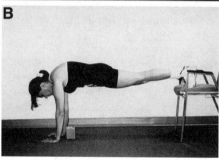

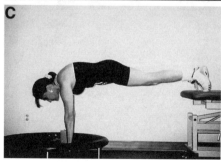

FIGURE 1.—Demonstration of the push-up progression. **A,** Demonstration of condition 1, the push-up with a plus; **B,** Demonstration of condition 2, the push-up with a plus with the feet elevated 45.7 cm; **C,** Demonstration of condition 3, the push-up with a plus with the feet elevated 45.7 cm and the hand placed on a minitrampoline. (Courtesy of Lear LJ, Gross MT: An electromyographical analysis of the scapular stabilizing synergists during a push-up progression. *J Orthop Sports Phys Ther* 28:146-157, 1998).

electrical activity of the scapular stabilizing synergists was assessed electromyographically.

Methods.—An electric goniometer and surface electrodes were attached to the upper extremities of 16 healthy volunteers (9 men), aged 23 to 33, with no previous upper extremity problems. Volunteers performed 5 repetitions for each of 3 push-up progression tests (Fig 1). Electromyographic (EMG) data were analyzed for the serratus anterior, upper trapezius, and lower trapezius muscles.

Results.—When the push-up work performed was analyzed, push-up condition had a significant effect on both the serratus anterior and upper trapezius muscles but not on the lower trapezius muscle. Differences were significant at each level. Increases in EMG levels during testing were probably the result of muscle fatigue.

Conclusion.—Push-up progressions incorporated into upper extremity rehabilitation programs optimize muscle activation.

▶ This study indicates that using a push-up progression can increase strength of the scapular stabilizers, especially the serratus anterior and the upper trapezius. Different exercises must be used to increase the strength of the lower trapezius. The authors indicate that women may have more difficulty using these exercises than men because of general upper body strength.

F.J. George, A.T.C., P.T.

Effects of Theraband and Lightweight Dumbbell Training on Shoulder Rotation Torque and Serve Performance in College Tennis Players
Treiber FA, Lott J, Duncan J, et al (Georgia Prevention Inst, Augusta)
Am J Sports Med 26:510-515, 1998   8–5

Objective.—Few studies have examined the effects of strength training on the rotator cuff musculature and related functional performance in uninjured tennis players. Results of a 4-week resistance training regimen using elastic tubing (Theraband) on shoulder strength and serve performance in a group of college tennis players are presented.

Methods.—A functional assessment of serve performance and isokinetic shoulder rotation torque assessment using the Cybex 6000 Isokinetic Dynamometer was performed in 25 uninjured collegiate varsity tennis players (12 men) during the 1995 and 1996 fall preseasons. In addition to practice sessions 5 days a week, the group was randomly allocated to the shoulder resistance training group (n = 11, 5 women) or the control group (n = 11, 5 women). The resistance training group performed internal and external rotational torque exercises after Theraband exercises. Patients were reassessed within 2 days after completing the study. Maximum and average serve speeds, internal and external rotation peak torque, total work, torque acceleration energy at slow and fast speeds, ratios of external

TABLE 3.—Results of Functional Performance Evaluations at Pre- and Posttraining by Sex

Functional Performance Parameters	Pretraining		Posttraining	
	Men (Mean ± SD)	Women (Mean ± SD)	Men (Mean ± SD)	Women (Mean ± SD)
Peak velocity of serve (mph)	106.7 ± 8.8	83.8 ± 8.4[a]	109.6 ± 8.7	83.0 ± 8.2[a]
Average velocity of serve (mph)	101.4 ± 7.5	77.1 ± 8.1[a]	103.2 ± 9.5	79.5 ± 8.3[a]

[a] Men greater than women, $P <0.001$.
(Courtesy of Treiber FA, Lort J, Duncan J, et al: Effects of Theraband and lightweight dumbbell training on shoulder rotation torque and serve performance in college tennis players. *Am J Sports Med* 26:510-515, 1998.)

rotation to internal rotation for peak torque, and total work at both speeds were compared for both groups and both sexes.

Results.—Average peak velocity in the resistance training group increased by 6% from pretraining to posttraining, whereas average peak velocity decreased by 1.8% in the control group. The average serve velocity increased by 7.9% in the resistance training group and decreased by 2.3% in the control group. Average peak internal and external rotation torque increased significantly more in the resistance training group than in the control group (23.8% and 17.0% vs. 1.0% and 1.2%). Torque acceleration energy increased significantly more in the resistance training group than in the control group (22.1% vs. 0%). Compared with the control group, total work performed in the resistance training group increased significantly during internal rotation at both 120 and 300 degrees per second (10.7% and 31.6% vs. 1.1% and 7.0%). Total work performed in external rotation was significantly higher for the resistance exercise group than for the control group (16.5% vs. 0.7%). Sex had a significant effect (Table 3). Men had a greater external to internal rotation torque imbalance than women.

Conclusion.—Resistance training increases internal and external shoulder rotation torque and serve velocity in both male and female varsity tennis players, with men experiencing greater increases than women. Men had a greater external to internal rotation torque imbalance than women.

▶ This is a relatively simple and inexpensive exercise program, which was effective in increasing strength of the shoulder muscles and significantly increasing the velocity of the tennis serve.

F.J. George, A.T.C., P.T.

Composition and Dynamics of Articular Cartilage: Structure, Function, and Maintaining Healthy State
Cohen NP, Foster RJ, Mow VC (Columbia Univ, New York)
J Orthop Sports Phys Ther 28:203-215, 1998   8–6

Objective.—The composition, structure, and multiphasic nature of articular cartilage and its unique mechanical properties were described, and current studies of how a healthy state of articular cartilage may be maintained were reviewed.

Composition and Structure of Normal Articular Cartilage.—Normal cartilage is composed of chondrocytes and an extracellular matrix consisting primarily of collagen and proteoglycans. Articular cartilage is composed of a superficial zone with parallel collagen fibrils, a transitional or middle zone with less organized collagen fibrils, and a deep zone with collagen fibrils perpendicular to the joint surface. Proteoglycans consist mainly of chondroitin sulfate and keratin sulfate.

Material Properties of Articular Cartilage.—Articular cartilage is biphasic, consisting of fluid and a solid porous-permeable matrix that facilitates transfer of load and provides load-bearing abilities. The permeability, with its associated resisting drag force, decreases as compressive strain and hydraulic pressure increase. The viscoelastic behavior of articular cartilage is characterized by creep and stress relaxation. The biphasic nature of articular cartilage is responsible for its compressive properties that allow it to balance external loads. Tensile properties are typically nonlinear. When a tensile load is placed on the cartilage, the tensile behavior becomes linearly elastic. Under shear stress, the collagen deforms but is held in place by proteoglycans. Swelling when cartilage is damaged is the result of an increase in water content that leads to a loss of tensile stiffness. Swelling is caused by an ionic imbalance in which the ion concentration in the articular cartilage is higher than in the surrounding synovial fluid.

Maintaining a Healthy State.—Degenerative changes occur gradually as a result of increasing inability to bear loads. Risk factors include obesity, immobility of the joint, long-term repetitive activities, transarticular impact, and some sports.

Conclusion.—The design and composition of articular cartilage create viscoelastic properties that allow it to respond to deformational loads. Obesity, immobility of the joint, long-term repetitive activities, transarticular impact, and some sports can induce degenerative changes.

▶ The authors have stated that 3 major questions need to be addressed, and they are as follows: (1) What is the mechanism of mechanical loading that induces changes in the composition of articular cartilage? (2) What initiates degenerative changes in articular cartilage? (3) What specific repetitive activities cause injury to the articular cartilage? (See also Abstract 3–24.)

F.J. George, A.T.C., P.T.

Unilateral Postural Control of the Functionally Dominant and Nondominant Extremities of Healthy Subjects
Hoffman M, Schrader J, Applegate T, et al (Univ of Nevada, Las Vegas; Indiana Univ, Bloomington)
J Athletic Train 33:319-322, 1998   8–7

Background.—Theoretically, limb dominance can be determined on the basis of strength, functional use, personal preference, and other parameters. However, the literature is unclear on which parameters best indicate dominance. Whether a difference exists in unilateral postural stability between the functionally dominant and nondominant legs of a healthy population was investigated.

Methods.—Ten healthy volunteers (5 male, 5 female), aged a mean of 19 years, participated in the study. Functional leg dominance was determined by a battery of tests, including 3 assessments of leg dominance for functional activity. Two assessments of postural control—sway area (SA) and sway path length (SPL)—were performed for the dominant and nondominant legs of all volunteers.

Findings.—A subject × leg repeated-measures analysis of variance (ANOVA) of SA and SPL indicated that the SA value was not significant. The mean value for the dominant-leg SA measure was 9,737 mm^2, and that for the nondominant leg, 9,432 mm^2. The SPL value also did not differ significantly in the bilateral comparison. Mean SPL for the dominant and nondominant legs were 4,322 and 4,342 mm, respectively.

Conclusions.—In this group of healthy young adults, unilateral postural stability did not differ between the functionally dominant and nondominant legs. This finding is of particular interest to clinicians who commonly use single-leg postural control assessments to determine an athlete's level of progress during rehabilitation.

▶ Most lower-extremity rehabilitation programs include single-leg balancing excercises and testing protocols. This study indicates that leg dominance does not have an effect on postural stability. Therefore, comparisons between the injured and noninjured extremity can be made without regard to dominance.

F.J. George, A.T.C., P.T.

Quantification of Full-Range-of-Motion Unilateral and Bilateral Knee Flexion and Extension Torque Ratios
Welsch MA, Williams PA, Pollock ML, et al (Univ of Florida, Gainesville)
Arch Phys Med Rehabil 79:971-978, 1998   8–8

Objective.—Muscle imbalance can result in joint injury. Recent research has shown that standardized isometric testing can generate accurate and reliable information about reciprocal flexion/extension muscle strength. To assess whether isometric knee flexion and extension testing could provide accurate and reliable information about reciprocal flexion/extension muscle strength was evaluated to establish the reliability of isometric knee flexion/extension strength measures, to quantify the extent of measurement error that may occur as a result of gravity, to describe isometric strength curves through a full range of motion for both knee flexion and extension, and to describe the ratio of isometric knee flexion/extension strength through full range of motion in healthy adults.

Methods.—Maximum isometric knee flexion and extension strength and lower leg mass at rest were measured at 6, 24, 42, 60, 78, 96, and 108 degrees of knee flexion in 77 healthy volunteers (38 women) aged 18 to 50 years. Net muscular torque was calculated as the difference between maximum voluntary isometric torque (total torque) and torque values obtained at relaxation at each angle.

Results.—Unilateral and bilateral tests had a reliability of 0.88 to 0.98 and a standard error of the measurement percentage of 5.1% to 12.6%. Total torque and net muscular torque values were significantly different at all angles measured. Flexion/extension torque ratios were correlated with angle, ranging from 1.30 at 6 degrees to 0.31 at 108 degrees.

Conclusion.—Standardized isometric testing can quantify knee extension and flexion strength if lower leg mass is accounted for and can provide a measure of muscular imbalance.

▶ Many questions arise in the discussion of muscle imbalance. How important is muscle imbalance? Does it increase the incidence of injury? What is the best method of measuring muscle imbalance? When muscle balance is measured, should concentric ratios be evaluated or should concentric/eccentric ratios of antagonist muscles be evaluated? At what speed and at what angles should these ratios be evaluated? Should the results be used to determine whether progression is made in a rehabilitation program or for return to activity? The authors present a rationale for testing isometrically at numerous angles, correcting for muscle mass and the effects of gravity.

F.J. George, A.T.C., P.T.

Heavy-Load Eccentric Calf Muscle Training for the Treatment of Chronic Achilles Tendinosis

Alfredson H, Pietilä T, Jonsson P, et al (Univ Hosp of Northern Sweden, Umeå)

Am J Sports Med 26:360-366, 1998   8–9

Background.—No prospective studies have been published on eccentric calf muscle training in patients with Achilles tendinopathies. The short-term effect of heavy-load eccentric calf muscle training on tendon pain during activity, and on calf muscle strength, in patients with chronic Achilles' tendinosis selected for surgery was investigated prospectively.

Methods.—Fifteen recreational athletes, aged a mean of 44.3, were studied. All had chronic Achilles tendinosis with a long duration of symptoms, despite conventional nonoperative treatment. Calf muscle strength and extent of pain during activity were determined before onset of training and after 12 weeks of eccentric training. At baseline, all patients had pain that prevented running. In addition, the injured side had significantly lower eccentric and concentric calf muscle strength than did the uninjured side.

Findings.—After 12 weeks of training, all patients could resume preinjury levels of activity, including running. Pain during activity was significantly reduced. Calf muscle strength on the injured side was increased significantly and did not differ from that of the uninjured side (Fig 1).

Conclusions.—This method of eccentric calf muscle training in patients with chronic Achilles' tendinosis is easy to perform, results in fast recovery of concentric and eccentric calf muscle strength, and enables previous running activity. This intervention should be attempted before surgery is performed.

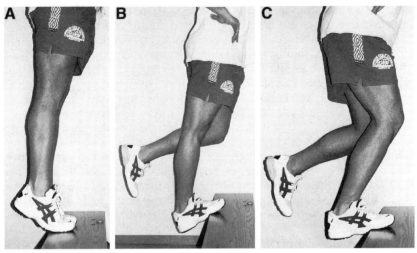

FIGURE 1.—From an upright body position and standing with all body weight on the forefoot and the ankle joint in plantar flexion lifted by the noninjured leg (**A**), the calf muscle was loaded eccentrically by having the patient lower the heel with the knee straight (**B**) and with the knee bent (**C**). (Courtesy of Alfredson H, Pietilä T, Jonsson P, et al: Heavy-load eccentric calf muscle training for the treatment of chronic Achilles tendinosis. *Am J Sports Med* 26:360-366, 1998.)

▶ The authors have described an interesting concept of using eccentric muscle contractions alone to rehabilitate chronic Achilles' tendinosis. All 15 patients who received this therapy returned to their preinjury running levels. All of the 15 patients receiving conventional therapy were referred for surgery. The statistical evidence of this study points strongly to the effectiveness of eccentric muscle contractions in rehabilitating these injuries.

F.J. George, A.T.C., P.T.

Postexercise Increase in Nitric Oxide in Football Players With Muscle Cramps
Maddali S, Rodeo SA, Barnes R, et al (Hosp for Special Surgery, New York)
Am J Sports Med 26:820-824, 1998   8–10

Background.—Skeletal muscle express high levels of nitric oxide, and in vitro studies have shown that the electrical stimulation of skeletal muscle preparations increases these levels. The in vivo changes that occur in serum nitric oxide concentrations after strenuous exercise causing severe generalized muscle cramps were evaluated.

Methods.—The subjects were 77 professional football players at a preseason training camp who provided baseline blood samples for determining levels of serum nitrite and other chemicals. During training, 25 subjects experienced generalized muscle cramps severe enough to require intravenous rehydration, while 52 subjects did not develop cramps. The 25 subjects with cramps provided a total of 40 serum samples for repeat measurements of serum nitrite and other chemical concentrations.

Findings.—The subjects who received intravenous rehydration for muscle cramps had a significantly higher percentage of body fat (14.7% vs 10.9%) and were significantly heavier (257 vs 237 pounds) than those who did not develop cramps. Compared with baseline values, postexercise serum samples in the subjects requiring intravenous rehydration showed signs of skeletal muscle breakdown (eg, 158% higher levels of alanine aminotransferase, 102% higher levels of lactate dehydrogenase) and dehydration (eg, 52% higher levels of protein, 12% higher levels of cholesterol). The most striking change occurred in serum nitrite concentrations, which almost quadrupled after exercise in these 25 subjects (from 0.11 to 0.41 µM). Furthermore, serum nitrite levels increased to a greater extent than did those of any other serum chemical (range 8% to 158%). Postexercise changes in serum nitrite did not correlate with changes in the other serum chemicals.

Conclusions.—During exercise strenuous enough to cause severe muscle cramps, nitric oxide synthesis increases dramatically. Whether this increase is due to the exercise or the muscle cramps is not known. Nonetheless, the increased nitric oxide synthesis is more than that which could be attributed to dehydration alone.

▶ Certainly an interesting article; however, the clinical significance remains somewhat obscure. Also, the exact source of the increased nitric oxide is not known. Another limitation is that postexercise nitrite measurements were not obtained from players without muscle cramps. Thus, it is not possible to state whether the increase was due to exercise, muscle cramps, or a combination of the 2.

J.S. Torg, M.D.

9 Women: Aging

Training and Injuries Amongst Elite Female Orienteers
Creagh U, Reilly TH (Liverpool John Moores Univ, England)
J Sports Med Phys Fitness 38:75-79, 1998   9–1

Background.—Orienteering is a cross-country endurance running event that lasts up to 90 minutes for elite female athletes. Most reported injuries occur during training, 57% resulting from overuse and 43% from trauma. Training levels and patterns of injury among elite female orienteers were investigated.

Methods.—Nineteen elite and 9 sub-elite athletes participated in the study. A questionnaire was administered eliciting data on training practices and injuries.

Findings.—Although the sub-elite orienteers trained less intensively than the elite orienteers in the off-season, the 2 groups did not differ in distribution or likely cause of injuries. Only 32% of the athletes trained predominantly on the road. The rest ran on off-road or mixed terrain. Sixty-eight percent of the participants reported injuries. Four percent had had upper-body injuries. Forty-three percent reported ankle injuries and 16%, knee injuries—the reverse of the injury pattern is typically seen in runners.

Conclusions.—Orienteering injuries are largely related to the rough terrain on which the athletes train and compete. This probably explains why orienteers had a higher number of ankle injuries than knee injuries.

▶ When two thirds of an elite group of orienteers report injuries that curtail training, there is reason to look for causative factors in hopes that further injuries can be prevented. The athletes seem to believe that overtraining and unsuitable footwear account for most of their injuries. Since both of these factors could be considered under the control of the coach, it would be interesting to see whether the coaches agree with the athletes' assessment of risk factors—and, if so, why corrective action isn't taken.

B.L. Drinkwater, Ph.D.

Association Between the Menstrual Cycle and Anterior Cruciate Ligament Injuries in Female Athletes

Wojtys EM, Huston LJ, Lindenfeld TN, et al (Univ of Michigan, Ann Arbor; Deaconess Hosp, Cincinnati, Ohio)
Am J Sports Med 26:614-619, 1998   9–2

Objective.—Female athletes have 4 to 8 times more anterior cruciate ligament (ACL) injuries than male athletes. It is possible that this increased injury rate in women is the result of the complex interactions between estrogen, progesterone, and relaxin. The variation in ACL injury rates during the female monthly cycle was investigated.

Methods.—A questionnaire was administered to 40 consecutive women with an acute ACL tear, and 28 of these women with a noncontact ACL injury were included in the study. Women with a history of irregular or missed cycles were excluded. Women were asked the date and mechanism of injury, the length of play before injury, whether the injury was sustained during practice or play, and whether the injury occurred during contact or noncontact, jumping, landing, or pivoting. Cycle length was divided into the follicular days (1 to 9), ovulatory days (10 to 14), and luteal days (15 to end). Observed and expected injury rates were calculated, and test-retest reliability of the questionnaire was established to validate results.

Results.—Injuries occurred while the women were playing basketball (29%), skiing (21%), soccer (14%), and other (36%). Injuries resulted after a jump in 30% of patients or pivoting, twisting, or deceleration in 23%. Significantly more injuries occurred during the ovulatory phase than were expected (29% observed vs. 18% expected), and significantly fewer occurred during the follicular phase than expected (13% observed vs. 32% expected). Test-retest reliability showed a kappa coefficient of 0.97.

Conclusion.—A significant association exists between the ACL injury rates in female athletes and the ovulatory phase of the menstrual cycle. Additional studies need to be conducted to establish the robustness of these results.

▶ There is no doubt that ACL injuries occur more frequently among female athletes than among males. Theories to explain this difference often focus on the menstrual cycle and the hormonal fluctuations that occur during the cycle. While there are many other male-female differences that can be explored, the role of estrogen and progesterone is a valid subject for research. However, the use of subject recall as to the day of cycle when the injury occurred and then the assumption that hormone levels can be predicted by the day of the cycle does not lend credence to the results. In all other physiologic studies examining the effect of cyclic changes in hormones, actual determination of the hormone levels are part of the protocol. The requirement should be no less when investigating the role female hormones play in ACL injuries.

B.L. Drinkwater, Ph.D.

The Relationship Between Serum Oestradiol Concentration and Energy Balance in Young Women Distance Runners

Zanker CL, Swaine IL (De Montfort Univ Bedford, England)
Int J Sports Med 19:104-108, 1998   9–3

Introduction.—Studies of the well-known reproductive dysfunction in some female distance runners suggest that ovarian suppression originates from a hypothalamic disturbance. The relationship between serum E_2 concentration and indices of energy balance (EB) (estimated EB, serum T_3, and serum IGF-1) was evaluated in 33 female distance runners with a variety of menstrual patterns and a range of activity levels.

Methods.—Mean age of runners was 27.2. Their menstrual status was: 16 eumenorrheic, 9 amenorrheic (Am), and 8 oligomenorrheic (Ol). All had been running regularly for at least 4 years at distances of 36 to 97 km/wk^{-1}. The mean daily EB was determined for each runner by subtracting dietary energy intake from estimated energy expenditure over 7 days. Energy expenditure was estimated using records of activity patterns. This evaluation was done during the week immediately after menstruation in women who were eumenorrheic.

Results.—Mean duration of amenorrhea in amenorrheic women was 4.8 years. Twenty-five of 33 women were in energy deficit. All women who were Am and 6 of 8 women who were Ol were in energy deficit. All Am and Ol women had serum E_2 concentrations below the normal reference range for eumenorrheic women who were during the early follicular phase of their menstrual cycles (Fig 1). There was a strong correlation between serum E_2 and estimated EB, serum total T_3, and serum IGF-1. The serum levels of T_3 and IGF-1 were strongly associated with estimated EB.

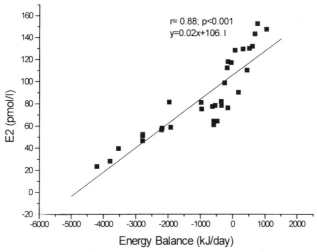

FIGURE 1.—Relationship between serum oestradiol (E_2) and energy balance for female runners (n = 33). (Courtesy of Zanker CL, Swaine IL: The relationship between serum oestradiol concentration and energy balance in young women. *Int J Sports Med* 19:104-108, 1998. Georg Thieme Verlag.)

Conclusion.—Strong correlations were found between serum E_2 concentration and indices of energy balance in female distance runners. These relationships have not been observed before and support the hypothesis that reproductive dysfunction is associated with an energy deficit. Even in the presence of energy deficit, all women reported that their body mass had been stable for 6 months before testing. Estimated EB and serum levels of T_3 and IGF-1 were more powerful predictors of serum E_2 concentration than body mass index or body fat was.

▶ Evidence that the menstrual irregularities observed in some female athletes are induced by an energy deficit continues to mount. If the evidence is correct, an appropriate intervention for oligo/amenorrheic athletes would be to convince these women to make small changes in both energy intake and energy expenditure in order to return energy balance to normal. This is easier said than done, of course, because many athletes will resist eating more or exercising less. However, the consequences of the persistent hypoestrogenic state on health, particularly bone health, can be devastating. We have found that a bone density test can be a great motivation. Seeing her bone density equivalent to that of women in their 60's, 70's or older brings home the seriousness of the problem.

B.L. Drinkwater, Ph.D.

Effects of Exercise and Estrogen Therapy on Lipid Profiles of Postmenopausal Women
Klebanoff R, Miller VT, Fernhall B (George Washington Univ, Washington, DC)
Med Sci Sports Exerc 30:1028-1034, 1998   9–4

Introduction.—The change from premenopausal to postmenopausal status is associated with unfavorable changes in the lipid profile and with increased risk of coronary artery disease. The effects of a moderate- to high-intensity exercise training program on blood lipid profiles were assessed in postmenopausal women who were or were not taking estrogen replacement therapy (ERT).

Methods.—Age range of 22 postmenopausal women was 45 to 61. Eleven participants were taking conjugated equine estrogen (or its equivalent in an oral estrogen preparation) 0.625 mg daily and 11 participants received no ERT. All women participated in graded exercise tests at baseline and at conclusion of a 12-week individualized training program that consisted of walking, stair-stepping, rowing, cycling, and aerobic dance. This supervised program met 3 times weekly, in addition to 1 unsupervised walking session each week. In the first 2 weeks of training, participants exercised at 65% to 70% of VO_{2max}, increased to 70% to 75% during weeks 3 and 4, and finally increased to 75% to 80% of VO_{2max} for the remaining program. Measures of body composition, diet, and lipoprotein lipid were taken at initiation and at completion of the exercise program.

Results.—There were 8 women on ERT and 10 women not on ERT who completed the trial. The VO_{2max} rose by 8% in both groups. Neither group changed their diet. The nonestrogen group had significantly higher baseline levels of LDL-C than the estrogen group. Significantly higher levels of triglycerides were observed in the estrogen group. Neither group had significant mean changes over time for total cholesterol, triglycerides, HDL-cholesterol, or LDL/HDL ratio. Individual changes in LDL-C and total cholesterol were strongly correlated with baseline weight in the nonestrogen group, but not in the estrogen group. There were significant associations between baseline body weight and individual changes in blood lipids for the group as a whole. All participants were divided into 2 groups based on body mass index (27 or less or greater than 27), regardless of ERT status. There was a significant reduction in total cholesterol in the 27 or less body mass index group, but not the greater than 27 body mass index group.

Conclusion.—Exercise intervention did not affect blood lipid profiles in postmenopausal women, regardless of ERT status. Body weight seemed to have modulating effects on changes in blood lipids with exercise training.

▶ It would be unfortunate if the initial results of this study led women to believe that exercise in the years following menopause has no positive effect on lipid profiles. To avoid misleading the reader, it is important to limit conclusions to the population studied. In this case, the mean body fat of the whole group averaged over 34%, body mass index greater than 28, and aerobic power 25.1 $mL \cdot kg^{-1} \cdot min^{-1}$. Fortunately the authors went beyond their original hypothesis and looked more closely at the effect of weight. Women with body mass index less than 27 did respond more favorably to the training program, which once again emphasizes the importance of maintaining a healthy weight throughout life.

B.L. Drinkwater, Ph.D.

Effects of Exercise Intensity and Training on Lipid Metabolism in Young Women
Friedlander AL, Casazza GA, Horning MA, et al (Univ of California, Berkeley)
Am J Physiol 275:E853-E863, 1998   9–5

Introduction.—Endurance training does not increase total lipid oxidation, measured at the same relative workloads, in men. These data are not available in women, however. The effects of exercise intensity and endurance training on lipid metabolism were assessed in 9 young women to determine whether exercise would increase their reliance on free fatty acid (FFA) oxidation during exercise, after 12 weeks of endurance training measured at both the same absolute and relative exercise intensities.

Methods.—Age range was 18 to 35 in healthy, nonsmoking, sedentary women with normal menstrual cycles who were not pregnant, lactating, or taking oral contraceptives. The women underwent 2 randomized stable isotope infusion trials, performed a minimum of 2 days apart, on a cycle ergometer for 1 hour at 45% and 65% of VO_{2peak} (45UT and 65UT, respectively). Two additional isotope trials were performed around 8 and 12 weeks of training: 1 at the same absolute workload (ABT), which elicited 65% of pretraining VO_{2peak} and 1 which elicited 65% of the postraining VO_{2peak}, the same relative workload (RLT). The women exercised with a personal trainer 5 days per week for 1 hour on the cycle ergometer and an additional hour on the weekend in any way they desired. Rates of FFA appearance (R_a) and disappearance (R_D) and oxidation (R_{oxp}) were measured.

Results.—Intensity effect on FFA R_a was not significant at pretraining; it was elevated after training at both the same ABT and RLT. Compared with 65UT, FFA R_d rose by 33% at the same ABT and 52% at the same RLT after exercise training. The metabolic clearance rate was notably increased after exercise training at the same ABT and RLT. The rate of R_{oxp} was significantly higher during exercise than at rest, unaffected by intensity pretraining, and significantly increased after training at the same ABT (58%) and RLT (117%).

Conclusion.—Women increased their reliance on lipid after endurance training, whether exercise was normalized to absolute or to relative power outputs. These data differ from earlier findings in men, which showed no rise in total lipid use at the same relative exercise intensity. The rise in FFA flux rates in women differs from earlier findings that men have reduced FFA R_d after training at the same ABT.

▶ When there are gender differences in physiologic studies, the search for an explanation often leads to the hormonal differences between women and men. In this study, the role of ovarian hormones was minimized by scheduling the trials during the midfollicular phase of the cycle. The authors' conclusions, therefore, apply only to that short period of the normal menstrual cycle. Conclusions about how higher levels of estrogen or the presence of progesterone affect lipid metabolism under similar conditions require further study.

B.L. Drinkwater, Ph.D.

HRT Preserves Increases in Bone Mineral Density and Reductions in Body Fat After a Supervised Exercise Program
Kohrt WM, Ehsani AA, Birge SJ Jr (Washington Univ, St. Louis)
J Appl Physiol 84:1506-1512, 1998   9–6

Background.—Although exercise training is known to increase bone mineral density (BMD) in older women, the extent to which this adaptation persists after reduction or discontinuation of exercise is not known. Previous research has shown that hormone-replacement therapy (HRT) augments exercise-induced BMD increases in older women. This study was

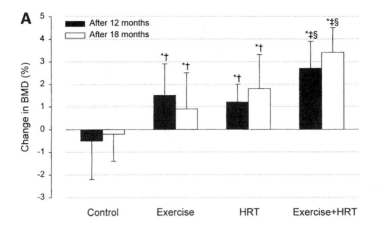

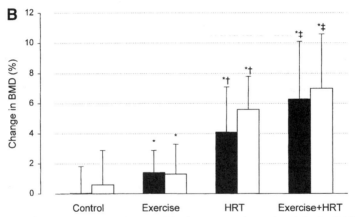

FIGURE 2.—Changes in total body (**A**) and lumbar spine (**B**) bone mineral density (*BMD*) after treatment (after 12 month) and follow-up (after 18 month) periods in control subjects and in response to exercise, Hormone replacement therapy (*HRT*), and exercise + HRT. *Asterisks* indicate significantly different from zero, P .05 or less; *single daggers* indicate significantly different from control, P .05 or less; *double daggers* indicate significantly different from exercise, P .05 or less; *section marks* indicate significantly different from HRT, P 0.05 or less. (Courtesy of Kohrt WM, Ehsani AA, Birge SJ Jr: HRT preserves increases in bone mineral density and reductions in body fat after a supervised exercise program. *J Appl Physiol* 84:1506-1512, 1998.)

undertaken to confirm these findings and to determine whether HRT preserves the adaptations after reduction or discontinuation of exercise.

Methods.—Fifty-four nonsmoking women, aged 60 to 72 years, completed the study. None of the women had used estrogen in the 2 years preceding study enrollment, and none were regular exercisers. The women were assigned to 1 of 4 groups: exercise alone, HRT alone, exercise plus HRT, or a control group. After the 11-month treatment phase, the women were followed for 6 months, during which HRT was continued.

Findings.—After treatment, mean total body BMD changes were −0.5% in the control group, 1.5% in the exercise group, 1.2% in the HRT group, and 2.7% in the exercise plus HRT group (Fig 2). Exercise plus HRT was more effective than HRT alone in increasing total body BMD and tended to be more effective at increasing BMD at the lumbar spine. The combined treatment was also more effective than exercise alone in increasing total body, lumbar spine, and trochanter BMD. During follow-up, exercise-induced gains in BMD were preserved only in women receiving HRT. In addition, HRT-attenuated fat accumulation, especially in the abdominal area, after the exercise program.

Conclusion.—HRT appears to be an important adjunct to exercise programs for preventing osteoporosis and illness related to abdominal obesity in older women. The concomitant use of HRT helps preserve the gains in BMD after an exercise program.

▶ The authors made every effort to avoid selection bias in spite of the fact that they were unable to randomize the women into treatment groups. However, it is up to the reader to decide whether the results from a nonrandomized trial are credible. Of more concern is the fact that neither the title nor the abstract mention that the participants were encouraged to continue exercising after the end of the 12 months of supervised activity. Although the amount of activity decreased, we still do not know precisely how much exercise is required to maintain gains in BMD and, therefore, how much it may have contributed to maintaining BMD. It is also evident from the error bars on the figures that there was considerable variability in the response of the women during the study and follow-up. Finally, results from a 6-month follow-up cannot predict what may occur over a longer period.

B.L. Drinkwater, Ph.D.

Effects of High-Intensity Resistance Exercise on Bone Mineral Density and Muscle Strength of 40-50-Year-Old Women

Dornemann TM, McMurray RG, Renner JB, et al (Univ of North Carolina, Chapel Hill)
J Sports Med Phys Fitness 37:246-251, 1997   9–7

Background.—Previous studies have suggested that muscle strength is significantly correlated with bone density. However, longitudinal studies have not reported such clear benefits of increased muscle strength. In the current study, the effects of a site-specific resistance-training regimen on bone mineral density (BMD) of the lumbar vertebrae, femoral neck, and distal radius were assessed in premenopausal women.

Methods.—Thirty-five women, aged 40 to 50 years, were assigned randomly to resistance training (RT) or a sedentary control group. Resistance training consisted of 6 months of high-intensity weight lifting 3 days a week, a regimen designed to place strain on the spine and hips.

Findings.—Women in the RT group significantly increased strength. Though analysis of variance of lumbar vertebrae BMD showed no significant difference between groups, there was a trend toward a group interaction effect. Vertebral BMD improved by a mean of 1.03% in the RT group and declined by a mean of 0.36% in the control group. Radial BMD declined in both groups, with no significant differences. Femoral BMD increased by about 1.2% in both groups.

Conclusions.—A short-term training program may maintain or improve BMD of the femoral neck and lumbar vertebrae in premenopausal women. Between-group differences in BMD were not significant at the femoral and radial sites, but a trend toward a difference was noted at the lumbar sites.

▶ It's tempting to be optimistic about exercise increasing bone density, but it's difficult to reconcile these authors' conclusions with the results of the study. If the resistance training was a significant factor, why was there a decrease in radial bone density when the arms were involved in a majority of the exercises? Did the training program actually "maintain or improve the BMD of the femoral neck and lumbar vertebrae" when the control group had the same small nonsignificant increase in femoral neck density as the training group did, and when there was no significant between-group difference in spinal BMD? This does not mean that resistance training cannot be effective in increasing bone density, but a six-month training period may be too short to effect a significant change.

B.L. Drinkwater, Ph.D.

Effect of Long-term Unilateral Activity on Bone Mineral Density of Female Junior Tennis Players

Haapasalo H, Kannus P, Sievänen H, et al (UKK Inst, Tampere, Finland)
J Bone Miner Res 13:310-319, 1998   9–8

Introduction.—Peak bone mass in early adulthood and the subsequent rate of bone loss are the primary determinants of bone mass in later life. The type, intensity, frequency, and duration of optimal exercise, and particularly the age-phase or developmental stage (Tanner stage) at which the effects of physical activity are most crucial on bone, are yet undefined. A cross-sectional investigation was conducted to determine at which Tanner stage the side-to-side bone mineral density (BMD) differences between the playing and nonplaying arms of tennis players become obvious, and to determine which training or background variables could explain interindividual differences in the response of bones to mechanical loading.

Methods.—Ninety-one 7 to 17-year-old female tennis players from the Finnish Tennis Federation and tennis clubs in southern Finland, who had trained on a regular basis longer than 1 year, underwent determinations of training history, Tanner stage, maximal isometric strength of the forearm extensors and flexors, grip strength, and areal BMD of both upper extremities (at 3 sites: proximal humerus, humeral shaft, and distal radius)

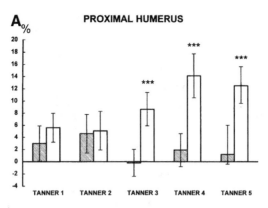

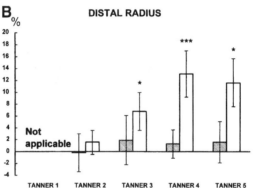

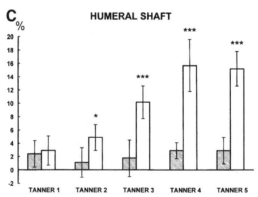

FIGURE 1.—The side-to-side BMD difference (%) in the upper extremities of controls (*shaded bars*) and players (*open bars*). The *bars* indicate the 95% confidence intervals. (Difference between controls and players *P less than .05, †less than .001.) **A,** Proximal humerus. In the ANOVA with Helmert contrasts, the player vs. control difference in the Tanner I (P = .041) and Tanner II (P less than .001) differed significantly from the average difference in the subsequent Tanner stages, whereas this was not the case in Tanner III (P=.49) and Tanner IV (P=.72). **B,** Humeral shaft. In the ANOVA with Helmert contrasts, the player versus control difference in the Tanner I (P less than .001) and Tanner II (P=.001) differed significantly from the average difference of the subsequent Tanner stages, whereas this was not the case in Tanner III (P=.066) and Tanner IV (P=.84). **C,** Distal radius. The ANOVA with Helmert contrasts revealed that in none of the Tanner stages did the player versus control difference contrast significantly with the average difference of the subsequent Tanner stages. The P-values were .071 for Tanner II, .067 for Tanner III, and .60 for Tanner IV. *Abbreviations:* BMD, bone mineral density; ANOVA, analysis of variance. (Courtesy of Haapasalo H, Kannus P, Sievänen H: Effect of long-term unilateral activity on bone mineral density of female junior tennis players. *J Bone Miner Res* 13:310-319, 1998. Reprinted by permission of Blackwell Science, Inc.)

and lumbar spine. Findings were compared with those in 58 similarly healthy girls from local schools.

Results.—In tennis players, the side-to-side differences were distinct and significant at all measured sites and Tanner stages except the distal radius in Tanner stage II. The Tanner stage III, IV, and V tennis players had significantly higher relative side-to-side BMD differences at every measured site than controls. For Tanner stage II, there was a significant difference between controls and players in the humeral shaft only. No significant differences were noted between players and controls for Tanner stage I (Fig 1). Significant differences were noted in lumbar spine BMD between players and controls in Tanner stage IV. There were no between-group differences in BMD of the nondominant distal radius at any Tanner stage. The total training hours and number of current training sessions per week were the only predictive variables that had a significant and systemic association with the relative side-to-side BMD differences in several measured sites. Not even strenuous tennis playing yielded a BMD benefit in girls in Tanner stage I.

Conclusion.—These and earlier findings suggest that the effect of unilateral activity on bone is greatest during a relatively short period in puberty, when rapid natural bone mineral accumulation and rapid longitudinal growth occur. Regular exercise is recommended during the pubescent years to maximize peak bone mass and prevent osteoporosis and related fractures in later life.

▶ The numerous studies from this Tampere group have directed attention to how important physical activity during adolescence is in helping children attain their genetically determined peak bone mass. It is reasonable to assume, as the authors do, that a higher peak bone mass is likely to diminish the risk of osteoporosis later in life. Yet in the United States, school physical education programs, the only avenue through which the majority of children can be assured of daily physical activity, have been disappearing at a rapid rate. Far from being a "frill", physical activity has been recognized by the Surgeon General of the United States and other medical professionals as essential to good health. When will school boards and educators discover this fact?

B. L. Drinkwater, Ph.D.

Women at Altitude: Changes in Carbohydrate Metabolism at 4,300-m Elevation and Across the Menstrual Cycle
Braun B, Butterfield GE, Dominick SB, et al (Veterans Affairs Health Care System, Palo Alto, Calif; Univ of Colorado, Denver; US Army Research Inst of Environmental Medicine, Natick, Mass)
J Appl Physiol 85:1966-1973, 1998   9–9

Introduction.—Exposure to high altitude may affect carbohydrate metabolism differently in men and women. Gender differences include adi-

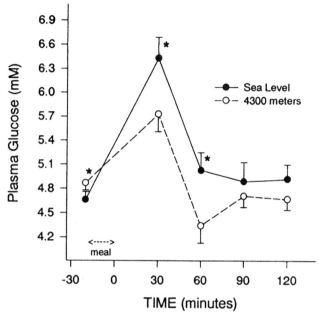

FIGURE 1.—Plasma glucose concentrations before and after a high-carbohydrate meal at sea level and at 4,300 m. Values are means ± standard error; n = 16. Women were studied in the same ovarian hormone condition at each elevation: 11 estrogen (E), 5 estrogen plus progesterone (E+P). *Significant differences at individual time points, P less than 0.05. (Courtesy of Braun B, Butterfield GE, Dominick SB: Women at altitude: Changes in carbohydrate metabolism at 4,300-m elevation and across the menstrual cycle. *J Appl Physiol* 85:1966-1973, 1998.)

posity, fat distribution, testosterone, and the direct and indirect effects of the ovarian hormones estrogen (E) and progesterone (P) on pathways of intermediary metabolism. It is possible that the blood glucose response (BGR) to a high-carbohydrate meal may be lower in women than men at high altitude relative to the response at sea level. The magnitude of the change in BGR to altitude may be reduced in the presence of E and P, relative to the presence of E alone. Glucose, insulin, and C-peptide response to a high-carbohydrate meal was assessed in young women in both phases (luteal and follicular) of the menstrual cycle, after 9 days at sea level and after 9 days of exposure to 4,300-m elevation at Pikes Peak.

Methods.—All women were nonsmokers, had regular menstrual cycles, and were in good health. The women were assessed for 12 days at sea level on 2 occasions, usually 6 weeks apart, and then were housed for 12 days at a laboratory at Pikes Peak. Sixteen women were evaluated in both E and E+P conditions at sea level and in either the E or E+P conditions at Pikes Peak. For each condition, blood was sampled on day 9 before, and every 30 minutes for 2 hours after a high-carbohydrate meal.

Results.—BGR peaked at a lower value and returned to baseline more slowly at 4,300 m than at sea level (Fig 1). Plasma insulin values were similar, but C peptide values were slightly higher at 4,300 m. The BGR returned to baseline more slowly in the E+P condition than in the E condition at sea level. Insulin and C peptide were similar during E and E+P conditions.

Conclusion.—The BGR to a high-carbohydrate meal was lower after 9 days at high altitude, than at sea level in young women. Effects of altitude were not dependent upon changes in plasma insulin concentrations. These effects may be related to differences in insulin secretion and clearance. The relative concentrations of ovarian hormones did not seem to modify the magnitude of change in BGR in women exposed to an altitude of 4,300 m.

▶ Now that women have successfully climbed most of the highest peaks in the Himalayas, including Mount Everest, studies of the female response to altitude hypoxia may be of practical value to climbers and skiers, as well as scientific interest to physiologists. However, although there are both logical and logistical reasons for doing research on Pikes Peak, responses at 4,300 m may be quite different from those at higher elevations and under different conditions. As the authors take care to note, their results are specific to the length of stay at altitude in this study. The nutritional needs of women climbing for several weeks at altitudes well above 4,300 m are also likely to be different.

B.L. Drinkwater, Ph.D.

The Female Athlete: The Triad of Disordered Eating, Amenorrhoea and Osteoporosis
West RV (George Washington Univ, Washington, DC)
Sports Med 26:63-71, 1998   9–10

Objective.—Although the importance of female athletes has grown during this century and has increased health and physical fitness through increased participation in physical activity, some female athletes are at risk of the development of 3 interrelated disorders: disordered eating, amenorrhea, and osteoporosis. The definition, identification, and treatment of this triad were discussed.

Definitions.—Disordered eating is most prevalent in sports that emphasize low body weight and includes fasting; laxative, diuretic, or diet pill use; and vomiting. These practices impair athletic performance, increase risk of injury, decrease ability to concentrate, and can lead to death. Amenorrhea, either primary or secondary, can result from acute weight loss or significant weight fluctuations that interfere with normal hormonal cycles or levels. Amenorrhea is particularly prevalent in females who begin intense training before puberty. Osteoporosis—inadequate bone formation or premature bone loss—is accelerated by estrogen deficiency, is increasingly common, and tends to be partially irreversible in women with amenorrhea. Bone mineral density is significantly lower in runners and significantly higher in gymnasts than in controls.

Screening.—Physical signs of disordered eating, follicle-stimulating hormone level determination, hormonal challenges, and imaging studies of the pelvis are useful in identifying and preventing the female triad.

Treatment.—Decreasing exercise intensity, weight gain, and increasing calcium intake are recommended. In adolescents, optimizing nutritional and calcium intake are important. Dietary patterns should be evaluated, exercise programs should be modified, and hormone therapy may be necessary in older females with amenorrhea.

Conclusion.—Some sports more than others put female athletes at risk of the female athlete triad. Prevention is the best treatment. Early diagnosis, education, and proper diet are imperative.

▶ The article emphasizes several important points regarding "the female athlete triad." First, the 3 components of this triad are synergistic and associated with significant morbidity and mortality. The prevalence of eating disorders may be as high as 62% in certain sports. All female athletes are at risk for developing this triad. Premature osteoporosis in women with amenorrhea is partially irreversible. A major problem with the bone loss associated with amenorrhea is that it occurs at a time when the young woman should be storing bone for the inevitable loss that occurs later in life.

J.S. Torg, M.D.

Bone Mineral Density and Menstrual Irregularities: A Comparative Study on Cortical and Trabecular Bone Structures in Runners With Alleged Normal Eating Behavior
Tomten SE, Falch JA, Birkeland KI, et al (Norwegian Univ, Oslo, Norway; Aker Hosp, Oslo, Norway)
Int J Sports Med 19:92-97, 1998   9–11

Objective.—Low bone mineral density (BMD) levels have been found in amenorrheic athletes relative to eumenorrheic athletes and even some sedentary and normal active individuals. BMD in the total body, lumbar spine, femoral neck, and lower leg was determined in a case-control study of 2 groups of long distance runners, those with menstrual irregularities (IR) and those with regular (R) menstrual cycles.

Methods.—BMD and biochemical and endocrine markers were determined in 13 runners, aged 18 to 40 years, with irregular menstrual cycles (5 oligomenorrheic and 8 amenorrheic) and 15 runners, aged 18 to 40 years, with normal menstrual cycles. All participants reported normal eating habits and were not using pathogenic weight-control methods. Total BMD was determined using dual X-ray absorptiometry. BMD was also determined at L2-L4, the femoral neck, the lower leg, and the arm. Blood was sampled during the follicular phase in regularly menstruating athletes and at any convenient time in IR athletes.

Results.—Serum estradiol, lutenizing hormone (LH), follicle-stimulating hormone (FSH), and free thyroxine (f-T_4) levels were significantly

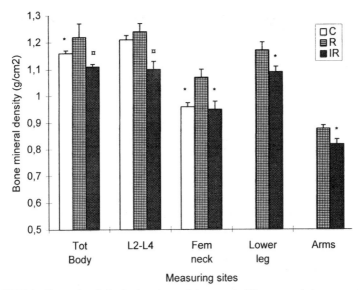

FIGURE 1.—Bone mineral density in eumenorrheic controls (C), eumenorrheic runners (R) and runners with menstrual irregularities (IR) in the total body, femoral neck, lumbar vertebrae, arms, and lower legs. *Horizontal limit bars indicate (Mean ± SEM). *P* less than .05 versus R, White bars) P < .05 versus C and R. (Courtesy of Tomten SE, Falch JA, Birkeland KI, et al: Bone mineral density and menstrual irregularities: A comparative study on cortical and trabecular bone structures in runners with alleged normal eating behavior. *Int J Sports Med* 19:92-97, 1998, Georg Thieme Verlag.)

lower in IR than in R athletes. BMD levels were significantly lower in IR athletes than in R athletes at all sites measured (Fig 1). Severity of past and present menstrual dysfunction was significantly related to BMD of the spine, femoral neck, and total body, but not in the lower leg. IR athletes had reduced BMD at all sites including the cortical structures of the arms and lower legs. Low BMD in the lower legs may be the result of failure to adapt to the increased mechanical load of running and may explain the increase incidence of stress fractures among IR athletes.

Conclusion.—The findings of low BMD levels in trabecular and cortical bone in athletes with menstrual irregularities and suggest a negative effect on bone tissue that may predispose these athletes to injury and perhaps to osteoporotic fractures later in life.

▶ In order to have a sample large enough for statistical evaluation, the authors combined oligomenorrheic and amenorrheic athletes into 1 group of 13 women. In this instance, the combination of menstrual irregularities did not minimize the negative effect on bone density. However, 1 of the important questions regarding oligomenorrhea and bone density remains unanswered. How many normal cycles per year are required to avoid bone loss and is the decrease related to the years of oligomenorrhea? The answer will require a large number of subjects and perhaps can only be answered by investigators combining their data.

B.L. Drinkwater, Ph.D.

Relation Between Bone Turnover, Oestradiol, and Energy Balance in Women Distance Runners

Zanker CL, Swaine IL (De Montfort Univ Bedford, UK)
Br J Sports Med 32:167-171, 1998   9–12

Objective.—Although weight-bearing exercise generally increases bone mass, exercise-associated amenorrhea in some young women leads to lower bone mineral density (BMD). Exercise-associated amenorrhea results from hypothalamic dysfunction that is thought to be induced by an energy deficit. The relations between biochemical markers of bone turnover, indices of nutritional status (estimated energy balance, serum triiodothyronine (T_3) concentration, and body mass index), and serum estradiol concentration in a group of young women distance runners with a variety of menstrual patterns and a range of activity levels were explored.

Methods.—Nutritional status was determined and biochemical analysis of fasting blood samples was performed in 33 young women distance runners, mean age 27.2 years, who were classified as eumenorrheic (n = 18), amenorrheic (n = 9), or oligomenorrheic (n = 6). Mean daily energy balance was defined as estimated energy expenditure minus mean daily energy intake measured during 1 week. Osteocalcin and bone-specific alkaline phosphatase (BAP) were measured in serum from fasting blood samples drawn between 9 and 10 AM during the early follicular phase. Level of deoxypyridinoline/creatinine (D_{pyr}/Cr) was determined from an early morning urine sample. Serum estradiol was measured using by ELISA.

Results.—All parameters were significantly lower in amenorrheic women than in the other 2 groups. No differences were noted in the BMIs, net energy balance, or serum T_3 levels of oligomenorrheic and eumenorrheic women. Oligomenorrheic women had significantly lower serum es-

TABLE 2.—Serum Levels of Estradiol, Total 3, 5, 3'-Triiodothyronine (T_3), Osteocalcin, Bone Alkaline Phosphatase (BAP) and Urine Deoxypyridinoline/Creatinine (D_{pyr}/Cr) Levels for the 33 Active Women. Values Are Indicated as Mean (SE)

	Amenorrhoeic (*n*=9)	Oligomenorrhoeic (*n*=6)	Eumenorrhoeic (*n*=18)	Normal Range
Oestradiol (pmol/L[1])	46.3 (5.5)†‡	72.2 (4.8)‖	110.7 (4.9)	80-180**
T_3 (nmol/L)	1.5 (0.1)†§	2.1 (0.2)	2.6 (0.2)	1.3-3.2
Osteocalcin (ng/ml)	7.3 (0.2)*‡	9.4 (0.3)‖	12.0 (0.2)	6.7-13.9
BAP (U/l)	11.4 (0.7)*‡	15.3 (0.8)‖	20.4 (0.6)	10.8-30.6
D_{pyr}/Cr (nmol/mmol Cr)	2.8 (0.8)†§	3.9 (0.9)¶	4.3 (0.6)	2.4-5.0

*Amenorrhoeic vs. oligomenorrhoeic, $P < 0.001$.
†Amenorrhoeic vs. oligomenorrhoeic, $P < 0.01$.
‡Amenorrhoeic vs. eumenorrhoeic, $P < 0.001$.
§Amenorrhoeic vs. eumenorrhoeic, $P < 0.01$.
‖Oligomenorrhoeic vs. eumenorrhoeic, $P < 0.001$.
¶Oligomenorrhoeic vs. eumenorrhoeic, $P < 0.05$.
**Follicular phase of menstrual cycle.

(Courtesy of Zanker CL, Swaine UK: Relation between bone turnover, oestradiol, and energy balance in women distance runners. *Br J Sports Med* 32:167-171, 1998.)

tradiol osteocalcin, BAP, and D_{pyr}/Cr levels than did eumenorrheic women (Table 2). T_3 Levels were similar for the oligomenorrheic and eumenorrheic women. Osteocalcin and BAP levels were significantly correlated with BMI and with serum estradiol levels in amenorrheic women only. Serum estradiol levels were significantly correlated with BMI in amenorrheic and oligomenorrheic women but not in eumenorrheic women. No correlation was observed between urine D_{pyr}/Cr and BMI, energy balance, or serum T_3 levels in any group.

Conclusion.—Amenorrheic and oligomenorrheic women had reduced bone turnover and reduced bone formation compared with eumenorrheic women. An association was noted between reduced bone formation and low BMI and low serum estradiol levels in amenorrheic women.

▶ The authors raise an important question for clinicians treating amenorrheic athletes. If bone turnover is already reduced in this population, is hormone replacement therapy (HRT), which is standard therapy for postmenopausal women, appropriate for young amenorrheic women? HRT after all acts by slowing down bone remodelling. If further studies replicate the finding of decreased bone turnover in amenorrheic athletes, the current treatment of choice will have to be reevaluated. As many of us have said all along, the first treatment option should be to convince the athlete that amenorrhea is a serious risk to her future health and that she should adjust her training and nutrition in an effort to resume normal menses. In many cases, this advice is not heeded and other options are necessary. Fortunately, when HRT has been prescribed for young adult women, further bone loss appears to be stopped if not reversed. Clearly we need to know much more about treating these young athletes.

B.L. Drinkwater, Ph.D.

Physical Activity and Osteoporotic Fracture Risk in Older Women
Gregg EW, for the Study of Osteoporotic Fractures Research Group (Univ of Vermont, Burlington; Univ of Pittsburgh, Pa; Univ of California, San Francisco; et al)
Ann Intern Med 129:81-88, 1998   9–13

Objective.—Reducing bone loss with physical activity and improving muscle strength, balance, mobility, and overall physical function may prevent osteoporotic fractures in older women. Baseline levels of physical activity and inactivity were measured in 9,704 nonblack women aged 65 years or more enrolled in the Study of Osteoporotic Fractures to determine the association of types, amounts, and intensity of physical activity with the risk of fracture in older women.

Methods.—Participants reported the frequency and duration of their participation in 33 physical activities during the past year including the number of city blocks or equivalent walked each day for exercise and the number of flights of stairs they climbed. The total physical activity index

TABLE 2.—Relative Risk for Hip Fractures Associated with Physical Activity

Variable	Patients %	Fractures n	Person-Years	Age-Adjusted Relative Risk (95% CI)	Multivariate-Adjusted Relative Risk (95% CI)*
Quintile of total physical activity					
Lowest (<340 kcal/wk)	20	132	13 388	1.00	1.00
Second (341-737 kcal/wk)	20	87	14 549	0.73 (0.55-0.95)	0.77 (0.58-1.02)
Third (738-1289 kcal/wk)	20	82	14 821	0.73 (0.55-0.97)	0.78 (0.59-1.04)
Fourth (1290-2201 kcal/wk)	20	65	14 997	0.60 (0.45-0.81)	0.64 (0.47-0.88)
Highest (>2201 kcal/wk)	20	58	15 100	0.58 (0.42-0.80)	0.64 (0.45-0.89)
P for trend				0.0002	0.003
Sport or recreational activity					
None	20	129	13 733	1.00	1.00
Low intensity	50	217	37 239	0.73 (0.58-0.90)	0.76 (0.61-0.95)
Moderate-to-vigorous intensity	30	80	22 390	0.55 (0.41-0.73)	0.58 (0.43-0.79)
P for trend				0.0001	0.0004
Hours of heavy chores per week					
<5	46	234	33 146	1.00	1.00
5-9	22	87	16 305	0.91 (0.71-1.17)	0.93 (0.72-1.20)
>9	32	103	23 814	0.78 (0.61-0.98)	0.78 (0.62-0.99)
P for trend				0.03	0.14
Hours sitting per day					
<6	33	119	24 464	1.00	1.00
6-8	40	151	29 634	0.99 (0.78-1.26)	0.98 (0.77-1.25)
>8	27	155	19 182	1.43 (1.12-1.82)	1.37 (1.08-1.76)
P for trend				0.003	0.01

*Controlled for age, weight, smoking, estrogen replacement therapy, dietary calcium, falls, alcohol intake, self-rated health, and functional difficulty.

(Courtesy of Gregg EW, for the Study of Osteoporotic Fractures Research Group: Physical activity and osteoporotic fracture risk in older women. *Ann Intern Med* 129:81-88, 1998.)

was calculated and expressed as kilocalories expended per week. Hours spent in heavy household chores and physical inactivity, measured as the number of hours per day the women spent sitting, were recorded. BMD was measured at the distal radius and calcaneus by single photon absorptiometry. Hip adductor strength was measured, and self-rated health, calcium intake, alcohol intake, use of medications including hormone replacement therapy, and medical conditions were recorded. Women were divided into quintiles according to physical activity level, and into 3 categories based on exercise intensity. Excluded from the study were women who reported difficulty walking 2 or 3 blocks, had gait abnormalities, required a walking aid, had fair or poor health or, had a history of diabetes, stroke, falls, or hip fracture, or who died within 3 years after baseline measurement.

Results.—The risk of hip fracture decreased with each increasing physical activity quintile level and with increasing intensity of energy expenditure. Hip fracture risk was lowest in women who engaged in moderate to vigorous activities and in at least 2 hours of sport or recreational activities per week (RR, 0.47) (Table 2). The hip fracture risk increased with the number of hours sitting per day. Although total physical activity was not associated with risk for vertebral fracture, the intensity of physical activity was, reducing the risk by 33% in women who engaged in moderate-to-vigorous exercise compared with sedentary women. Risk of hip fracture was not related to health or functional status, history of falling, or other health behaviors.

Conclusion.—Physical activity prevents hip fractures not only by increasing muscle strength and reducing bone loss but also in other ways that are not completely explained.

▶ This comprehensive study is the latest to demonstrate a positive relationship between physical activity and reduced risk of osteoporotic fractures. Even more compelling is the fact that the analysis controlled for a number of other factors which might have influenced the results such as age, health status, calcium intake, hormone replacement therapy, falls, and calcaneal bone density. The greatest benefit was seen in the reduced number of hip fractures. Physical activity had less effect on vertebral fractures and no effect on wrist fractures. Whether bone density would have played a larger role if it had been possible to measure it at the 3 sites, (hip, spine, and wrist) is uncertain at this time. What the study does very effectively is provide evidence that even low-intensity activities such as walking, gardening, and dancing have a significant effect on risk. For those of us who enjoy more vigorous activities, it's nice to know that the greatest reductions in risk were among women who participated on a regular basis in moderate to vigorous activities.

B.L. Drinkwater, Ph.D.

Physical Activity and Osteoporotic Fracture Among Older Women
Turner LW, Leaver-Dunn D, DiBrezzo R, et al (Univ of Arkansas, Fayetteville; Univ of Alabama, Tuscaloosa)
J Athletic Train 33:207-210, 1998   9–14

Objective.—Although physical activity is known to have a beneficial effect on the prevention of osteoporotic fractures in older women, little information is available on the order of importance of physical activity in relation to other risk factors, and on specific exercise guidelines. The importance of physical activity in the occurrence of osteoporotic fracture and the impact of exercise frequency on osteoporotic fracture among a national sample of women aged 50 years or more was investigated.

Methods.—The study included 2,325 women, mean age, 68.8 years, who participated in the Third National Health and Nutrition Examination Survey, Phase 1. Of the total women, 59% were white, 22% were black, 18% were Hispanic, and 2% were of other ethnicity. Age, race, biologic mother's osteoporotic status, biologic mother's hip fracture status, body mass index (BMI), physical activity, smoking status, alcohol use, and dairy product intake were recorded.

Results.—Race, age, BMI, and inactivity, but not biologic mother's osteoporosis and hip fracture status, were significant predictors of osteoporotic fractures. Activity 2 or more times per week significantly reduced the incidence of hip fracture. Inactive women were 84% more likely to experience a fracture than women who were active 2 or more times per week.

Conclusion.—Physical activity was more important than heredity, smoking status, alcohol use, and dairy product intake in determining risk of fracture. Physical activity 2 or more times a week minimizes fracture risk.

▶ The data from the third National Health and Nutrition Examination Survey (NHANES III) fill in some of the gaps in the previous study by Gregg et al. The participants included Black, Hispanic, and Asian women as well as Caucasian women and women aged 50 years and older. On the other hand, the data lack the depth and precision evident that was possible in a study devoted only to osteoporosis. Nevertheless, inactivity was once again a significant risk factor for fracture. One is left to assume that ethnicity was not a factor in determining the protective effect of activity, although no data examining the interaction of race and activity were presented.

B.L. Drinkwater, Ph.D.

Training in Pregnant Women: Effects on Fetal Development and Birth
Kardel KR, Kase T (Univ of Oslo, Norway; Moss Hosp, Oslo, Norway)
Am J Obstet Gynecol 178:280-286, 1998   9–15

Introduction.—More women are desiring to exercise during pregnancy; however; the course of pregnancy and the health of the fetus appear to depend on a woman's prior physiologic adaptation to exercise and her adaptation to the exercise regimen during pregnancy. There is still no comprehensive understanding of the effects of different intensities of exercise on the fetus and the mother. The intensity of women's activity was studied retrospectively before conception, during pregnancy, and after delivery.

Methods.—There were 42 women who were well-trained athletes who performed intense exercise before conception with a large part of the body's muscle mass involved. During pregnancy and until 6 weeks after delivery, they followed either a high- or medium-intensity exercise program. The effect of the 2 different intensity levels of exercise during pregnancy on the fetus and mother were recorded, as were the onset and length of labor, birth weight, and Apgar score.

Results.—In duration of labor, birth weight, or 1- and 5-minute Apgar scores, there were no differences between the high- and medium-intensity exercise groups. A significantly greater maternal weight gain during pregnancy and a significantly earlier onset of labor correlated with the higher level of exercise for those women who gave birth to girls but not for those women who gave birth to boys. Because higher placental weight was found to be an effect of exercise during pregnancy, one might conclude that exercise has an increased nutritive effect on the fetus.

TABLE 2.—Maternal Complications During Pregnancy and
Use of Anesthesia During Labor

Parameter	MEG ($n = 21$)	HEG ($n = 21$)
Edema (0-3)		
None	17	11
Grade 0.5: Very little	0	1
Grade 1.0: Little (duration)	4 (1-6 wk)	8 (1-7 wk)
Grade 2.0: Moderate	0	1
Proteinuria (0 to 4+)		
None	15	17
Grade 1.0 (trace)	6 (only once)	4 (only once)
Anesthesia		
No anesthesia and no analgesic	2	1
Opiates	14	10
Inhalation anesthesia (nitrous oxide)	6	8
Epidural anesthesia	2	6
Pudendal nerve block	3	6
Paracervical block	0	1
Narcosis	2	0

Note: Values represent the number of cases in each training group that were affected.
Abbreviations: MEG, medium-intensity exercise group; *HEG,* high-intensity exercise group.
(Courtesy of Kardel KR, Kase T: Training in pregnant women: Effect on fetal development and birth.
Am J Obstet Gynecol 178:280-286, 1998.)

Conclusion.—During pregnancy, healthy and well-conditioned women exercised without compromising fetal growth and development, as judged by birth weight, and without complicating the course of pregnancy or labor (Table 2). Future studies should conduct a comparison with a non-exercising group. These findings may also have limited value for the general population.

▶ Recent studies on exercise and fetal health suggest that exercise by physically fit women with uncomplicated pregnancies has no adverse effect on fetal growth. However, the amount and intensity of exercise differs among active pregnant women, and there is little evidence to determine how much exercise might be excessive and possibly harmful to the fetus. The aim of this study was to examine the effect of 2 different intensities of exercise during pregnancy on the mother and the fetus and the effect of the exercise on the onset and length of labor, birth weight, and Apgar score. The research subjects were highly active women who continued to exercise throughout pregnancy. In comparing the high-intensity and medium-intensity exercise groups with other populations, the authors found that placental weights and birth weights were higher in this group and that there were no complications related to the exercise regimen. The study is limited in the following ways: there is no comparison with a nonexercising group and this was an exceptionally healthy group who had exercised heavily before becoming pregnant.

M.J.L. Alexander, Ph.D.

Customary Physical Activity and Physical Health Outcomes in Later Life
Bath PA, Morgan K (Univ of Sheffield, England)
Age Ageing 27-S3:29-34, 1998   9–16

Purpose.—Previous studies of physical activity patterns in older adults have suggested that the elderly are selectively active or inactive in certain task-specific domains. Broad-based customary physical activity (CPA) scores have proven to have clear cross-sectional utility and longitudinal validity, but their performance has not been compared with traditional, single activity–based indices of habitual activity. The relationship between CPA and subsequent mortality and health care utilization outcomes was assessed in older adults.

Methods.—The longitudinal study included a random sample of 1,042 general practice patients aged 65 years or older. CPA levels were determined by questionnaire. The effects of physical activity on 12-year all-cause and disease-specific mortality were analyzed. Eight-year change in utilization of general practitioners and social services was also related to CPA. The analysis was adjusted for baseline age, health and smoking status, and weight.

Findings.—The patients were divided into high, intermediate, and low physical activity levels. Among men, 12-year mortality was significantly increased in the intermediate and low physical activity groups, with adjusted hazard ratios of 1.53 (95% confidence interval [CI], 1.10 to 2.14) and 1.75 (95% CI, 1.24 to 2.48), respectively. For women, being in the

TABLE 3.—Physical Activity in 1985 and Service Use Month Prior to 1993 Interview Among Survivors

Service Used	Sex	n	Risk Factor	Adjusted OR*	97% CI	P
General practitioner	Male	121	'Intermediate-activity' group†	1.61	0.66-3.95	0.30
			'Low-activity' group†	0.80	0.27-2.39	0.69
	Female	219	'Intermediate-activity' group†	1.18	0.62-2.25	0.43
			'Low-activity' group†	1.38	0.63-3.03	0.43
	All	342	< 10 min total walking per day‡	0.82	0.51-1.33	0.42
District nurse	Male	121	'Intermediate-activity' group†	0.91	0.30-2.80	0.88
			'Low-activity' group†	1.47	0.44-4.93	0.53
	Female	219	'Intermediate-activity' group†	1.64	0.72-3.73	0.24
			'Low-activity' group†	3.43	1.38-8.52	<0.01
	All	342	<10 min total walking per day‡	1.21	0.69-2.12	0.51
Home help	Male	121	'Intermediate-activity' group†	3.08	0.64-14.90	0.16
			'Low-activity' group†	6.10	1.06-34.99	<0.05
	Female	219	'Intermediate-activity' group†	2.75	1.27-5.96	<0.05
			'Low-activity' group†	1.70	0.63-4.61	0.30
	All	342	<10 min total walking per day‡	0.79	0.42-1.49	0.47

*Adjusted for age group, sex, health status, smoking status, and weight category and service use as measured at baseline.
†Relative to "high-activity" group.
‡Relative to ≥ 10 minutes total walking per typical day.
Abbreviations: CI, confidence interval; OR, odds ratio.
(Courtesy of Bath PA, Morgan K: Customary physical activity and physical health outcomes in later life. *Age Aging* 27-S3:29-34, 1998, by permission of Oxford University Press.)

low activity group carried a mortality hazard ratio of 1.73 (95% CI, 1.28 to 2.33). For both sexes, a low level of physical activity was significantly related to higher utilization of health and social services at 8 years' follow-up (Table 3). Men in the low physical activity group were more likely to die of respiratory diseases.

Conclusion.—Physical activity by older adults has a significant effect on subsequent all-cause and disease-specific mortality, and utilization of health and social services. These associations hold even after adjustment for baseline health and smoking. Although total duration of walking is still a useful index of health in later life, more broadly based measures of CPA are more sensitive predictors of health outcomes.

▶ A few years ago, we demonstrated by retrospective questioning[1] that physical activity at the age of 50 years had a substantial effect in protecting seniors against institutionalization, and (by inference) associated health care costs. The study of Bath and Morgan makes a similar point, showing by means of a 12-year longitudinal study that even after adjusting for 3 very important variables (age, initial health, and smoking habits), physical activity in a large sample of adults who initially were aged 65 years or more was associated with a substantially reduced mortality rate and a reduced demand for health and personal care.

R.J. Shephard, M.D., Ph.D., D.P.E.

Reference

1. Shephard RJ, Montelpare W: Geriatric benefits of exercise as an adult. *J Gerontol* 1988; 43:M86-M90, 1988.

Body Fat and Skeletal Muscle Mass in Relation to Physical Disability in Very Old Men and Women of the Framingham Heart Study
Visser M, Harris TB, Langlois J, et al (Natl Inst on Aging, Bethesda, Md; Harvard Med School, Boston; Tufts Univ, Boston; et al)
J Gerontol 53A:M214-M221, 1998   9–17

Introduction.—Cross-sectional investigations have revealed that persons with heavier body weight and higher body mass index are more disabled than persons of medium body weight and body mass index. No trials have specifically evaluated the relation between muscle mass and disability or the association between body mass and disability. A cross-sectional investigation of the Framingham Heart Study was performed to determine for the first time the relationship of total and regional body composition to self-reported physical disability status.

Methods.—The association between skeletal muscle and percent body fat and self-reported physical disability was evaluated in 753 men and women aged 72 to 95. Participants underwent measurements of whole body dual x-ray absorptiometry radiograph scan, dual-energy absorpti-

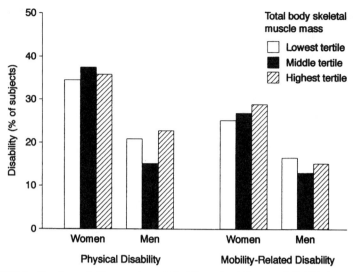

FIGURE 1.—Prevalence of self-reported overall disability and mobility-related disability in women and men, aged 72 to 95, by level of total body skeletal muscle mass. (Courtesy of Visser M, Harris TB, Langlois J, et al: Body fat and skeletal muscle mass in relation to physical disability in very old men and women of the Framingham Heart Study. *J Gerontol* 53A:M214-M221, 1998. Republished with permission of the Gerontological Society of America, 1030 15th Street, NW, Suite 250, Washington, DC. Reproduced by permission of the publisher via Copyright Clearance Center, Inc.)

ometry (to determine body composition), grip strength, fat distribution, and self-reported physical disability status and self-rated health. Potential confounders were also assessed.

Results.—There was no significant correlation between total body and lower extremity muscle mass and disability in men or women (Fig 1). However, there was a strong positive association between percent body fat and disability. This increase in risk could not be explained by age, education, physical activity, smoking, alcohol use, estrogen use in women, muscle mass, or health status.

Conclusion.—Low skeletal mass was not correlated with self-reported physical disability. Older adults with a high percent body fat had significantly higher levels of disability. This information could be useful in planning intervention programs focused on reducing the risk for disability.

▶ In older adults, low skeletal muscle mass and high body fat are often associated with physical disability. Over 700 men and women had their body composition assessed by dual energy x-ray absorptiometry and their disability scored by a questionnaire. The authors report a higher disability risk for subjects with a high body mass index and high body weight. The disability could be due to inactivity caused by overweight, or due to chronic disease associated with high body weight. No association was observed between skeletal muscle mass and disability, but low weight and low muscle mass subjects were underrepresented in the study. Some inaccuracy in dual energy x-ray absorptiometry measurements in obese subjects may have affected the results. This study is 1 of the first to show that body composition is strongly associated with physical disability in very old age, and to suggest that exercise intervention programs may reduce the risk for disability.

M.J.L. Alexander, Ph.D.

Techniques to Evaluate Elderly Human Muscle Function: A Physiological Basis
Hunter S, White M, Thompson M (Univ of Sydney, New South Wales, Australia; Univ of Birmingham, England)
J Gerontol 53A:B204-B216, 1998   9–18

Introduction.—Elderly people often exhibit muscle weakness and a slowing in muscle velocity. The rate of variation in this strength decrement can vary greatly among individuals (Fig 1). The objective quantification of these properties requires reliable and practical tests to evaluate muscle contractile characteristics. A review was conducted to explain suitable voluntary and involuntary tests and measurements used to assess elderly muscle function. The value, limitations, and physiological background of such measurements were assessed to aid in the choice of appropriate methods for the evaluation of elderly muscle function.

Methods.—The weaker and slower contractile properties of elderly muscles can be analyzed by a variety of voluntary and electrically evoked techniques. Reliable tests using voluntary contractions can be used to evaluate the integrity of the central and peripheral neuromuscular system

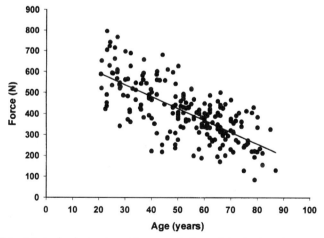

FIGURE 1.—Maximal voluntary isometric contractile force of the dominant knee extensor in 220 healthy community-dwelling Australian women aged 20 to 87. A linear trend accounts for 96% of the systematic variation with age. (Courtesy of Hunter S, White M, Thompson M: Techniques to evaluate elderly human muscle function: A physiological basis. *J Gerontol* 53A:B204-B216, 1998. Republished with permission of the Gerontological Society of America, 1030 15th Street, NW, Suite 250, Washington, DC 20005. Reproduced by permission of the publisher via Copyright Clearance Center, Inc.)

in young and elderly persons. Techniques that use electrically evoked contractions make it possible for the muscles in elderly persons to be evaluated independently of volitional effort and central inhibition. A comparison of test performances using a voluntary vs. electrically evoked test can ascertain whether the site of failure or weakness is proximal to the neuromuscular junction or is within the muscle itself. Motor nerve stimulation may be useful in evoking involuntary contractions, but percutaneous stimulation may be more practical with large muscle groups when the physician is analyzing isometric contractile behavior.

Conclusion.—These voluntary and involuntary tests and measures contribute to a body of knowledge about the characteristics and limitations of elderly muscle function. Reliable and reproducible muscle properties can be measured in elderly persons when time is taken to familiarize the patients with the techniques and protocols.

▶ This comprehensive review describes some of the most reliable and practical tests to measure muscle contraction in older adults. Some of the common techniques described to measure maximum voluntary strength include the hand-grip dynamometer and the force transducer. The results from these techniques may be inaccurate because of the subjects' inability due to poor neural function to produce a maximum force contraction. Electrical muscle stimulation can be used to evoke a supramaximal twitch and rates of contraction and relaxation time. Maximal voluntary dynamic strength can be measured by having the patient lift a maximal weight or by observing maximal torque on an isokinetic dynamometer. This excellent review describes the problems and limitations associated with evaluating muscle function in older adults, and cautions practitioners to ensure that tests of muscle function are valid.

M.J.L. Alexander, Ph.D.

Grip Strength Changes Over 27 Yr in Japanese-American Men
Rantanen T, Masaki K, Foley D, et al (NIH, Bethesda, Md; Kuakini Med Ctr, Honolulu, Hawaii)
J Appl Physiol 85:2047-2053, 1998   9–19

Objective.—Grip strength is a reproducible, accurate, and inexpensive way to measure the change in muscle strength with age. The extent of change in grip strength in Japanese-American men, aged 45 to 68 years at baseline, over a follow-up period of 27 years, and the age, body weight changes, and morbidity as predictors of grip-strength change were studied.

Methods.—Hand-grip strength, body weight, height, upper arm circumference, triceps skinfold, and health history were obtained in 8,006 Japanese-American men living in Hawaii who responded to a questionnaire and agreed to participate in the study at baseline. Upper arm lean area (A_l) was estimated. At final follow-up, tests were repeated in 3,741 participants.

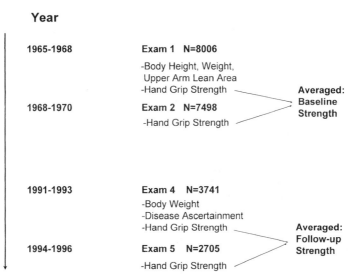

FIGURE 1.—Design of study; *n*, no. of study participants in each exam period. (Courtesy of Rantanen T, Masaki K, Foley D, et al: *J Appl Physiol* 85:2047-2053, 1998.)

Results.—At the baseline examination, older men had significantly lower grip strength, body weight, height, and BMI and smaller A_l than younger men. Age-adjusted height, body weight, body mass index, and A_l were significantly correlated with grip strength. Men who died before follow-up had a lower grip strength and body weight than survivors. Men with greater grip strength at baseline also had greater grip strength at follow-up (Fig 1). Grip strength decreased at an average annual rate of 1%. Among men with chronic diseases, average annual grip strength declined by 1.5%. The risk of grip-strength disability was 8 times higher for men in the lowest grip-strength tertile at baseline and 2 times higher for men in the middle tertile compared with those in the highest tertile. After adjusting for age, height, and baseline grip strength, men who lost 5 kg or less were 5 or 6 times more likely to have grip-strength disability at follow-up.

Conclusion.—Maintaining body weight and health are important to maintaining grip strength in men as they age.

▶ Muscle strength decreases with increasing age, and hand-grip strength has often been used as an indicator of overall muscle strength. Previous studies have reported that hand-grip strength increases up to the 30s, then starts to decrease with accelerated speed after the 40s. This large study of more than 3,000 men of Japanese ancestry aged 71 to 96 years reported a consistent decrease in grip strength of 1% per year, with greater losses in older age groups. Weight loss and illnesses such as stroke, diabetes, heart disease, and arthritis were associated with steeper strength decreases. Maintenance of body weight and a healthy lifestyle to prevent diseases of old age will assist in maintenance of strength to perform activities of daily living.

M.J.L. Alexander, Ph.D.

Longitudinal Changes in Selected Physical Capabilities: Muscle Strength, Flexibility and Body Size
Bassey EJ (Univ of Nottingham, England)
Age Ageing 27-S3:12-16, 1998   9–20

Objective.—Loss of physical capabilities with aging is possibly related to decreasing levels of physical activity. Longitudinal changes in maximal voluntary strength of the handgrip muscles, maximal range of movement in the shoulder joint, body weight, and skeletal size were measured, and the associations between the changes in muscle strength and both customary physical activity and health outcomes were investigated.

Methods.—Handgrip strength, shoulder joint movement, and body weight were measured in 347 individuals at baseline and at 4 and 8 years. Health outcomes were assessed from the Nottingham Longitudinal Study (NLSAA) health index score, the Life Satisfaction Index (LSI), the Brief Assessment of Social Engagement (BASE), the Symptoms of Anxiety and Depression (SAD) scale, and on a 5-point self-assessment scale.

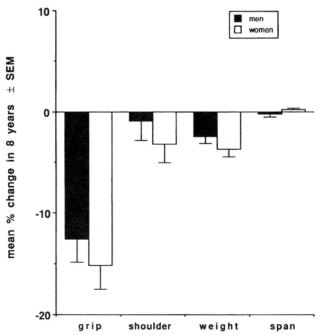

FIGURE 1.—Percentage changes in objective measurements over 8 years in men and women. (Courtesy of Bassey EJ: *Age Ageing* 27-S3:12-16, 1998. By permission of Oxford University Press.)

Results.—The average ages of men and women at final assessment were 79.9 and 81.2 years, respectively. Handgrip strength declined significantly in both men and women by 8 and 37 N, respectively, but the loss was greater in women older than 75 compared with women younger than 75 (22% vs 10%, respectively) (Fig 1). Weight declined significantly in both men and women by 1.7 and 2.5 kg, respectively. The number of health problems increased from 3 to 5 in men and from 5 to 7 in women. LSI and BASE scores declined significantly (20%) in both sexes. Physical activity scores declined from 960 to 355 minutes per day for men and from 840 to 415 minutes per day for women. Changes in physical activity and effort scores were significantly correlated with each other but not with health or psychological indices except for effort scores and BASE in men. Changes in health, age, and weight in men were correlated with 8-year changes in grip strength. Changes in the SAD, age, and effort scores in women were correlated with 8-year changes in grip strength.

Conclusion.—Loss of grip strength with age was significantly related to decline in physical activity and an increase in SAD. These findings reinforce the need for encouraging physical activity and treating depression in the elderly.

▶ Consistent losses in physical capabilities occur with aging; such losses are often associated with deterioration in physical and mental health. A group of 350 older subjects older than age 73 (mean age 80 years) from a previous longitudinal study on aging were tested for functional losses 8 years later. The 4 measurements recorded in this study included grip strength, shoulder range of motion, body weight, and demispan (distance between fingertips and sternal notch). The results showed that there was little or no loss of body weight or shoulder range of motion and a modest loss of muscle strength of less than 2%. The rate of loss of muscle strength was twice as fast in the older women; however, some individuals in the younger half of the age distribution improved in strength. Loss of body mass in men was associated with strength losses. This study provides primarily descriptive data of 4 easily measured physical variables that were maintained fairly well over time. Possibly use of more sophisticated testing protocols would provide more useful information describing changes in physical capabilities in older subjects.

M.J.L. Alexander, Ph.D.

Adverse Changes in Fibre Type Composition of the Human Masseter Versus Biceps Brachii Muscle During Aging
Monemi M, Eriksson P-O, Eriksson A, et al (Umeå Univ, Sweden)
J Neurol Sci 154:35-48, 1998   9–21

Objective.—Muscle fiber composition varies with the type of muscle. With aging, changes in muscle fibers lead to functional impairment. The age-related changes in muscle fiber types and fiber diameter were investi-

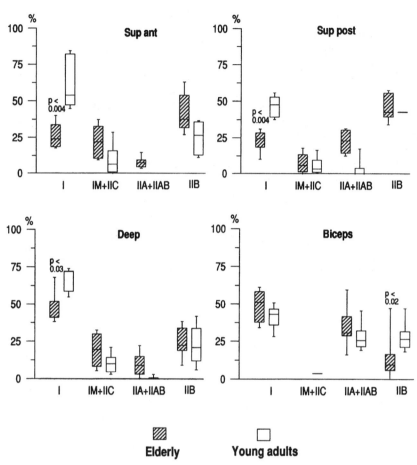

FIGURE 4.—Fiber type proportion (%) in the anterior (*Sup ant*) and posterior (*Sup post*) regions of the superficial portion and the deep (*Deep*) portion of the human masseter, and the biceps brachii (*Biceps*) muscles from elderly and young adult (Eriksson, 1982; Eriksson and Thornell, 1983) individuals. Data for young adult biceps was reevaluated for the proportion of type IIAB fibers. Note significantly lower proportion of type I fibers in all masseter regions in the elderly. Note also significantly lower proportion of type IIB fibers in the old biceps. *Box-and-whisker plots*, showing median, quartiles, and minimum and maximum values. (Courtesy of Monemi M, Eriksson P-O, Eriksson A, et al: Adverse changes in fiber type composition of the human masseter versus biceps brachii muscle during aging. *J Neurol Sci* 154:35-48, 1998. Reprinted by permission of the publisher, copyright by Elsevier Science Inc.)

gated in masseter muscle of elderly human individuals by using morphologic and enzyme-histologic methods.

Methods.—Muscle fibers from specimens from the anterior (sup ant) and posterior (sup post) area of the superficial portion and the deep portion of the human masseter muscle and the biceps muscle of elderly persons and young adults were classified on the basis of staining pattern for myofibrillar ATPase, as type I, type IM, type IIC, type IIA, type IIAB, or type IIB. Muscle fiber diameter and cross-sectional area were determined by means of morphometric analysis.

Results.—There was no correlation between fiber composition of masseter muscle and age or dental health. Whereas all muscle fiber types were detected in all specimens, elderly persons had significantly more type IM and II fiber types and significantly less type I fibers in all areas. Type IIA and IIAB fibers, found in virtually all regions of elderly masseter muscle, were typically absent or rare in young adult masseter muscle. Fiber diameters in the sup ant and sup post of elderly masseter muscle were significantly smaller than the corresponding muscle fiber diameters in young adults (Fig 4). Coefficients of variation of fiber diameters in elderly masseter muscle were larger than for masseter muscle in young adults. The only significant difference in elderly muscle fiber types for biceps muscle was that the proportion of type IIB fibers was smaller than for young adult biceps.

Conclusion.—The difference between age-related changes in masseter and biceps muscles indicates that aging affects different muscles in different ways, which are probably related to differences in genetic control, functional performance, and nerve and hormonal influences.

▶ The masseter muscle of young adult subjects had a predominance (63%) of Type I (slow-twitch) fibers; while older subjects had a predominance (67%) of Type II (fast-twitch) and Type IM (slow glycolytic) fibers. This finding suggested that there is a shift during aging from slow to fast motor units in the masseter muscle. This may be due to a selective loss of the slow twitch motoneurons innervating Type I fibers, followed by a reinnervation of these fibers from nearby fast-twitch motoneurons. The biceps brachii muscles showed either an unchanged fiber–type composition or an age-related decrease of the Type II fiber population. This difference between aging of the masseter and biceps muscles suggests that muscular alterations during aging are specific to individual muscles. Is this difference apparent in healthy, fit, older adults as well as in normal subjects?

M.J.L. Alexander, M.D.

Age-related Alterations in Muscular Endurance
Bemben MG (Univ of Oklahoma, Norman)
Sports Med 25:259-269, 1998   9–22

Objective.—The age-related decline in muscular strength is well demonstrated, but few studies have focused on the effects of aging on muscular endurance. Animal and human studies of this issue have given conflicting results, resulting from differences in study design, statistics, and control of such variables as physical activity and diet. Current knowledge regarding age-related changes in muscular endurance were reviewed.

Morphologic Changes.—Some past studies have suggested that muscular endurance is maintained or even improved with increased age. This finding has been related to a decreasing proportion of type II muscle fibers with age. However, recent studies using whole-muscle cross-sections, as opposed to muscle biopsies, have questioned this selective loss of type II muscle fibers. Despite this controversy, a shift to predominantly type I (slow-twitch) muscle fibers remains the most likely explanation for maintenance of muscular endurance with aging. Muscle atrophy is a well-documented effect of aging, although it is unclear whether this effect is inevitable or the result of decreased physical activity. Several lines of evidence support the hypothesis that reduced muscle fiber numbers is an inevitable part of aging. However, the effects of aging on muscle fiber size remain unclear. Few studies have examined the effects of aging on muscle blood flow and capillarity, and the resultant effects on endurance.

Metabolic Changes.—Past studies have suggested that the oxidative capacity of aged skeletal muscle is similar to that of young muscle, with maintenance of enzymes involved in the Krebs cycle and β-oxidation. However, recent investigators have found a significant age-related reduction in oxidative capacity, which might impact muscular endurance. The previous studies may have failed to account for the effects of physical activity level.

Training Effects.—Provided with an adequate intensity and duration of endurance training, aged muscle appears to adapt in a way similar to young muscle. Training can improve oxidative capacity and muscle capillarity as well. Endurance training for the elderly appears to produce hypertrophy of type I and type IIa muscle fibers but no change in the overall percentages of these fiber types. Endurance and strength training appear to have differing effects in aged muscle.

Discussion.—Despite the shortcomings of the research, considerable knowledge has been gained into the effects of aging on skeletal muscle endurance. The positive effects of training on muscular endurance in the elderly has important health implications, including bone health and risk of falls. Research is needed to establish the most effective type of training for older adults. Such a program must balance the risks of inactivity against those of exercise while addressing social needs and the need to modify training intensity, duration, and frequency.

▶ It is generally agreed that aging produces declines in muscular strength and endurance. It was determined that the muscles of the lower extremity (dorsiflexors and plantarflexors) were better able to maintain muscle endurance than the muscles of the upper extremity. It has been suggested that there is selective loss of type II fibers during aging, but this issue of selective loss of fiber type is controversial. This loss would produce improvement or maintenance of endurance because of increases of type I fibers, but fiber atrophy occurs with aging so this would also alter endurance.

Recent studies have also reported a significant decline in the oxidative capacity of skeletal muscle, although this change can be reversed with endurance training. The author concluded with the need for development of the most effective type of training for the elderly that carefully balances the risk for inactivity with the risk of exercise.

M.J.L. Alexander, Ph.D.

Spatial-Temporal Analysis of Mobility Over the Adult Age Range Using the Postural-Locomotor-Manual Test

Samson MM, Crowe A, Duursma SA, et al (Utrecht Univ, The Netherlands)
J Gerontol 53A:M242-M247, 1998   9–23

Purpose.—In older adults, reduced performance in motor tasks can be related to aging and to pathologic conditions, and it is important to differentiate between these 2 factors. The recently developed Postural-Locomotor-Manual Test (PLM-test) provides a useful measure of certain aspects of motor performance (Fig 1). However, questions still remain about the use of this test, including the relationship between age and test performance and speed at which the test should be performed. These issues were addressed in a study of PLM-test performance by subjects, aged from young adulthood to elderly.

Methods.—The research subjects were 95 men and 122 women, aged 19 to 90 years. All subjects were healthy, had no evidence of cognitive disorders, and were able to walk unassisted. The test was performed using an optoelectronic technique with computerized analysis. Each subject performed the PLM maneuver at their "preferred" speed and at a "fast" speed. In addition to test-retest coefficient of variability, the effects of age and sex on test performance were analyzed.

Results.—Analysis of test-retest coefficient of stability showed between-measurement correlations of 0.90 for the fast-speed condition and 0.70 for the preferred-speed condition. All phases of the procedure, and the total movement time, were slower in older subjects than in younger subjects.

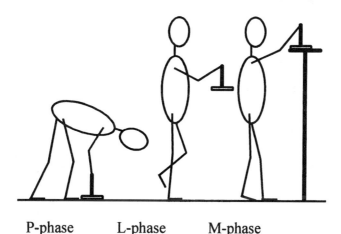

P-phase   L-phase   M-phase

FIGURE 1.—In the Postural-Locomotor-Manual Test, subject picks up object from the floor, walks forward at "preferred" or "fast" speed without pausing, and places object on a chin-high shelf. *Abbreviations*: *P-phase*, postural phase; *L-phase*, locomotor phase; *M-phase*, manual phase. (Courtesy of Samson MM, Crowe A, Duursma SA, et al: Spatial-temporal analysis of mobility over the adult range using the Postural-Locomotor-Manual Test. *J Gerontol* 53A:M242-M247, 1998. Republished with permission of The Gerontological Society of America, 1030 15th Street, NW, Suite 250, Washington, DC 20005. Reproduced by permission of the publisher via Copyright Clearance Center, Inc.)

Women showed a more rapid slowing, starting at about age 50 years, whereas men showed a more gradual decline.

Conclusions.—The findings support the use of the PLM-test as a noninvasive and relatively simple evaluation of motor performance. Test performance differs significantly between older and younger adults. Separate reference values should be used for men and women. This and previous studies suggest that subjects should be instructed to perform the test maneuver as fast as possible.

▶ Performance testing of mobility of older adults is an important aspect of evaluating functional performance. There have been a number of simple tests of mobility and performance developed over the past few years, with varying degrees of difficulty for the subjects performing them. The Postural-Locomotor-Manual Test (PLM-test) consists of 3 phases: (1) subject picks up an object from the floor, (2) subject walks forward a couple of paces, and (3) subject places the object on a shelf at chin height. The test can either be performed at a freely chosen speed or as fast as possible. Results of this study suggested that older subjects were slower than younger subjects, and there is a wide range of values for subjects of similar age. Females were found to have a change in slope of the regression line after the age of 50 years, indicating that test time increases dramatically after that age. Males have a more gradual increase in test times over the adult age range. The test is sold as a commercial package with markers that are attached to the subjects and are tracked by an optical tracking device. The test may have some value because of the norms available that allow comparisons of pathologic populations with normal subjects, but the cost of the testing equipment is not known.

M.J.L. Alexander, Ph.D.

Age-related Changes in the Ability to Side-Step During Gait
Gilchrist LA (Univ of North Carolina, Greensboro)
Clin Biomech 13:91-97, 1998   9–24

Background.—Previous studies suggest that older adults have a decreased ability to avoid obstacles at short notice during gait. In this respect, ability to sidestep is particularly important. The ability of younger women to side-step in response to a visual cue was compared with that of older women.

Methods.—The study included 17 young women (mean age, 27 years) and 16 older women (mean age, 70 years), who performed a 5-m walking test, along a path divided into 3 parallel lanes. On the third step, the subjects received a visual cue on a computer monitor, which prompted them to stay in the center lane or move to the right or left lanes as quickly as possible. Foot-switches attached to the shoes, infrared beams, and videotaping were used to gather data on the accuracy and speed of the side-step (Fig 1).

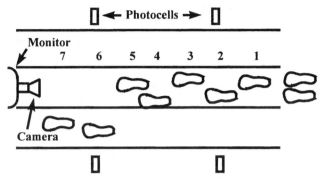

FIGURE 1.—A schematic of a response for a contralateral shift. Step numbers are shown; a "step" began with the heel contact of one foot and ended with the heel contact of the other foot. The visual cue appeared during step 3. Steps 4 and 5 would be considered "extra" steps. One error would be noted (step 4). (Courtesy of Gilchrist LA: Age-related changes in the ability to side-step during gait. *Clin Biomech* 13:91-97, 1998. Reprinted from *Clinical Biomechanics*, vol no. 13, pp 91-97, copyright 1998, with kind permission from Elsevier Science Ltd, The Boulevard, Langford Land, Kidlington 0X5 1GB UK.)

Results.—The sideways shift was achieved in just 1 extra step in only 26% of trials for older women versus 58% of trials for younger women. The 2 groups were similar in speed and foot placement accuracy for 1 of the 2 shift directions. However, older women reduced speed by approximately 3% when shifting in the other direction, whereas younger women made the shift with no significant reduction in speed. In the steps after the sidestep, older women made errors in foot placement in 22% of trials, compared with 3% for younger women.

Conclusions.—Older women appear less able to perform a simple side-step maneuver in response to a visual cue than younger women. Older women also have more difficulty in making subsequent steps, after the sidestep. Reduced ability to sidestep is an age-related reduction in balance and agility; its amenability to correction remains to be determined.

▶ This study examined the ability to alter the intended direction of travel at relatively short notice, which is essential for full mobility. When an obstacle suddenly appears, last-minute adjustments have to be made in the gait pattern. Older adults have less strength, less control over postural muscle activity, and less control over upper-limb motions which may affect movements of the lower limb. Young and older women were tested while travelling down a walkway and were asked to sidestep upon presentation of a visual cue. The older women were less able to adjust to the sidestep motion, and tended to take an extra step or to make more errors in foot placement following the sidestep. Further investigation will determine whether an intervention strategy will slow this decline in performance in older subjects.

M.J.L. Alexander, Ph.D.

Treadmill Exercise Testing in an Epidemiologic Study of Elderly Subjects

Hollenberg M, Ngo LH, Turner D, et al (Univ of California, San Francisco; Veterans Affairs Med Ctr, San Francisco)
J Gerontol 53A:B259-B267, 1998   9–25

Background.—Few data exist regarding the level of physical fitness and exercise capacity in older people, particularly those more than 70 years old. The oxygen consumption of a large group of older subjects, some who were healthy and some who had chronic diseases associated with aging, was examined.

Methods.—A community-based, longitudinal, epidemiologic study of physical fitness in elderly people identified 3,057 people greater than or equal to 55 years old living in Sonoma, Calif. Of these, 2,092 (68.4%) agreed to participate in the study, and of these volunteers, 1,101 were free of known heart disease and could perform stress treadmill testing. These 1,101 people (438 men and 663 women, aged 55 to 94 years, (mean age, 67 years) also had no cerebrovascular disease or musculoskeletal impairment. About a quarter of them did have disease conditions, including diabetes mellitus, renal or liver disease, asthma, bronchitis, emphysema, and malignancy. Treadmill exercise testing was performed according to the Cornell protocol to determine cardiorespiratory parameters, including oxygen consumption ($\dot{V}O_2$), respiratory gas exchange ratio (RER; oxygen consumption divided by carbon dioxide production), oxygen consumption at peak exercise (peak $\dot{V}O_2$), and heart rate. The minimum threshold workrate was set at greater than or equal to 2 minutes of exercise at an RER greater than or equal to 1.0. Maximal exercise was determined as an RER greater than or equal to 1.1.

Findings.—Of the 1,101 people, 174 of 663 women (26.2%) and 46 of 438 men (10.5%) failed to meet the minimum threshold workrate. Factors significantly associated with the failure to meet the minimum threshold workrate included a history of shortness of breath with walking, current smoking (for men), a peak expiratory flow rate less than 5 L/sec), and a history of cancer (for men). The minimum threshold workrate was met by 489 women (73.8%) and 392 men (89.5%). Furthermore, 218 of these 489 women (32.9%) and 231 of these 392 men (52.7%) were able to achieve the maximal threshold workrate. For those who achieved at least the minimum threshold workrate, women averaged 10.0 ± 4.0 minutes of exercise and men averaged 13.2 ± 4.6 minutes. The duration of exercise, peak $\dot{V}O_2$, and heart rate decreased linearly with age for men and women (when adjusted for lean body mass), and for the healthy and those with a disease condition. At all ages, peak $\dot{V}O_2$ was better in the healthy than in those with a disease condition (Fig 2).

Conclusions.—Most of these elderly people (74% of women and 90% of men) could meet the minimum threshold workrate of greater than or equal to 2 minutes of exercise at an RER greater than or equal to 1. Moreover, a third of the women and half the men could meet or surpass

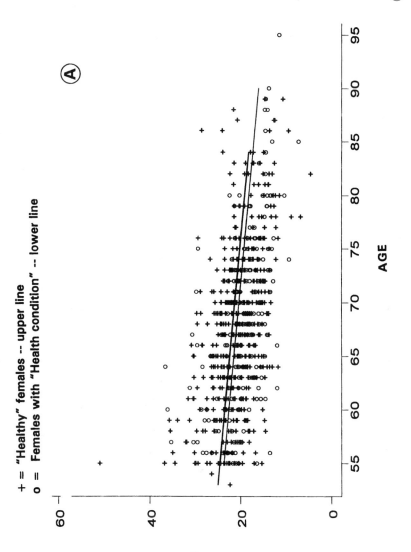

(Continued)

FIGURE 2 (cont.)

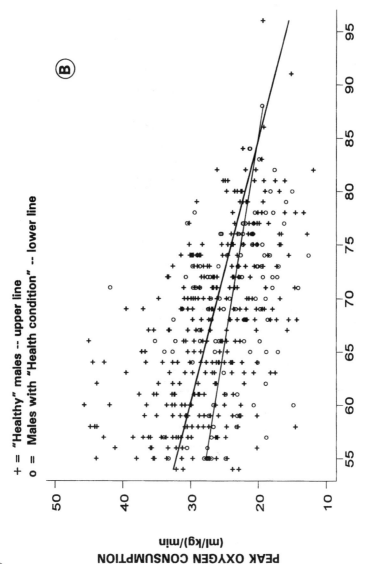

FIGURE 2.—Peak oxygen consumption. Effect of age on peak oxygen consumption adjusted for total body mass ($\dot{V}O_2$/kg/min) in women (A) and men (B) who are healthy (+) or who have a disease condition (o). The *dark, upper line* represents those who are healthy without any disease condition; the *light, lower line* represents those with a disease condition. (Courtesy of Hollenberg M, Ngo LH, Turner D, et al. Treadmill exercise testing in an epidemiologic study of elderly subjects. *J Gerontol* 53A: B259-B267, 1998. Republished with permission of the Gerontological Society of America, 1030 15th Street, NW, Suite 250, Washington, DC 20005. Reproduced by permission of the publisher via Copyright Clearance Center, Inc.)

the maximum threshold workrate (RER greater than or equal to 1.1). These cross-sectional data establish age-adjusted standards for oxygen consumption in healthy elderly men and women, as well as in those with a disease condition other than cerebrovascular or cardiac disease.

▶ Hard data on the physical condition of the very old is quite limited, so this article by Hollenberg and associates is welcome. The presented graphs might suggest a slower deterioration of aerobic function than previously assumed;[1] indeed, the loss of peak aerobic power between 65 and 85 years of age seems to proceed more slowly than in younger adults. Although the authors claim their data are representative, the figures are for a volunteer sample living on the West coast of the United States, where fitness levels are generally somewhat higher than in areas with a more continental climate. Moreover, there is probably a substantial survivor effect, since the proportion of the very old who were well enough to participate in treadmill testing was much smaller than in the young old. Nevertheless, it is encouraging that even at 85 years, a substantial fraction of the North American population can retain more than the minimum of aerobic power (probably around 12 to 14 mL.kg/1minute-=1) needed for independent living.

R.J. Shephard, M.D., Ph.D., D.P.E.

Reference

1. Shephard RJ: Aging, Physical Activity and Health. Champaign, Ill: Human Kinetics Publishers, 1997.

Expanded Blood Volumes Contribute to the Increased Cardiovascular Performance of Endurance-trained Older Men

Hagberg JM, Goldberg AP, Lakatta L, et al (Univ of Maryland, Baltimore; Natl Inst on Aging, Baltimore, Md; Johns Hopkins Med Institutions, Baltimore, Md)
J Appl Physiol 85:484-489, 1998   9–26

Background.—As one ages, maximal oxygen intake ($\dot{V}O_{2max}$) declines, but endurance training can improve it. Studies suggest that these benefits are caused by an increase in left ventricular end-diastolic volume (LVEDV) and, thus, preload. Left ventricular filling can be improved by expanding plasma volume, and young endurance-trained athletes have higher plasma volumes than their sedentary peers. Older endurance-trained athletes were compared with their sedentary peers to determine any differences in intravascular volumes between the groups.

Methods.—The subjects were 7 endurance-trained men (mean age, 56.0 years) and 12 age-matched lean, sedentary men. The $\dot{V}O_{2max}$ was measured by progressive treadmill exercise, and all subjects underwent blood volume determinations before an exercise protocol. The exercise protocol consisted of an upright cycle ergometer test that began at a work rate of 25 W

TABLE 4.—Hemodynamic Variables at Rest and During Peak Cycle Ergometer Exercise In the Master Athletes and the Lean Sedentary Men

Variable	Master Athletes ($n = 7$)	Lean Sedentary Men ($n = 12$)
Rest		
Heart rate, beats/min	51 ± 10*	62 ± 10
Systolic BP, mmHg	126 ± 11	135 ± 16
Diastolic BP, mmHg	76 ± 6	82 ± 12
LV end-diastolic volume index, mL/m²	85.4 ± 12.3†	73.8 ± 12.9
LV end-systolic volume index, mL/m²	29.5 ± 9.1	26.9 ± 9.1
Stroke volume index, mL/m²	56.1 ± 6.4*	47.0 ± 8.1
Cardiac index, l·min⁻¹·m²	2.9 ± 0.6	2.9 ± 0.3
Peak exercise		
Work rate, W	200 ± 20*	156 ± 22
Heart rate, beats/min	145 ± 10	153 ± 17
Systolic BP, mmHg	210 ± 29	206 ± 20
Diastolic BP, mmHg	88 ± 9	101 ± 19
LV end-diastolic volume index, mL/m²	90.6 ± 10.6†	77.1 ± 17.4
LV end-systolic volume index, mL/m²	154. ± 6.6	20.0 ± 11.3
Stroke volume index, mL/m²	75.2 ± 8.4*	57.3 ± 13.1
Cardiac index, 1·min⁻¹·m²	10.9 ± 1.4*	8.7 ± 1.6
Change from rest to peak exercise		
LV end-diastolic volume, mL	10.6 ± 21.2	6.4 ± 15.7
LV end-systolic volume, mL	−25.4 ± 17.0†	−13.2 ± 14.1
Stroke volume, mL	35.5 ± 9.5*	19.6 ± 14.2

Note: Values are means ± standard deviation.
Significantly different from older, lean, sedentary men; *P less than .05; †P less than .07-.08.
Abbreviations: n, number of subjects; LV, left ventricular; BP, blood pressure.
(Courtesy of Hagberg JM, Goldberg AP, Lakatta L, et al: Expanded blood volumes contribute to the increased cardiovascular performance of endurance-trained older men. J Appl Physiol 85:484-489, 1998.)

and increased by 25 W every 3 minutes until exhaustion. Cardiac, red cell, and plasma volumes were determined during exercise.

Findings.—At rest, the master athletes had significantly greater $\dot{V}O_{2max}$ than the sedentary men (3.60 ± 0.43 vs 2.60 ± 0.28 L/min) and also significantly greater plasma volume (45.9 ± 8.0 vs 38.3 ± 5.0 mL/kg), red cell volume (29.7 ± 2.6 vs 25.9 ± 3.5 mL/kg), and total blood volume (75.6 ± 9.7 vs 64.2 ± 7.2 mL/kg). During exercise, the master athletes had a significantly higher LVEDV index (90.6 ± 10.6 vs 77.1 ± 17.4 mL/m²), stroke volume index (75.2 ± 8.4 vs 57.3 ± 13.1 mL/m²), and cardiac index (10.9 ± 1.4 vs 8.7 ±1.6 L/min/m²) (Table 4). For all subjects combined, there was a significant correlation between $\dot{V}O_{2max}$ and plasma, red cell, and total blood volumes. Also, peak exercise stroke volume was significantly associated with plasma, red cell, and total blood volumes.

Multiple regression analysis indicated 3 independent predictors of peak exercise stroke volume and $\dot{V}O_{2max}$: fat-free mass, plasma volume, and total blood volume. Furthermore, the changes in LVEDV and stroke volume correlated significantly with the plasma and total volumes.

Conclusion.—Older endurance-trained athletes had greater $\dot{V}O_{2max}$ than their sedentary peers, and this difference was associated with significantly expanded intravascular volumes in these athletes (particularly plasma and total blood volumes). The improvement in cardiovascular parameters in these endurance-trained men during peak exercise correlated significantly with the expanded intravascular volumes. Thus, this mechanism likely played a role in their improved cardiovascular performance.

▶ There is a surprisingly large difference in aerobic power between master athletes and the sedentary population (51.3 vs. 34.2 mL/kg/min) at ages 56–58 years). Because the study has a cross-sectional design, a part of this difference may be constitutional. Nevertheless, the data do make the point that there are persons nearing the age of retirement who have better aerobic power than a young adult, illustrating the injustice in setting age ceilings to employment that demands a substantial $\dot{V}O_{2max}$. The fact that the high $\dot{V}O_{2max}$ is associated with an increased plasma volume emphasizes the point that many of the gains expected from training can develop quite rapidly through a change in fluid balance, rather than through structural changes. This is a point that Holmgren[1] made many years ago in distinguishing between regulatory and dimensional aspects of training.

R.J. Shephard, M.D., Ph.D., D.P.E.

Reference

1. Holmgren A: Commentary. *Can Med Assoc J* 96:794, 1967.

Energy Requirements and Physical Activity in Free-Living Older Women and Men: A Doubly Labeled Water Study
Starling RD, Toth MJ, Carpenter WH, et al (Univ of Vermont, Burlington)
J Appl Physiol 85:1063-1069, 1998   9–27

Background.—The determinants of daily energy needs and physical activity have not been established in noninstitutionalized elderly persons. Determinants of daily total energy expenditure (TEE) and free-living physical activity in elderly women and men were reported.

Methods.—Fifty-one women, mean age 67, and 48 men, mean age 70, were included. Doubly labeled water and indirect calorimetry were used in the analysis. Data on resting metabolic rate (RMR), body composition, peak oxygen consumption, leisure time activity, and plasma thyroid hormone were obtained.

Findings.—After adjustment for body composition, women and men did not differ in mean TEE (2,306 and 2,456 kcal/day respectively), RMR (1,463 and 1,378 kcal/day, respectively), and physical activity energy expenditure (612 and 832 kcal/day, respectively). In a subgroup of 70 women and men, RMR and peak oxygen consumption accounted for about two thirds of the variance in TEE. This equation was cross-validated in the remaining subjects, with no differences between predicted and measured TEE. Peak oxygen consumption, fat-free mass, and body mass

TABLE 5.—Pearson Product Correlations Between PAEE and Various Independent Variables for 99 Women and Men

Variable	Unadjusted PAEE, kcal/day	Adjusted PAEE, kcal/day	Measured PAL Ratio, kcal/day
Age, yr	0.10	−0.09	−0.06
Body mass, kg	0.34*	0.09	0.18*
Body fat, %	−0.10	−0.14	−0.16
Fat mass, kg	0.04		0.01
Fat-free mass, kg	0.39*		0.12
LTA, kcal/day	0.21*	0.20*	0.18*
Vo_{2peak}, L/min	0.43*	0.31*	0.23*

Adjusted PAEE is covaried for fat and fat-free mass, as previously suggested.
*$P < 0.05$.
(Courtesy of Starling RD, Toth MJ, Carpenter WH, et al: Energy requirements and physical activity in free-living older women and men: A doubly labeled water study. *J Appl Physiol* 85:1063-1069, 1998.)

were the best predictors of physical activity energy expenditure in both sexes (Table 5).

Conclusions.—In noninstitutionalized elderly persons, resting metabolic rate and peak oxygen consumption are important independent predictors of energy requirements. Cardiovascular fitness and fat-free mass moderately predict physical activity in this population.

▶ Many physical activity questionnaires show a rather poor correlation with objective measurements of physical activity; for example, the present study found a correlation of only 0.21 between the very time-consuming Minnesota Leisure-time Activity Survey and estimates of energy expenditure based on doubly labeled water. Thus, using such indices as aerobic power and body fatness as surrogate measures of physical activity has become a growing trend. In support of this tactic, correlations with susceptibility to cardiovascular disease are much stronger for measures of aerobic power than questionnaire assessments of physical activity.[1] Starling and associates take one of the more reputable objective methods of assessing habitual energy expenditure and show strong correlations of this index with aerobic power and fat-free mass. However, it leaves one important question unanswered. Is aerobic power a cause or a consequence of physical activity?

The measurement of habitual activity by doubly labeled water is too expensive to use beyond small samples. Thus, we must ask whether it is possible to adopt such surrogates as aerobic power and fat–free mass when estimating the food needs of older individuals. As always with biological predictions, the main problem is a substantial standard error of the estimate. Even with a substantial sample of elderly people, the error is about 2 MJ/day (460 kcal/day). Unfortunately, the scatter is so large that no useful prediction is obtained in individual cases.

R.J. Shephard, M.D., Ph.D., D.P.E.

Reference

1. Blair SN. Effects of moderate physical activity on cardiovascular disease mortality independent of risk factors, in: AS Leon: *Physical Activity and Cardiovascular Health*. Champaign, IL, Human Kinetics Publishers, 1997.

Creatine Supplementation and Age Influence Muscle Metabolism During Exercise

Smith SA, Montain SJ, Matott RP, et al (Boston Univ; United States Army Research Inst of Environmental Medicine, Natick; Mass; Harvard Med School, Boston)
J Appl Physiol 85:1349-1356, 1998   9–28

Background.—Previous studies have shown that during moderate- to–high-intensity exercise, muscle fatigue may be caused, at least in part, by a decrease in the availability of phosphocreatine (PCr). Elderly people have lower resting levels of PCr, and this deficit may contribute to the generalized muscle weakness that occurs with aging. The effects of creatine supplementation on muscle PCr metabolism in younger and middle-aged healthy subjects were examined.

Methods.—Healthy young subjects (less than 40 years of age; 3 men and 1 woman) and middle-aged subjects (more than 50 years of age, 3 men and 1 woman) were recruited. The groups were similar in their level of physical activity and dietary habits. The subjects underwent 2 trials, with a 7-day washout period between trials. First, they took placebo (granulated sugar; 0.3 gm/kg/day) in a flavored powdered drink mix for 5 days, then they took creatine monohydrate (0.3 gm/kg/day) in a flavored powdered drink mix for 5 days.

After 5 days of using the supplement, subjects performed single-leg knee extension exercises from a supine position inside an MRI system. They performed two 2-minute exercise bouts, with 3 minutes of recovery in between, then performed a third exercise bout in which they exercised to exhaustion (1 to 2 minutes). Phosphorus-31 spectra during exercise were analyzed every 10 seconds to assess pH and the relative concentrations of inorganic phosphate and PCr, PCr hydrolysis, and the rate of PCr resynthesis.

Findings.—During the first (placebo) trial, the middle-aged subjects had significantly lower PCr at rest and during recovery than the younger subjects (resting rates, 35.0 ± 5.2 vs. 39.5 ± 5.1 mmol/kg). The middle-aged subjects also had significantly lower initial PCr resynthesis (18.1 ± 3.5 vs. 23.2 ± 6.0 mmol/kg/min). Phosphocreatine supplementation improved resting and recovery PCr in both groups, such that levels in the middle-aged group no longer differed significantly from those in the younger subjects (middle-aged subjects, 30% increase, to 45.7 ± 5.5 mmol/kg; younger subjects, 15% increase, to 45.7 ± 7.5 mmol/kg).

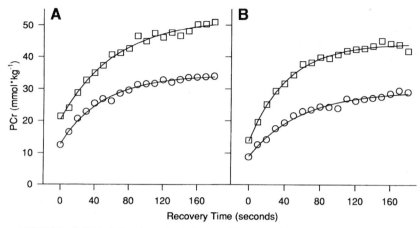

FIGURE 4.—Individual phosphocreatine (*PCr*) (mmol/kg wet weight) vs. time (seconds) results during recovery 1 for a representative young (**A**) and middle-aged (**B**) subject. *Circles* indicate placebo trial; *squares* indicate creatine trial. (Courtesy of Smith SA, Montain SJ, Matott RP, et al., Creatine supplementation and age influence muscle metabolism during exercise. *J Appl Physiol* 85:1349-1356, 1998.)

Also, PCr supplementation caused a significant increase in the PCr resynthesis rate in the middle-aged group, again to a point at which there were no significant differences between the 2 groups (24.3 ± 3.8 vs. 24.2 ± 3.2 mmol/kg/min) (Fig 4). Phosphocreatine supplementation enabled both groups of subjects to exercise longer before exhaustion (combined times to exhaustion, from 118 ± 34 to 154 ± 70 seconds), and the 2 groups had similar degrees of improvement in endurance.

Conclusion.—Compared with younger subjects, middle-aged subjects had lower initial levels of PCr availability and resynthesis, but PCr supplementation significantly improved these measures. Both groups of subjects enjoyed improved muscle endurance after PCr supplementation, although there were no differences in the magnitude of improvement in endurance between the 2 groups.

▶ The potential value of PCr in enhancing high-intensity, intermittent exercise performance has attracted a great deal of attention in recent months,[1,2,3] and, as with any other performance-enhancing substance, controversy has arisen regarding the ethics of its use and the potential dangers of self-administration. Benefit is thought to arise through an increase of muscle PCr reserves and a faster interbout resynthesis of the PCr needed for muscle contraction. Resting PCr levels are low, and resynthesis rates are slow in the elderly,[4] and this suggests that there may be a legitimate place for creatine in treating the muscle weakness of seniors. The present data show that older adults reap greater benefit than those who are younger in terms of PCr resynthesis. The time to fatigue was also increased by the PCr, but (at least with the relatively small sample that was tested) this variable showed no difference between young and older individuals.

R.J. Shephard, M.D., Ph.D., D.P.E.

References

1. Balsom PD, Soderlund K, Sjodin B, et al: Skeletal muscle metabolism during short duration high-intensity exercise: Influence of creatine supplementation. *Acta Physiol Scand* 154:303-310, 1995.
2. Earnest CP, Snell PG, Rodriguez R, et al: The effect of creatine monohydrate ingestion on anaerobic power indices, muscle strength and body composition. *Acta Physiol Scand* 153:207-209, 1995.
3. Greenhaff PL, Bodin K, Soderlund K, et al: Effect of oral creatine supplementation on skeletal muscle phosphocreatine resynthesis. *Am J Physiol* 266:E725-E730, 1994.
4. McCully KK, Fielding RA, Evans, WJ, et al: The relationship between in vivo and in vitro measurements of metabolism in young and old human calf muscle. *J Appl Physiol* 75: 813-819, 1993.

The Effect of Lifelong Exercise on Psychomotor Reaction Time: A Study of 38 Pairs of Male Monozygotic Twins

Simonen RL, Videman T, Battié MC, et al (Univ of Jyväskylä, Finland; Univ of Helsinki; Univ of Alberta, Edmonton, Canada; et al)
Med Sci Sports Exerc 30:1445-1450, 1998   9–29

Background.—Controversy exists regarding whether regular physical activity increases psychomotor reaction times in the elderly. Reaction times have a strong genetic dependency. One study reported that genetics accounted for more than 85% of the variance in reaction times. These authors studied the lifelong physical activity habits of identical male twin pairs to determine whether reaction times were affected by habitual physical exercise.

Methods.—The 38 identical male twin pairs (mean age, 49; range, 35–69) had discordant levels of physical activity. The subjects were divided into 2 groups of pairs. The first group of 29 pairs (mean age, 50) included 1 twin who exercised occasionally (mean, 1.6 times/week; intensity, 1.5 on a 4-point scale; duration, 1.2 hours) and 1 twin who exercised frequently (mean, 4.0 times/week; intensity, 2.0; duration, 1.3 hours). The second group of 9 pairs (mean age, 47) included 1 twin who exercised infrequently (mean 0.7 times/week; intensity, 1.5; duration, 1.5 hours) and 1 twin who exercised regularly (mean, 2.9 times/week; intensity, 1.2; duration, 1.3 hours).

Medical (smoking status, alcohol consumption, etc.) and physical activity histories were obtained. Visual reaction times were measured by a simple choice method and then by a 7-choice method, first on the index finger of the dominant hand, then on the first toe of the (bare) ipsilateral foot, then on the first toe of the contralateral foot. The 5 fastest decision, movement, and reaction (decision plus movement) times at each of the 3 sites were averaged and compared.

Findings.—In the first group of twin pairs, the frequent exercisers had some faster psychomotor reaction times than the occasional exercisers, but the results were not consistent for either the hand or the foot (Table 3).

TABLE 3.—Group Hand and Ipsilateral and Contralateral Foot Simple and Choice Reaction Times and Reaction Time Differences

Reaction Time	Frequent vs Occasional					Regular vs Infrequent				
	M	SD	M	SD	Mean Diff.	M	SD	M	SD	Mean Diff.
Hand										
Simple										
Decision Time	231	(23)	236	(29)	−4	230	(37)	247	(35)	−16
Movement time	187	(55)	186	(47)	+2	163	(46)	171	(39)	−8
Reaction time	432	(61)	434	(60)	−2	404	(72)	426	(63)	−21
Choice										
Decision time	345	(57)	372	(59)	−26*	336	(75)	346	(51)	−9
Movement time	212	(48)	220	(64)	−8	185	(45)	190	(39)	−5
Reaction time	586	(86)	615	(100)	−30	543	(97)	564	(46)	−20
Ipsilateral foot										
Simple										
Decision time	287	(36)	287	(38)	0	266	(24)	286	(23)	−20†
Movement time	266	(85)	282	(70)	−16	242	(64)	239	(60)	+3
Reaction time	571	(108)	593	(98)	−22	528	(74)	540	(82)	−13
Choice										
Decision time	359	(50)	364	(48)	−5	355	(49)	378	(84)	−24
Movement time	304	(90)	315	(77)	−11	254	(58)	252	(64)	+2
Reaction time	697	(115)	713	(107)	−16	648	(96)	661	(78)	−12
Contralateral foot										
Simple										
Decision time	293	(44)	302	(51)	−9	283	(29)	283	(29)	−0
Movement time	254	(64)	277	(74)	−23	265	(84)	231	(62)	+34
Reaction time	560	(91)	594	(13)	−35	571	(110)	527	(83)	+44
Choice										
Decision time	357	(50)	364	(44)	−7	340	(48)	360	(62)	−21
Movement time	288	(73)	324	(90)	−36	280	(77)	248	(69)	+31
Reaction time	676	(105)	727	(116)	−51†	655	(98)	642	(99)	+13

Note: Reaction times are given in milliseconds. Standard deviations are in parenthesis.
P values indicate the adjusted predicted differences (not shown) that remained statistically significant after controlling for occupational physical loading.
*$P < 0.01$.
†$P < 0.05$.
(Courtesy of Simonen RL, Videman T, Battié MC, et al. The effect of lifelong exercise on psychomotor reaction time: A study of 38 pairs of male monozygotic twins. Med Sci Sports Exerc 30(9):1445-1450, 1998.)

After controlling for occupational loading, the frequent exercisers had significantly improved hand choice decision times (26 msec faster) and contralateral foot choice reaction times (51 msec faster). In the second group of twin pairs, there were no significant differences in reaction times between the regular and infrequent exercises, even after controlling for occupational physical demands.

Conclusion.—The data from these twin pairs suggest that the only type of physical activity that might affect reaction times is lifelong frequent exercise, and even then, the improvement in reaction times is slight. Regular exercise (almost 3 times a week for 1.3 hours at an intensity of 1.2 on a 4-point scale) had no effect on reaction times. Although studies report that frequent, vigorous physical activity can improve psychomotor speed, further examination is needed to determine whether that improvement in reaction times has any effect on long-term health.

▶ One of the benefits frequently claimed for regular exercise in older members of the population is a speeding of reaction time, with, by implication, a reduction in the number of accidents and falls.[1,2] However, even in this age group, benefit has not always been demonstrated.[3] This report, based on the exercise habits of a substantial sample of monozygotic twins, shows almost no difference between regular and infrequent exercisers in this respect. Certainly, it seems unwise to promise large gains in reaction speed to an elderly person who decides to engage in an exercise program.

R.J. Shephard, M.D., Ph.D., D.P.E.

References

1. Lupinacci NS, Rikli RE, Jones CJ, et al: Age and physical activity effects on reaction time and digit symbol substitution performance in cognitively active adults. *Res Q Exerc Sport* 64:144-150, 1993.
2. Spirduso WW, Clifford PJ: Replication of age and physical activity effects on reaction and movement time. *J Gerontol* 33:26-30, 1978.
3. Roberts BL Effects of walking on reaction and movement time among elders. *Percept Mot Skills* 71:131-140, 1990.

The Effects of Resistance Training on Well-Being and Memory in Elderly Volunteers
Perrig-Chiello P, Perrig WJ, Ehrsam R, et al (Univ of Berne, Bern, Switzerland; Univ of Basle, Switzerland)
Age Ageing 27:469-475, 1998   9–30

Background.—Although physical exercise clearly has health benefits for elderly people, whether it benefits cognition or well-being is more controversial. The differences in study methods reported in the literature make resolving this controversy more difficult. In this randomized, placebo-controlled study, the authors compared the effects of resistance training on objective measures of cognition and well-being, and examined the long-term (1 year) effects of the intervention on these parameters.

Methods.—Twenty-eight elderly men and 18 elderly women (mean age 73 years) volunteered from a larger ($n = 442$) Interdisciplinary Ageing (IDA) study. They were randomized to the resistance training group ($n = 23$) or the control group ($n = 23$). Resistance training consisted of 8 weeks of 8 different resistance exercises on machines. Muscle strength determinations (leg extensor power) and psychological tests (well-being, competence/control, and memory and cognitive speed) were performed 1 week before the study, 1 week after its end, and 12 months after the intervention. Psychological well-being was assessed by a questionnaire that measured the meaning of life, self-attentiveness (including self-centered thoughts and anxiety about the future), and the absence of complaints. Self-reported physical well-being was scored on a 3-point scale. Control beliefs were assessed by a questionnaire that measured self-efficacy beliefs, internal control, social-external control, and fatalistic-exter-

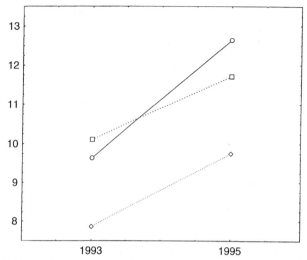

FIGURE 2.—Free recall (word remembered) in 1993 and 1995 for the training ○ and control □ groups and in the whole Interdisciplinary Ageing Study population ◇. (Courtesy of Perrig-Chiello P, Perrig WJ, Ehrsam R, et al: The effects of resistance raining on well-being and memory in elderly volunteers. *Age Ageing* 27:469-475, 1998 by permission of Oxford University Press.)

nal control. Memory and recognition were assessed by free recall of an 8-word list with 8 distractors. Cognitive speed was assessed through a digit-symbol test to characterize hand-eye coordination, attention, and information processing speed. At 1 year after training, because of another program offered immediately after the first one, there were 33 people in the training group and 19 in the control group.

Findings.—Compared with the control group, the training group had significantly improved muscle strength immediately after training. Their immediate and delayed recall (P = NS) and immediate and delayed recognition (P less than 0.01) were also better than the control group, and they reported significantly improved self-attentiveness. At 1 year after training, muscle strength remained significantly better in the training group than in the control group. Furthermore, the training group had significantly improved free recall compared with both the controls and the IDA enrollees (Fig 2).

Conclusions.—Physically, those who engaged in a training program had better muscle strength up to 12 months after training. Although the training program did not affect most measures of well-being, they had improved self-attentiveness and less anxiety immediately after the training program. Furthermore, both short- and long-term free recall were improved in the training group.

▶ Perhaps the most intriguing aspect of the article by Perrig-Chiello and associates is the finding that after 1 year of participation in a program of resistance training, free memory recall was better than in control subjects who did not participate in the training program. The impact of regular exercise upon the cerebral function of the elderly remains a controversial topic. There have been occasional strong advocates of benefit, such as Dustman and associates,[1] but the majority of reports have found little change in mental performance. Divergent responses to training have been explained in terms of task specificity, need for deterioration of function to show benefit, the use of ineffective exercise programs, and a ceiling of benefit once a certain aerobic power has been attained.[2,3] If there is indeed an effect, possible mechanisms include an exercise-induced increase in blood pressure, the passage across the blood-brain barrier of chemicals important to mood state, neural transmission and cerebral performance, a lessening of anxiety, and increases in arousal and self-esteem. Nevertheless, studies are rarely randomized, and as Perrig-Chiello and associates are careful to point out, it is difficult to discount such factors as the greater motivation of those who enroll and persist in exercise programs, and the new interest in life contributed by involvement in such a program.

R.J. Shephard, M.D., Ph.D., D.P.E.

References

1. Dustman RE, Emmerson R, Shearer D: Physical activity, age and cognitive–neuropsychological function. *J Aging Phys Activ* 2:143-181, 1994.
2. Shephard RJ, Leith L: Physical activity and cognitive changes with aging. In: Howe ML, Stones MJ, Brainerd CJ (eds). Cognitive and Behavioral Performance Factors in Atypical Aging (pp. 153-180). New York: Springer Verlag, 1990.
3. Shephard RJ: Aging, physical activity and health. Champaign, Ill: Human Kinetics Publishers, 1997.

Physical Fitness, Physical Activity, and Functional Limitation in Adults Aged 40 and Older
Huang Y, Macera CA, Blair SN, et al (Univ of South Carolina, Columbia; Cooper Inst for Aerobics, Dallas)
Med Sci Sports Exerc 30:1430-1435, 1998   9–31

Objective.—Physical activity improves fitness and prevents functional limitations. The association between fitness, physical activity, and functional limitation was assessed in middle-aged and older adults.

Methods.—Baseline fitness levels were assessed, between 1980 and 1988, for 3,495 men and 1,175 women older than 40, by using total time on a treadmill. Their functional status was assessed by questionnaire in 1990.

Results.—At follow-up, 350 (7.1%) individuals reported having at least 1 physical limitation. The prevalence of physical limitation was twice as high in women as in men. There was a strong inverse relationship between initial physical fitness and functional limitation in both men and women (Table 2). Men and women who were moderately or highly fit at baseline had a lower prevalence of functional limitations later than did persons who were less fit regardless of age, length of follow-up, body mass index,

TABLE 2.—Prevalence of Functional Limitation by Physical Fitness and Activity

	Overall	40-49	50-59	60+
			Age at Baseline (yr)	
Men	(N = 3495)	(N = 1859)	(N = 1199)	(N = 437)
Physical fitness				
Low	12.0	6.6	13.6	24.3
Moderate	4.0	2.9	3.8	9.4
High	2.7	2.7	1.2	7.1
Test for linear trend	*	*	*	*
Physical activity				
Sedentary	8.0	4.9	10.3	14.9
Moderate	5.9	3.8	5.3	15.1
Active	3.6	2.6	3.5	9.5
Test for linear trend	*	—	*	—
Women	(N = 1175)	(N = 645)	(N = 386)	(N = 140)
Physical fitness				
Low	23.1	18.1	22.6	45.5
Moderate	11.9	8.0	13.4	25.9
High	7.0	7.0	3.0	18.4
Test for linear trend	*	*	*	*
Physical activity				
Sedentary	15.0	11.8	15.3	31.0
Moderate	12.5	9.1	11.9	28.6
Active	11.1	9.2	10.1	22.2
Test for linear trend	—	—	—	—

P value of comparisons among three fitness/activity groups: * < 0.05; — > 0.05.
(Courtesy of Huang Y, Macera CA, Blair SN, et al: Physical fitness, physical activity, and functional limitation in adults aged 40 and older. *Med Sci Sports Exerc* 30:1430-1435, 1998.)

alcohol consumption, and presence of chronic disease. The association between physical activity and physical limitation was significant for men but not for women.

Conclusion.—Physical activity in men and women is associated with less functional limitation later in life.

▶ In my view, the ability of regular physical activity to delay the age-related loss of biological function is one of the most important dividends of a regular physical activity program. The present paper indicates the development of a large difference in the prevalence of functional limitation between fit and unfit, and between active and inactive subjects over 8 years of follow-up, although it could be argued that a part of this apparent benefit reflects undetected or incipient illness in the unfit individuals at their first examination. It is particularly striking that the average age at which limitations are being observed is less than 60 years! Given current longevity statistics, this means that those who are showing functional limitation are likely to be burdened with this for many years before they die.

R.J. Shephard, M.D., Ph.D., D.P.E.

The Relationship of Running to Osteoarthritis of the Knee and Hip and Bone Mineral Density of the Lumbar Spine: A 9 Year Longitudinal Study

Lane NE, Oehlert JW, Bloch DA, et al (Univ of California, San Francisco; Stanford Univ, Calif)
J Rheumatol 25:334-341, 1998   9–32

Background.—Running has become a very popular form of exercise among middle-aged and older adults. This trend has raised concerns that running might lead to accelerated development of osteoarthritis (OA) in weight-bearing joints. Cross-sectional studies suggest that runners have increased lumbar spine bone mineral density (BMD) more than nonrunners, but no increase in radiographic evidence of OA exists. This longitudinal study examined the relationships between running, hip and knee OA, and BMD in older adult runners.

Methods.—The 9-year study included 28 members of a "50-Plus" runners' club, age 60–77, at follow-up. They were matched to 27 nonrunner controls for age, education, and occupation. A rheumatologic examination and radiographs of the knees were completed in 1984, 1986, 1989, and 1993. Hip radiographs were obtained in 1993. Quantitative computed tomography (QCT) of the first lumbar vertebrae was performed in 1984, 1986, 1989, and 1993. The 1984 and 1993 knee radiographs were compared in pairwise fashion. The hip radiographs were read in blinded fashion by 2 independent examiners.

Results.—Both runners and nonrunners demonstrated significant progression in knee osteophytes and total knee radiographic scores. The nonrunners showed progressive joint space narrowing. Radiographic scores tended to be higher in the runners; however, there were no significant differences between groups in 1984 or 1993. The runners and nonrunners were similar in terms of radiographic signs of hip OA. At all intervals, the runners had greater lumbar spine BMD values, although the rate of change in these values did not differ.

Conclusions.—Older adult runners and nonrunners show similar evidence of hip OA and progression of knee OA. Although runners have higher lumbar spine BMD values, the 9-year changes in lumbar spine BMD are similar in runners and nonrunners. Although the results need confirmation in a longitudinal, case-control study of sufficient power, they suggest that running into old age does not hasten the development of joint OA.

▶ We cover this time-honored debate regularly; in 1996, we commented on 8 relevant studies.[1] This report, from the longstanding Stanford study of the 50-Plus Runners Association (and a nonrunning control group) agrees with majority opinion, that on the whole, running helps preserve youth and vigor and does not cause or accelerate osteoarthritis. A diehard critic could argue, however, that perhaps runners who got osteoarthritis from their running were forced to quit running (because of the arthritis) before reaching the age of 50 and so could not have been included in this study. A related review concludes that sports that subject joints to repetitive high levels of impact and torsional loading increase the risk of articular cartilage degeneration and the resulting clinical syndrome of osteoarthritis, but moderate habitual exercise does not increase the risk of osteoarthritis.[1]

E.R. Eichner, M.D.

References

1. 1996 YEAR BOOK OF SPORTS MEDICINE, pp 318-319.
2. Buckwalter JA, Lane NE: Athletics and osteoarthritis. *Am J Sports Med* 25:873-881, 1997.

Subject Index

A

Abduction
moment arms of rotator cuff, comparison of two methods of computing, 275

Abrasions
management, 138
standardized, healing of, effects of selected dressings on, 139

ABT-761
effects on exercise-induced bronchoconstriction and urinary LTE_4 in asthmatics, 165

N-Acetylcysteine
lymphocyte proliferation and natural killer cell activity responses to exercise and, 209

Achilles tendinitis
in runners, 297

Achilles tendinosis
chronic, heavy-load eccentric calf muscle training for treatment, 312

Achilles tendon
blood supply of, 106
force, individual muscle contributions to, 289
injuries, 106
ultrasound in differential diagnosis, 121
rupture
acute, in badminton players, 114
acute, surgical repair, early full weightbearing and functional treatment after, 110
repair, cross-stitch, early active motion and weightbearing after, 109
subcutaneous, clinical diagnosis, 108
surgically repaired, MRI during healing of, 113

Acromioclavicular
joint abnormality, active compression test in diagnosis, 44

Active
compression test in diagnosis of labral tears and acromioclavicular joint abnormality, 44

Activity
physical (see Physical, activity)

Adductor
muscle activity during grand-plié in ballet and modern dancers, 265
-related groin pain, long-standing, effect of active training on, in athletes, 4

Adolescent
athlete, meniscal repair in, 98
female, physical activity in, and later breast cancer risk, 170
knee pain in, anterior, natural history of, 89
tennis players, female, effects of unilateral activity on bone mineral density of, 323

Age
adult age range, Postural-Locomotor-Manual Test for spatial-temporal analysis of mobility over, 347
grip strength decrease with, in men, 340
meniscus repair in patients age 40 and older, clinical results, 85
muscle metabolism during exercise and, 357
-related alterations in muscular endurance, 345
-related changes in ability to side-step during gait, 348
static vs. dynamic predictions of protective stepping after waist–pull perturbations and, 267

Aging, 315
fiber type composition changes in masseter vs. biceps brachii muscle during, adverse, 343
physical capabilities change with, 342

Airway
obstruction and exertional dyspnea, 168

Alar
ligament, mechanical properties at slow and fast extension rates, 300

Alcohol
intoxication and snowmobile injuries, 20

Allograft
patellar tendon, reconstruction of lateral collateral ligament of knee with, 103

Altitude
training, individual variation in response to, 253
women at, 325

Amenorrhea
osteoporosis and disordered eating, in athletes, 327

Anabolic
steroids, effect on healing of muscle contusion injury (in rat), 7

Anatomical
factors in snapping of medial head of triceps and recurrent dislocation of ulnar nerve, 63

Author Index